SEXUAL
PHARMACOLOGY
FAST
FACTS

A NORTON PROFESSIONAL BOOK

SEXUAL
PHARMACOLOGY
FAST
FACTS

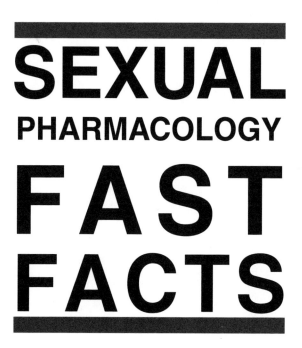

Robert Taylor Segraves, M.D., Ph.D.

Richard Balon, M.D.

W. W. Norton & Company
New York • London

Library of Congress Cataloging-in-Publication Data

Segraves, Robert Taylor, 1941–
    Sexual pharmacology : fast facts / Robert Taylor Segraves,
Richard Balon.
        p.   cm.
    "A Norton professional book."
    Includes bibliographical references and index.
    ISBN 0-393-70354-1 (pbk.)
    1. Reproductive toxicology.   2. Generative organs—Effects of drugs on.
3. Drugs—Side effects.   4. Sexual disorders—Chemotherapy.   I. Balon,
Richard.   II. Title.
RA1224.2.S446   2003
616.6′5071—dc21   2002044486

W. W. Norton & Company, Inc., 500 Fifth Avenue, New York, N.Y. 10110
www.wwnorton.com

W. W. Norton & Company Ltd., Castle House, 75/76 Wells St.,
London W1T 3QT

1   2   3   4   5   6   7   8   9   0

Dedications

To my wife, Kathleen, and my sons, Sherrod and Brendan, who have provided me with great happiness and support.

R.T.S.

To my wife, Helena Balon, M.D., for all her help.

R.B.

Contents

Introduction

Sexual side effects of pharmacological agents are often an unspoken cause of treatment noncompliance. Controlled studies in the United States, the United Kingdom, and Spain have been consistent in finding that approximately 75% of patients who experience sexual side effects from prescribed medications do not volunteer this information. In some studies, patients were even discontinued or modified their treatment because of sexual side effects without informing their physicians of the problem. Clearly, many patients are either embarrassed to bring up the topic of sexual dysfunction or feel that their physician is uninterested.

Reluctance to discuss sexual difficulties with physicians probably varies by age group, region, religion, and cultural subgroup. With changes in societal norms regarding sexuality, many younger patients may feel less embarrassment than their parents in discussing sexual problems with physicians. Many patients who previously would not have inquired about sexual problems associated with drugs may now utilize the Internet to obtain background information and then feel more comfortable confronting the physician armed with this new information.

Unfortunately, other forces can offset the changes that would permit a more open exchange about the sexual side effects of drugs. In some managed care environments, the physician may be forced to treat a large number of patients in a brief period of time. This brief period may not give patients sufficient time to relax and establish a sense of comfort with the physician in order to bring up personal matters such as sexual dysfunction. Some physicians have attempted to accommodate the competing demands for briefer patient visits and good patient care by administering questionnaires, which the patient is asked to complete in the waiting room. It is unclear whether these questionnaires adequately compensate for the diminished time allowed to establish a comfortable physician–patient relationship. To date, clinical studies relying on spontaneous patient self-report of drug-induced sexual side effects consistently underestimate their prevalence.

Many physicians do not have easy access to reliable information concerning the sexual side effects of pharmacological agents. Many texts in all areas of medicine, including psychiatry and obstetrics and gynecology, do not include information about the sexual side effects of drugs. Most physicians use the *Physicians' Desk Reference* (*PDR*) as their major source of information concerning drug side effects. The information in the *PDR* is based on clinical trials conducted by pharmaceutical companies and monitored by the U.S. Food and Drug Administration. Clinical trail data typically base adverse drug event information on the spontaneous reports of patients. For this reason, side effect data in the *PDR* frequently underreflect the true incidence of sexual side effects. A convenient and reliable source of information concerning the prevalence of sexual dysfunction associated with pharmacological agents is not currently available. Examples of misinformation concerning drug-induced sexual side effects contained in the *PDR* is illustrated in Table I.

The purpose of this text is to provide practicing physicians with rapid access to available data concerning the sexual side effects of various pharmacological agents. Hopefully, we provide this data in a format that allows physicians of all specialties and subspecialties to rapidly access data relevant to their practices.

The organization of this book is such that any chapter can be read alone. This structure is utilized to allow the busy practitioner to turn rapidly to the relevant section for a clinical decision. For this reason,

Table I   Incidence of abnormal ejaculation according to the *PDR* and subsequent trials using direct inquiry by physician.*

Drug	*PDR*	Subsequent Studies
fluoxetine (Prozac)	2–7%	44–75%
paroxetine (Paxil)	13–28%	up to 58%
sertraline (Zoloft)	14%	up to 45–67%

* The *PDR* lists only male sexual dysfunction for Prozac and Zoloft. Paxil is listed as causing female orgasm problems in 2–9% of patients. Subsequent studies found sexual dysfunction in both male and female patients at approximately the same rate for all three drugs.

some material is repeated in different sections. For example, anticonvulsants are increasingly utilized in psychiatry as mood stabilizers, so a discussion of anticonvulsant side effects occurs under a section on mood stabilizers as well as a section on neurological drugs. References are listed at the end of each chapter; in the interest of presenting uncluttered, easy-to-access material, references are not cited in the text.

Initial chapters present a brief review of the (1) physiology of sexual function, (2) prevalence of sexual dysfunction in the general population, and (3) means of identifying drug-induced sexual dysfunction. Subsequent chapters are grouped by classes of drugs, allowing physicians rapid access to clinically relevant information. Separate chapters address the sexual side effects of antidepressants, antianxiety drugs, antipsychotic agents, antihypertensives, urological agents, cardiovascular drugs, and other classes of drugs. The chapters focus on the common sexual side effects that may be the unspoken causes of treatment noncompliance, such as inability to ejaculate, anorgasmia, difficulty in reaching orgasm, erectile dysfunction, and lubrication failure. When the data are available, information concerning spontaneous erections, spontaneous orgasm, and priapism is included. Reports of decreased libido are often difficult to interpret. For that reason, data concerning libido are reported only if the evidence clearly supports a diagnosis of disturbed libido as a drug side effect. Incidence of drug-induced sexual dysfunction is taken from studies using direct inquiry by the physician. When data are available from placebo-controlled double-blind studies and/or large clinical series that used direct inquiry, an estimate of incidence is listed. When adequate data are unavailable, sexual side effects are listed as *highly probable*, *possible*, or *unlikely*. When data are available for both sexes, it will be listed. When data are available only for males, only that data will be listed in tables. Final chapters address the pharmacological treatment of sexual disorders.

INTRODUCTION

1. General Information

PREVALENCE OF SEXUAL DYSFUNCTION IN THE GENERAL POPULATION

National Health and Social Life Survey

The National Health and Social Life Survey provides the largest and most well-conducted survey of sexual behavior in the United States. This survey assessed a variety of sexual behaviors in a probability sample of 1,749 women and 1,410 men ages 18–59. A face-to-face interview was utilized, in which respondents were asked specifically about the presence of any sexual problems in the preceding 12 months. Forty-three percent of women and 31% of men complained of sexual difficulties in that time period.

Female subjects listed the following complaints:

Pain with coitus	14.4%
Sex not pleasurable	21.2%
Unable to reach orgasm	24.1%
Lacked interest	33.4%
Anxiety about performance	11.5%
Climaxed too soon	10.3%
Trouble with lubrication	10.4%

Male subjects listed these complaints:

Pain with coitus	3.0%
Sex not pleasurable	8.1%
Unable to reach orgasm	8.3%
Lacked interest	15.8%
Anxiety about performance	17.0%
Climaxed too soon	28.5%
Cannot keep erection	10.4%

Trouble with lubrication increased with age in women; dyspareunia did not increase with age. Trouble with erections tripled in men ages 18–59. The finding that 10% of women complained of reaching climax too soon is discrepant with other studies and suggests a methodological flaw in the interview.

Massachusetts Male Aging Study

Another recent cross-sectional population study, the Massachusetts Male Aging Study, assessed erectile function in a population-based sample of men, ages 40–70, living in Boston suburbs. The prevalence of total erectile failure increased 5–15% from ages 40–70. The prevalence of any form of erectile impairment for the total population was 52%. However, this 52% rate included minimal impotence, which was constant across all ages. Minimal impotence may represent occasional failures of no medical significance.

Studies of Female Sexuality

Numerous surveys of women seeking routine gynecological care have indicated that the most frequent sexual problems are lack of interest, difficulty with orgasm, and inadequate lubrication. One survey of women seeking routine gynecological care found that 87% of the patients had problems with low sexual desire, 83% had difficulty reaching orgasm, and 75% complained of inadequate vaginal lubrication.

Other surveys indicated that problems with urinary incontinence during coitus is frequently associated with sexual dysfunction. In one study of women seeking treatment at a gynecology clinic, less than 1% of women having this problem spontaneously reported it to their physicians; direct inquiry was necessary. Several surveys have indicated that 29–68% of women with coital urinary incontinence also report sexual dysfunction. Successful treatment of the urinary incontinence has been found to reverse sexual dysfunction in only a minority of such patients. Female sexual problems in population surveys tend to correlate with self-reports of marital difficulties, anxiety, and depression.

Tables 1.1a and 1.1b summarize the findings of these general population studies.

Table 1.1a Prevalence of female sexual dysfunction

Arousal disorder	10%
Dyspareunia	14%
Hypoactive sexualo desire disorder	33%
Orgasm disorder	24%

Table 1.1b   Prevalence of male sexual dysfunction

Dyspareunia	3%
Erectile disorder	10%
Hypoactive sexual desire disorder	16%
Orgasm disorder	8%
Premature ejaculation	28%

Population Studies in Other Countries

A recent survey of a stratified population in the United Kingdom also found that sexual problems were more common in women than men, 34% of men and 41% of women reported sexual problems. The median age of respondents was 50. Erectile problems and premature ejaculation were the most common male complaints; vaginal dryness and infrequent orgasm were the most common female complaints.

A survey of Danes born in Rigshspitalet in 1959–1961 (ages 31–33 at time of survey) found that approximately one-fourth of the population experienced sexual problems. The most common female complaint was reduced sexual desire; the most common male sexual dysfunction was premature ejaculation. In another Danish population study, a representative sample of Danish citizens, ages 18–88, were studied. The most common female complaint was reduced sexual desire; the most common male disorder was erectile dysfunction.

Population studies of erectile dysfunction in Japan, Italy, and Malaysia have revealed similar results to the Massachusetts Male Aging Study, with the incidence of erectile problems increasing with age and the presence of hypertension, diabetes mellitus depression, and smoking. Preliminary analysis of this data indicates that the prevalence of erectile problems in Japan may be higher than in the United State and Europe. Population studies in Pakistan, Turkey, Denmark, Egypt, Nigeria, Finland, and Morocco have also found that the incidence of erectile problems increases with age.

RISK FACTORS FOR ERECTILE FAILURE

In the Massachusetts Male Aging Study, age was the major predictor of erectile failure. Other conditions associated with erectile failure included heart disease, diabetes mellitus, and cardiovascular medications. Serum dehydroepiandrosterone and high-density lipoprotein were inversely correlated with erectile failure. Smoking has also been identified as a risk factor for erectile dysfunction. Further analysis of the data from the Male Massachusetts Aging study indicated

Table 1.2 Risk factors for erectile disorder

Cardiovascular disease
Depression
Diabetes mellitus
Hyperlipidemia
Low dehydroepiandrosterone
Prostate surgery
Sedentary life style
Smoking
Submissive personality style

that men with blue-collar employment had higher risk of developing erectile dysfunction than men with white-collar jobs. Erectile failure was more common in men with depressive symptoms.

The original population in the Massachusetts Male Aging Study was re-examined 8 years later. This prospective study found that risk factors for impotence included obesity and sedentary lifestyles. Changes in smoking and alcohol consumption did not change the risk of erectile failure. Smoking at baseline doubled the risk of impotence at follow-up. Passive exposure to cigarette smoking also was associated with impotence. Questionnaire measures indicating a submissive personality style were associated with a higher incidence of impotence at follow-up.

A probability sample of South Australian men was studied for the presence of erectile dysfunction. Age was positively correlated with the presence of erectile problems. Erections inadequate for coitus were reported by 3% of men ages 40–49 and by 64% of men ages 70–79. High triglyceride levels, blood pressure medication, and non-cancer-related prostate surgery were independent predictors of erectile problems. A history of vigorous exercise was negatively related to the presence of erectile dysfunction. Studies in Finland have found that smoking and alcohol consumption are correlated with a higher risk of impotence.

Table 1.2 summarizes risk factors for erectile failure.

CORRELATES OF SEXUAL PROBLEMS IN FEMALES

In general, sexual problems tend to cluster in relation to self-reported social problems in women and physical problems in men. A number of population surveys have shown that the major correlates of female sexual dysfunction are marital discord, anxiety, and depression. Negative affect and marital adjustment appear to be high predictors of dyspareunia in females. A recent French study reported that approximately 11% of French women suffer from anorgasmia and that the

Table 1.3 Correlates of female sexual dysfunction

Anxiety
Depression
Marital discord
Urinary incontinence

frequency of anorgasmia was negatively correlated with the degree of expressed love for the partner.

Table 1.3 summarizes correlates of sexual problems in females.

PSYCHIATRIC COMORBIDITY

Hypoactive sexual desire disorder is more common in patients with major depressive disorder, panic disorder, obsessive–compulsive disorder, anorexia nervosa, and schizophrenia. Erectile disorder frequently accompanies major depressive disorder. Increased libido, more frequent sexual activity, and more extramarital relationships may be associated with the manic phase of bipolar disorder. Recent studies have found that, in patients with anorexia nervosa, sexual drive increases with weight gain. Patients with bulimia report greater sexual interest and a lower age of first coitus than women with anorexia. Women with schizophrenia report low rates of sexual interest and satisfaction. Studies indicate that they are more likely to have been raped or to have engaged in prostitution than controls.

Table 1.4 summarizes comorbid psychiatric conditions.

MEDICAL COMORBIDITY

Numerous diseases have been reported to be associated with sexual dysfunction. Diseases that interfere with the vascular, neurologic, or endocrinological integrity of the reproductive system can cause sexual dysunction. Some of the most common medical causes of sexual dysfunction are diabetes mellitus and multiple sclerosis. Erectile problems have been reported as the initial symptom indicator of multiple sclerosis in some patients. Vascular disease is clearly a common cause of erectile dysfunction. Hyperlipidemia is a risk factor for impotence,

Table 1.4 Psychiatric comorbidity and sexual dysfunction

Anorexia nervosa
Major depressive disorder
Obsessive–compulsive disorder
Panic disorder
Schizophrenia

Table 1.5　**Sexual dysfunction associated with diseases and secondary for medical intervention and trauma**

Diseases	Medical intervention/Trauma
Alcoholism	Abdominal aneurysmectomy
Cerebral vascular accident	Abdominoperitoneal surgery
Chronic obstructive pulmonary disease	Aorto–iliac surgery
Diabetes mellitus	Aorto–inguinal surgery
Hyperlipidemia	Cystoprostectomy
Hyperprolactinemia	Genitourinary cancer surgery
Hypertension	Lumbar disk disease
Hypogonadism	Head injury
Hypothyroidism	Pelvic fracture
Major depressive disorder	Penile fracture
Multiple sclerosis	Perineal prostatectomy
Multiple system atrophy	Perineal trauma
Parkinson's disease	Proctocolectomy
Polyneuropathy	Retroperitoneal node dissection
Renal failure	Spinal cord injury
Systemic lupus	Suprapubic prostatectomy
Temporal lobe epilepsy	

and there is evidence that untreated hypertensive disease can be associated with an increased prevalence of erectile dysfunction.

A number of endocrinopathies may be associated with decreased libido, including hypogonadism and hyperprolactinemia in males; the exact relationship of hypogonadism to decreased libido in females in less clear. There is suggestive evidence that hypothyroidism may cause decreased libido in both sexes. A knowledge of the diseases that can influence sexual function is important when a differential diagnosis is needed. Clinicians frequently encounter situations in which the underlying disease and its treatment both contribute to impaired sexual function. In these cases, an etiological diagnosis may be extremely difficult. Table 1.5 contains a partial list of diseases associated with sexual problems.

IATROGENIC SEXUAL DYSFUNCTION

Any procedure that destroys or damages innervation pathways to the genitalia may result in sexual dysfunction. Common procedures associated with sexual dysfunction include aorto–iliac surgery, radical prostatectomy, cystecomy, retroperitoneal resection, cord injury, and pelvic radiation. Physicians are now becoming aware that many of the interventions in oncology result in permanent sexual impairment. Because cancer treatment frequently involves surgery, radiation, and combination chemotherapy, it can be difficult to identify the intervention responsible. Table 1.5 contains a partial list of medical interventions and trauma associated with secondary sexual dysfunction.

CHARACTERISTICS OF DRUG-INDUCED SEXUAL DYSFUNCTION

The diagnosis of drug-induced sexual dysfunction is based on the sexual history. The differential diagnosis may be relatively easy if the difficulty starts shortly after beginning a new drug or after a dose increase. In such a case, inquire if the problem is present in all sexual situations or has a situational component (e.g., only when the spouse partner is the initiator). A situational component would suggest an interpersonal etiology as opposed to a drug side effect. Depression, anxiety disorders, marital discord, and other stressors also need to be ruled out. Most often, an off-drug trial and a rechallenge will establish the diagnosis. If the side effect is drug-related, a change in medication often will restore sexual function, contribute to treatment compliance, and enhance quality of life.

Unfortunately, most clinical situations are embedded with numerous factors that make diagnosis and treatment complicated. It is not uncommon to have patients who are afflicted by multiple diseases, any one of which can cause sexual dysfunction, and who are taking numerous medications—which may also cause sexual impairment. The situation is often further complicated by marital discord, alcohol abuse, and general life stress. In such cases, try to establish a relationship between the onset of the problem and the introduction of a new pharmacological agent. Often, a precise etiology is extremely difficult to identify. An even more complicated situation occurs when the drug-induced sexual problem has a delayed onset, so that establishing a temporal relationship between the introduction of a drug and the sexual problem is impossible. Examples of delayed-onset drug-induced sexual dysfunction include carbamazepine- and estrogen-induced increases in serum hormone binding globulin, decreasing the availability of serum free testosterone. Complicated clinical situations reinforce the importance of routine reviews eliciting baseline sexual function prior to new treatments, and recording this information clearly in the medical chart. Table 1.6 summarizes characteristics of drug-induced sexual dysfunction.

Table 1.6   Characteristics of drug-induced sexual dysfunction

Dissipates with drug discontinuation or dose reduction
Not better explained by physical illness or environmental stress
Onset with drug initiation or dose increase
Present in all sexual situations
Reappears with reintroduction of the drug

NEURAL ORGANIZATION OF SEXUAL BEHAVIOR

The neural organization of sexual behavior can be understood as organized by several general principles:

1. Spinal reflex mechanisms are largely organized in the spinal cord.

2. The spinal sexual centers are under supraspinal control.

3. There are extensive interconnections between supraspinal sites.

4. Gonadal hormones have influences at the cord and central nervous system.

Neurophysiology of Ejaculation

Ejaculation is conceptualized as an integrated series of spinal cord reflexes that are triggered when sensory stimuli, primarily from the glans penis, reach threshold levels. Supraspinal structures influence this threshold value. Sensory stimuli travel (1) in the pudendal nerve to the sacral cord and (2) via the hypogastric plexus to the ganglia of the paraventricular lumbrosacral sympathetic chain. Once a threshold value is reached, contractions of the vas deferens, seminal vesicles, and prostatic smooth muscle occur. Stimulation of the urethral bulb by the ejaculate elicits reflex closure of the bladder neck (preventing retrograde ejaculation) and rhythmic contractions of the perineal muscles (resulting in expulsion of the ejaculate). Efferent fibers mediating ejaculation arise from the thoracolumbar cord and join the lumbar sympathetic ganglia. Descending nerves encircle the aorta and come together below the bifurcation of the aorta to form the hypogastric plexus. Preganglionic fibers of the hypogastric nerve synapse intersect with short adrenergic fibers that innervate the organs involved in orgasm. Alpha-1 adrenergic receptors appear to mediate ejaculation. These same organs also have a rich cholinergic innervation, although the function of these fibers is not totally clear. In lower animals, it has been shown that there is some cross-innervation of the peripheral sympathetic nervous system at the level of the pelvic plexus.

Supraspinal structures involved in integrating the complex sequence of events involved in ejaculation include the (1) medial preoptic area, (2) paraventricular nucleus, (3) nucleus paragigantocellularis, and (4) possibly the periaqueductal gray of the midbrain. Electrical stimulation of the medial preoptic area elicits ejaculation in lower animals. The medial preoptic nerve has connections with both the periaqueductal gray and the paraventricular nucleus, both of which have connections to the spinal cord. Serotonin in the lateral hypothalamus appears to inhibit ejaculation, and fibers from this area also descend to the spinal cord.

G
E
N
E
R
A
L

I
N
F
O
R
M
A
T
I
O
N

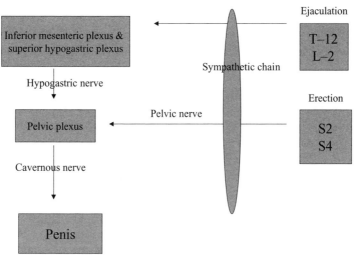

Figure 1.1   Spinal innervation of the genitalia

Another center involved in mediating ejaculation is the nucleus paragigantocellularis, from which inhibitory serotonergic fibers descend to spinal centers. It is hypothesized that the medial preoptic area inhibits action of the nucleus paragigantocellularis. This nucleus has also been proposed as one site at which serotonergic antidepressants act to delay ejaculation. (Figure 1.1 is a simplified schematic of the ejaculatory reflex. Figure 1.2 is a representation of the structures involved in mediation of erection.)

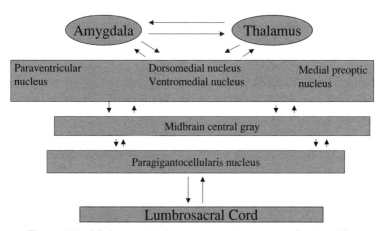

Figure 1.2   Higher central nervous system areas involved in
erectile functioning

Neurophysiology of Erection

Erection (and presumably vaginal lubrication) are spinal reflexes under supraspinal control. The major efferent pathway mediating erection is the S2–S4 area of the cord. The spinal reflexes cause relaxation of the trabecular smooth muscle, dilation of the helcine arteries, expansion of the lacunar spaces, and compression of the venules against the tunica albuginea, resulting in erection. Vasodilatory fibers from T12–L4 also may be involved, although their role is poorly understood. The neurotransmitter involved in the erectile response from S2–S4 does not appear to be cholinergic or adrenergic, although terminals of both systems are abundant in erectile tissue.

Cholinergic nerves may be involved in the erectile process via several mechanisms. First, adrenergic nerves, which tend to decrease tumescence, receive inhibitory interneuronal cholinergic modulation. This prejunctional regulation may decrease adrenergic tone, thereby facilitating erection. Cholinergic nerves also facilitate the vasodilation response mediated by the non-cholinergic, non-adrenergic neurotransmitter (nitric oxide, discussed below). Stimulation of the peripheral beta-2 adrenergic receptor also has been shown to facilitate penile erection. Detumescence is mediated by stimulation of the peripheral alpha-1 adrenergic receptor, which causes constriction of the penile arteries and trabecular smooth muscle. (Figure 1.3 is a schematic representation of the peripheral nervous system concerned with erection and detumescence.)

The intracellular mechanisms mediating erection appear to involve both cylic GMP and AMP systems. Nitric oxide has been proposed to be the non-cholinergic, non-adrenergic neurotransmitter of penile erection. Nitric oxide is released from the endothelium and activates guanylate cyclase, producing cyclic guanosine monophosphate (cyclic GMP), which produces relaxation of arterial walls and the trabecular

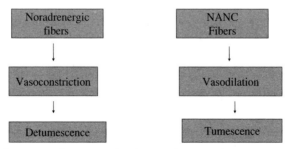

**Figure 1.3   Local mechanisms of penile detumescence
and tumescence**

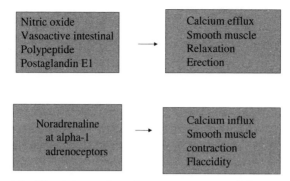

Figure 1.4   Physiology of penile tumescence and detumescence

muscle through a cascade of events. Cyclic GMP is inactivated by phosphodiesterase type 5, which sildenafil inhibits. Vasoactive intestinal polypeptide and prostaglandins E1 and E2 stimulate adenyl cyclase, which leads to the formation of cyclic AMP and the relaxation of penile arterial walls. It is hypothesized that similar mechanisms operate in the human female. Many of the same neurotransmitters involved in erection have been identified in the vaginal wall and/or clitoris. (The physiology of erection is illustrated in Figure 1.4 and the action of sildenafil in Figure 1.5.)

The supraspinal sites involved in erection have been identified in animal studies employing a variety of techniques, including ex copula reflexes, changes in intracavernous pressure, activation of the urethrogenital reflex, c-fos staining of the transcription factor, and pseudorabies virus transneuronal tracing. A number of brainstem, pons, and hypothalamic nuclei send direct projections to the spinal nuclei that control erection. Descending fibers of 5HT project from the nucleus paragigantocellularis to the pelvic efferents, where interneurons

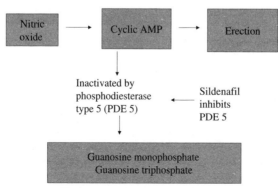

Figure 1.5   Action of sildenafil

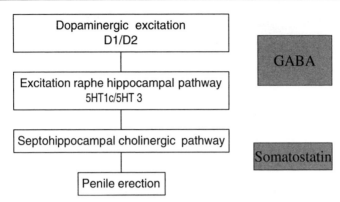

Figure 1.6   Penile erection in the rat. (Maeda 1994a, 1995b; Matsuoka 1996.)

have an inhibitory influence on the erectile response. There is a direct hypothalamic–spinal–oxytocin pathway from the paraventricular nucleus of the hypothalamus to the spinal cord. Apomorphine is believed to work by activating these oxytocinergic fibers. In lower animals, apomorphine injected into the medial preoptic area inhibits erection, whereas injection of the same drug into the paraventricular nucleus stimulates erections. Dopaminergic fibers communicate directly with oxytocinergic fibers. In primates, the dopamine D2 receptor is believed to mediate erection.

Numerous higher central nervous system areas involved in erectile functioning include the hypothalamus, midbrain gray, medulla, and amydala. In many mammals, sexual behavior is androgen-dependent. It is believed that testosterone acts on the brain via androgen receptors. The highest concentrations of androgen receptors are found in the medial preoptic area, ventromedial nucleus of the hypothalamus, medial amygdala, and lateral septum. Of these areas, the medial preoptic area appears to be the most sensitive to testosterone. There are extensive interconnections between most of these areas.

Positron emission tomography study of the response to erotic visual stimuli in the human male has suggested that sexual arousal is accompanied by bilateral activation of the inferior temporal lobe, right insula, right inferior frontal cortex, and left anterior cingulate cortex. One model of the central control of erectile functioning derived from animal research hypothesizes that dopaminergic excitation causes excitation of the raphe hippocampal serotonergic pathway, which in turn activates the septohippocampal cholinergic pathway (Figure 1.6).

Neurophysiology of the Female Sexual Response

Many of the hypotheses concerning human sexuality are derived from animal studies, and individual investigators have tended to concentrate on one sex or the other. Investigation of male sexual behavior has concentrated on measures of erection and ejaculation, whereas studies of female sexuality have tended to focus on lordosis behavior. Clearly, the human female sexual behavior and behaviors studied in female animal models are quite different and may have different neural pathways.

The spinal substrate of the female sexual response has been studied in other species and is partially known. Vasocongestive events in either sex can be elicited by genital stimulation transmitted by the pudental nerve or by supraspinal stimuli. Genital stimulation in female rats can elicit rhythmic vaginal and uterine contractions as well as activation of the cavernous, hypogastric, and pelvic preganglia. This response is similar to orgasm in the human. Similar responses can be elicited in both sexes. Clitoral engorgment and vaginal vasocongestion are mediated by vasodilatory fibers in the cavernous nerve. In the male, stimulation of the dorsal nerve of the penis results in increased intracavernous pressure. To date, similar experiments have not been performed with stimulation of the clitoral nerve.

Studies in cats have revealed interneurons in the medial gray of the sacral cord that respond to pelvic visceral and perineal stimulation. Retrograde tracing of viruses injected into the vagina and clitoris reveals labeled neurons in the central gray of the spinal cord and near the intermediolateral cell column of the cord. Sensory information from pelvic regions is relayed to supraspinal areas by the spinothalamic and spinoreticular pathways. Cortical evoked potentials from stimulation of the clitoral nerve confirm cortical representations deep in the midline interhemispheric fissure.

The nucleus paragigantocellularis is felt to exert inhibitory control over sexual reflexes in both sexes. Virus injection in the clitoris results in labeled areas in the nucleus paragigantocellularis. Neurons in this nucleus receive genital sensory information in the male and female. Other brainstem serotonergic nuclei—the raphe nuclei, pallidus, magnus, and pyramidal region—project to the lumbrosacral cord. Adrenergic projections to the cord can be traced to the locus coeruleus. These nuclei were identified by injecting labeled pseudorabies virus into the clitoris and uterus.

The periacqueductal gray (midbrain central gray) has connections with number of different pathways, and direct stimulation of this area elicits sexual responses. This area does not project directly to the cord but has connections with brainstem sites, including the nucleus paragigantocellularis and the medial preoptic area of the hypothalamus.

Fos labeling of the amygdala and bed nucleus of stria terminalis is strongly affected by vaginocervical stimulation. The medial amygdala is believed to be involved in sexual motivation in the male. It is unclear if it has a similar function in the female. The medial preoptic area in the male is hypothesized to be involved in mate selection, but its function in the female is unknown.

Sexual stimulation leads to clitoral and vaginal smooth muscle relaxation, which is followed by increased blood flow and engorgment of the clitoris and vagina. Although the clitoris does become engorged, it does not become rigid. Pelvic nerve stimulation leads to increased vaginal blood flow. As in the male, ingestion of sildenafil or phentolamine increases genital vasocongestion. Evidence of peripheral neurotransmitters in the female sexual response has been identified in the human vagina. These neurotransmitters include neuropeptide Y, vasoactive intestinal polypeptide (VIP), nitrous oxide synthase (NO), calcitonin gene-related peptide, and substance P. VIP and NO appear to be the major neurotransmitters regulating relaxation of the vaginal smooth muscle. Adrenergic fibers appear to be the major influence regulating smooth muscle contraction in the vagina and clitoris. Both alpha-1 and alpha-2 receptors appear to be involved in the rabbit. Supraspinal control of the spinal reflexes involves the nucleus paragigantocellularis, the periaqueductal gray, the medial preoptic area, the ventral medial nucleus, the paraventricular nucleus, and the amygdala. Orgasm is associated with central thalamic depolarization and contraction of the pelvic floor and of the smooth muscle of the vagina and uterus.

Sexual behavior in the female rat is dependent on gonadal steroid activation of receptors in the hypothalamus. Several peptinergic transmitters, including alpha-melanotrophin, gonadotropin releasing hormone, and oxytocin, have a stimulatory effect on sexual behavior and also release noradrenaline. Noradrenaline has been hypothesized to mediate the effects of alpha-melanotrophin via beta receptors.

Other Neurotransmitters Involved in Sexual Activity

A number of other neurotransmitter systems are involved in the modulation of sexual activity. Gamma-aminobutyric acid receptors in the paraventricular nucleus have an inhibitory modulator effect on reflex pathways involved in erectile functioning. Oxytocinergic pathways from the paraventricular and supraoptic area of the hypothalamus

Table 1.7 Effects of neurotransmitters on sexual function

ACTH	excitatory
Alpha melanocye	excitatory
Endothelium E–1	excitatory
Gamma-aminobutyric acid	inhibitory
Nitric oxide	excitatory
Opiod	inhibitory
Oxytocin	excitatory
Prostaglandins	excitatory

project to spinal centers and probably influence sacral autonomic outflow. Oxytocin injected into the lateral cerebral ventricle, the paraventricular nucleus, or the hippocampus is a potent inducer of penile erection. Injection of oxytocin receptor antagonists in the lateral ventricle reduces erection in laboratory animals. Opioid stimulation centrally prevents penile erections, and morphine injected into the paraventricular nucleus impairs copulation in laboratory animals. Evidence suggests that nitric oxide may act in the medial preoptic area and paraventricular nucleus to modulate the actions of other CNS neurotransmitters involved in sexual function. Peptides such as adrenocorticotropic hormone and alpha-melanocyte hormone have been associated with erection in laboratory animals. Recent work has shown that alpha-melanocyte hormone can induce erections in humans.

It is widely accepted that nitric oxide and VIP are involved in the relaxation of the corpus cavernosum smooth muscle; endothelin E-1 induces contractions in different penile smooth muscles. Prostaglandins and thromboxanes, locally active hormones, are present in penile tissue and may have a role in producing the contraction involved in orgasm.

Table 1.7 lists neurotransmitters and their functions in sexual activity.

ENDOCRINE FACTORS

Male Sexuality

From studies with hypogonadal men, it is clear that testosterone is necessary for libido. In fact, in hypogonadal men, libido, ejaculatory demand, and ejaculatory volume are all decreased; the addition of exogenous testosterone returns these sexual components to normal levels. Many men with hypogonadism have erectile difficulties, which are believed to be due to attempts at coitus with minimal libido, rather than a direct effect of a low testosterone level on erectile function itself.

Table 1.8 Androgens and libido

In males, a threshold amount of testosterone is necessary for normal sexual function
In eugonadal men, supraphysiological levels of testosterone have minimal effect
In females, supraphysiological levels of testosterone increase libido
In females, it is unclear whether a threshold level of testosterone is necessary for libido
In females, hypoestrogenism increases the liklihood of dyspereunia

Secretion of testosterone by the testes is under feedback control of the hypothalamus and pituitary gland. The hypothalamus secretes gonadotrophin-releasing hormone (GnRH), which stimulates pituitary production of luteinizing and follicle stimulating hormone. In turn, these hormones stimulate the testes to produce spermatozoa and to secrete testosterone, dihydrotestosterone, and small amounts of estradiol. Circulating testosterone has an inhibitory effect on GnRH secretion. It is believed that this inhibition is caused by estradiol, which is formed from CNS testosterone by aromatization. Dihydrotestosterone also has inhibitory effects on LH and FSH secretion. Approximately 5 grams of testosterone are produced per day in a pulsatile manner. In normal males, about 2% is free (unbound), about 30% is bound to the sex hormone-binding globulin, and the rest is bound to albumin. Free and albumin-bound testosterone are referred to as bioavailable testosterone. It is clear that abnormally low testosterone is associated with decreased libido. It is not clear that supraphysiological levels of testosterone augment libido in males. However, the lowest limit of testosterone that permits normal function is unknown. Normative values set by deviations from a statistical mean may not always be relevant to an individual patient.

Table 1.8 summarizes endocrine factors involved in male and female sexuality.

Female Sexuality

The relationship of endocrine factors to female sexuality is less well understood, although the endocrinology of female reproduction has been well documented. There is clear evidence that supraphysiological levels of androgens increase libido in the human female; it is less clear whether a minimum level of androgen is necessary to support libido, and whether variations in androgen within normal levels are related to changes in libido. Estrogen is clearly necessary to support vaginal integrity and lubrication. Hypoestrogenism can increase the liklihood of dyspareunia. The precise effect of progesterone on female sexual function is unclear.

Follicle stimulating hormone (FSH) levels begin to rise just before menses, stimulating the granulosa cells of ovarian follicles to produce estradiol. Estradiol exerts a negative feedback on the production of

FSH.When estadiol hits a critical threshold level, it exerts positive feedback on the production of luteinizing hormone (LH). There is a preovulatory peak of LH, FSH, and estradiol. The LH surge results in the production of progesterone, which replaces the production of estradiol by the granulosa cells. Progesterone enhances endometrium receptivity to implantation of the embryo.The levels of these hormones decline during the luteal phase, while the levels of progesterone peak in the mid-luteal phase. To date, no studies have demonstrated a consistent relationship between phase of the menstrual cycle and sexual activity in the human female, other than the decrease in activity during menses for religious and cultural reasons. Although some investigators have reported such relationships, they frequently are not replicated in subsequent investigation.

MECHANISMS OF DRUG-INDUCED SEXUAL DYSFUNCTION

Given that most pharmacological agents have unintended as well as targeted effects, the possible mechanisms of drug-induced sexual dysfunction are myriad. Many drug side effects on sexual behavior occur because the drug interferes with neurotransmission, either peripherally or centrally.

Many drugs in common usage have significant anticholinergic side effects. Cholinergic receptors are present in the corpora cavernosa and in organs mediating ejaculation. In animal models, CNS cholinergic transmission is necesssary for normal erectile function. In addition, cholinergic activity may modulate adrenergic tone.To date, the role of cholinergic fibers in the genitals remains unclear. Parasympathetic activity may facilitate penile tumescence by inhibiting the release of noradrenaline through stimulation of muscarinic receptors on adrenergic nerve terminals and by releasing nitric oxide or VIP.

Peripheral alpha-adrenergic blockade has been shown to retard ejaculation and facilitate erection. Adrenergic activity appears to be responsible for penile detumescence. Many psychiatric drugs, including tricylic antidepressants and antipsychotic drugs, have significant alpha-adrenergic blockade as a side effect. In the central nervous system, noradrenergic activity appears to facilitate sexual functioning.

Drugs influencing serotonergic neurotransmission may influence sexual function by affecting the inhibitory fibers to sexual centers in the cord. The adverse sexual effects of serotonin appear to be mediated by the 5HT2A receptor. These effects, in turn, may be mediated by effects at the level of the nucleus paragigantocellularis; lesions on this nucleus block the effect of fluoxetine on ejaculation. Serotonin is present in spinal, peripheral, and supraspinal sites. In general, serotonin has an inhibitory effect on most aspects of sexual behavior. However, there are multiple serotonin receptors. Serotonin can have both facilitative and inhibitory effects on sexual behavior, depending on the receptor subtype and its location. Serotonin 5HT1A agonists can inhibit erection and promote ejaculation; serotonin 5HT1C agonists faciltate penile erection. Drugs blocking the 5HT2 receptor would be expected to have fewer sexual side effects; both nefazodone and mirtazapine block the 5HT2 receptor.

Drugs that block the D1 and or D2 dopaminergic receptors elevate serum prolactin; elevated serum prolactin is associated with sexual dysfunction. The effect of dopamine receptor activation may vary, given the anatomical location of the receptor. For example, activation of the D1 receptor in the medial preoptic area facilitates erectile functions, whereas stimulation of the D2 receptor in the paraventricular nucleus has a similar effect. Paraventricular dopaminergic receptor activation involves oxytocinergic neurotransmission.

There is considerable "cross-talk" between neuropathways. Stimulation of 5HT2 may inhibit mesolimbic dopaminergic pathways, and presynaptic cholinergic receptors are present on many adrenergic neurons. Adrenergic neuronal activity may inhibit serotonergic activity; this observation is compatible with the clinical observation that bupropion and amphetamines reverse serotonergic antidepressant-induced anorgasmia. Another possible mechanism is inhibition of nitric oxide synthase; paroxetine inhibits this enzyme, and this inhibition has been proposed as the mechanism by which SSRIs may influence sexual behavior.

Drugs that directly affect antiandrogenic function, either by supressing LH and/or FSH secretion or decreasing bioavailable testosterone by increasing serum hormone binding globulin, are affecting hormonal systems that influence sexual function.

Table 1.9 summarizes the mechanisms of drug-induced side effects.

Table 1.9 Mechanisms of drug-induced sexual side effects

Antiandrogenic effect
Anticholinergic effects
Antiestrogenic effect
Alpha-adrenergic effects
Beta-adrenergic effects
Dopaminergic effects
Hyperprolactinemia
Inhibition of nitric oxide synthase
Serotonergic effects
Suppression of gonadotrophin release

OBTAINING A BASELINE OF SEXUAL ACTIVITY PRIOR TO DRUG THERAPY

It is critical to obtain a baseline measure of sexual function prior to starting a new pharmacological treatment. Many patients may erroneously attribute a sexual difficulty to a given drug. Patients with multisystemic diseases who are on multiple agents and who are also experiencing marital discord or symptoms of depression may find it extremely difficult to determine retrospectively the etiology of a sexual complaint.

It is recommended that baseline sexual function be established in all patients. Studies have demonstrated that most patients do not resent such inquiries and, in fact, respect their physicians for being concerned about their sexual lives. Most clinicians regard direct inquiry as preferable to the use of questionnaires.

A sexual history may be initiated in various ways that do not interrupt the flow of the patient history. In new patients, sexual questions can easily be included in the review of systems. In depressed patients, one might inquire about sexual appetite after inquiring about disturbances of sleep or appetite. When pertinent, one may state that it is important to establish a baseline of sexual function because certain medications may interfere with it.

In general, inquire if there is any sexual difficulty, then follow up with brief, specific questions about problems with libido, erection, lubrication, orgasm, ejaculation, or pain. Often, patients answer negatively to a general inquiry about sexual function but report problems when more specific questions are asked. If a patient appears unduly distressed by sexual questions, it is always an option to delay this part of the interview to a subsequent session.

A baseline assessment may serve medicolegal purposes if a patient subsequently claims that a treatment caused sexual impairment, when your medical record clearly indicates abnormal sexual function prior to treatment.

REFERENCES

Ahlenius S, Larsson K. Opposite effects of 5-methoxy-N,N-di-methyl-tryptamine and 5-hydroxytryptophan on male rat sexual behavior. *Pharmacol Biochem Behav.* 1991;38(1):201–205.

Ahlenius S, Hillegaart V, Hjorth S, Larsson K. Effects of sexual interactions on the in vivo rate of monoamine synthesis in forebrain regions of the male rat. *Behav Brain Res.* 1991;46(2):117–122.

Aiello-Zaldivar M, Luine V, Frankfurt M. 5,7-DHT facilitated lordosis: effects of 5-HT agonists. *Neuroreport.* 1992;3(6):542–544.

Allen D, Renner K, Luine V. Naltrexone facilitation of sexual receptivity in the rat. *Horm Behav.* 1985;19:98–103.

Andersson K. Neurotransmitters: central and peripheral mechanisms. *Int J Impot Res.* 2000;12(suppl 4):26–33.

Andersson K, Holmquist F. Regulation of tone in cavernosal smooth muscle. *World J Urology.* 1994;12:249–261.

Andersson KE. Pharmacology of penile erection. *Pharmacol Rev.* 2001;53:417–450.

Arato M, Frecska E, Tekes K, MacCrimmon D. Serotonergic interhemispheric asymmetry: gender difference in the orbital cortex. *Acta Psychiatr Scand.* 1991;84(1):110–111.

Arajo A, Durante R. The relationship between depressive symptoms and male erectile dysfunction:cross-sectional results from the Massachusetts Male Aging Study. *Urology.* 1998;60:458–465.

Aytac L, McKinlay J, Krane R. The likely worldwide increase in erectile dysfunction between 1995 and 2025 and some possible consequences. *BJU International.* 1999;84:50–56.

Azadzoi K, Payton T, Krane R, Goldstein I. Effects of intracavernosal trazodone hydrochloride:animal and human studies. *J of Urology.* 1990;144:1277–1282.

Babichev V, Adamskaya E, Ozol' L, El'tseva T. Neuromodulator role of luliberin in the regulation of sexual behavior in the male rat. *Neurosci Behav Physiol.* 1991;21(4):330–334.

Balon R, Yeragani V, Pohl R, Ramesh C. Sexual dysfunction during antidepressant treatment. *J Clin Psychiatry.* 1993;54:209–212.

Barclay S, Harding C, Waterman S. Correlations between catecholamine levels and sexual behavior in male zebra finches. *Pharmacol Biochem Behav.* 1992;41(1):195–201.

Bazzett T, Eaton R, Thompson J, Markowski P, Lumley L, Hull E. Dose dependent D2 effects on genital reflexes after MPOA injections of quineloraine and apomorphine. *Life Sci.* 1991;48:2309–2315.

Benelli A, Zanoli P, Bertolini A. Effect of clenbuterol on sexual behavior in male rats. *Physiol Behav.* 1990;47:373–376.

Benelli A, Arletti R, Basaglia R, Bertolii A. Male sexual behavior: further studies on the role of alpha 2-adrenoceptors. *Pharmacol Res.* 1993;28(1):35–45.

Bitran D, Hull EM. Pharmacological analysis of male rat sexual behavior. 1987;11(4):365–389.

Brambilla F, Guerrini A, Guastalla A, Rovere C, Riggi F. Neuroendocrine effects of haloperidol therapy in chronic schizophrenia. *Psychopharmacology.* 1974;44:17–22.

Brown H, Salamanca S, Stewart S, Uphouse L. Chlordecone (Kepone) on the night of proestrus inhibits female sexual behavior in CDF-344 rats. *Toxicol Appl Pharmacol.* 1991;110(1):97–106.

Bortolotti A, Parazzini F. The epidemiology of erectile dysfunction and its risk factors. *Int J Andrology.* 1997;20:312–334.

Chew K, Earle C, Stuckley B, Jamrozik K, Keough E. erectile dysfunction in general medial practice:prevalence and clinical correlates. *Int J Impot Res.* 2000;12:41–45.

Clark JT. Suppression of copulatory behavior in male rats following central administration of clonidine. *Neuropharmacology.* 1991;30:373–382.

Dallo J, Lekka N, Knoll J. The ejaculatory behavior of sexually sluggish male rats treated with (-)deprenyl, apomorphine, bromocriptine and amphetamine. *Pol J Pharmacol Pharm.* 1986;38:251–255.

Dieckmann KP, Huland H, Gross AJ. A test for the identification of relevant sympathetic nerve fibers during nerve sparing retroperitoneal lymphadenectomy. *J Urol.* 1992;148(5):1450–1452.

Doherty P, Wisler P. Stimulatory effects of quineloraine on yawning and penile erection. *Life Sci.* 1994;54:507–514.

Dornan WA, Katz JL, Ricaurte GA. The effects of repeated administration of MDMA on the expression of sexual behavior in the male rat. *Pharmacol Biochem Behav.* 1991;39(3):813–816.

Dourish CT, Hutson PH. Bilateral lesions of the striatum induced with 6-hydroxydopamine abolish apomorphine-induced yawning in rats. *Neuropharmacology.* 1985;24:1051–1055.

Dunn K, Croft P, Hackett G. Sexual problems:a study of the prevalence and need for health care in the general population. *Family Practice.* 1998;15:519–524.

Dunn K, Croft P, Hackett G. Association of sexual problems with social, psychological, and physical problems in men and women a cross sectional population survey. *J Epidemiol Community Health.* 1999;53:144–148.

Eaton RC, Markowski VP, Lumley LA, Thompson JT, Moses J, Hull EM. D2 receptors in the paraventricular nucleus regulate genital responses and copulation in male rats. *Pharmacol Biochem Behav.* 1991;39:177–181.

Fernandez-Guasti A, Escalante A, Hong E, Agmo A. Behavioural actions of the serotonergic anxiolytic indorenate. *Pharmacol Biochem Behav.* 1990;37:83–88.

Fernandez-Guasti A, Escalante A, AS, Hillegaart V, Larsson K. Stimulation of 5-HT1A and 5-HT1B receptors in brain regions and its effects on male rat sexual behaviour. *Eur J Pharmacol.* 1992;210:121–129.

Fernandez-Guasti A, Roldan-Roldan G, Larsson K. Anxiolytics reverse the acceleration of ejaculation resulting from enforced intercopulatory intervals in rats. *Behav Neurosci.* 1991;105(2):230–240.

Fernandez-Guasti A, Hanssen S, Archer T, Jonsson G. Noradrenaline-serotonin interactions in the control of sexual behavior in the male rat: DSP4-induced noradrenaline depletion antagonizes the facilitatory effect of serotonin receptor agonists, 5-MeODMT and lisuride. *Brain Res.* 1986;377(1):112–118.

Ferrari FGD. Influence of idazoxan on the dopamine D2 receptor agonist-induced behavioural effects in rats. *Eur J Pharmacol.* 1993;250:51–57.

Fibiger HC, Nomikos GG, Pfaus JG, Damsma G. Sexual behavior, eating and mesolimbic dopamine. *Clin Neuropharmacol.* 1992;15(suppl 1 Pt A):566–567.

Foreman M, Fuller R, Nelson D, Calligaro D, Kurz K, Misner J, Garbrecht W, Parli C. Preclinical studies on LY237733, a potent and selective serotonergic antagonist. *J Pharmacol Exp Ther.* 1992;260(1):51–57.

Feldman H, Goldstein I. Impotence and its medical and psychosocial correlates: results of the Massachusetts Male Aging Study. *J URL.* 1994;151:54–61.

Ghezzia A, Baldini S, Zibetti A. Sexual dysfunction in male multiple sclerosis patients in relation to clinical findings. *J Neurol.* 1996;3:462–466.

Gordon D, Groutz A, Sinai T, Wiezman A, Lessing J, David M, Aizenberg D. Sexual function in women attending a urogynecology clinic. *Int Urogynecol J.* 1999;10:325–328.

Gereau RT, Kedzie KA, Renner KJ. Effect of progesterone on serotonin turnover in rats primed with estrogen implants into the ventromedial hypothalamus. *Brain Res Bull.* 1993;32(3):293–300.

Gonzalez M, Leret M. Extrahypothalamic serotonergic modification after masculinization induced by neonatal gonadal hormones. *Pharmacol Biochem Behav.* 1992;41:329–332.

Gonzalez M, Leret M. Role of monoamines in the male differentiation of the brain induced by androgen aromatization. *Pharmacol Biochem Behav.* 1992;41:733–737.

Gorzalka BB, Mendelson SD, Watson NV. Serotonin receptor subtypes and sexual behavior. *Ann N Y Acad Sci.* 1990;600:435–436.

Gower AJ, Berendsen HG, Princen MM, Broekkamp CL. The yawning-penile erection syndrome as a model for putative dopamine autoreceptor activity. *Eur J Pharmacol.* 1984;103:81–87.

Heaton J. Central neurophramacological agents and mechanisms in erectile dysfunction: the role of dopamine. *Neurosci Biobehav Rev.* 2000;24:561–569.

Heaton J, Varrin S. Metoclopramide decreases apomorphine-induced yawning and penile erection. *Pharmacol Biochem Behav.* 1991;38:917–920.

Hierons R, Saunders M. Impotence in men with temporal lobe lesions. *Lancet.* 1996;2:761–763.

Hillegaart V. Functional topography of brain serotonergic pathways in the rat. *Acta Physiol Scand.* 1991;598(suppl):1–54.

Hillegaart V, Ahlenius S. Region-selective inhibition of male rat sexual behavior and motor performance by localized forebrain 5-HT injections: a comparison with effects produced by 8-OH-DPAT. *Behav Brain Res.* 1991;42:169–180.

Ho M, Hsu H, Young F, Hsu C, Peng M. Improvement of sexual behavior in aged rats by p-chlorophenylalanine and methysergide. *Kao Hsiung I Hsueh Ko Hsueh Tsa Chih.* 1992;8:342–348.

Hull EM, Pahek EA, Bitran D, Holmes GM, Warner RK, Band LC, Bazzett T, Clemens LG. Brain localization of cholinergic influence on male sex behavior in rats: agonists. *Pharmacol Biochem Behav.* 1998;31:169–174.

Hull EM, Bitran D, Pahek EA, Holmes GM, Warner RK, Band LC, Clemens LG. Brain localization of cholinergic influence on male sex behavior in rats: antagonists. *Pharmacol Biochem Behav.* 1988;31:175–178.

Hull EM, Eaton RC, Moses J, Lorrain D. Copulation increases dopamine activity in the medial preoptic area of male rats. *Life Sci.* 1993;52(11):935–940.

Hull E, Eaton R, Markowski V, Moses J, Lumley L, Loucks J. Opposite influence of medial preoptic D1 and D2 receptors on genital reflexes:implications for copulation. *Life Sci.* 1992;51:1705–1713.

Hunter A, Hole D, Wilson C. Studies into the dual effects of serotonergic pharmacological agents on female sexual behaviour in the rat: Preliminary evidence that endogenous 5HT is stimulatory. *Pharmacol Biochem Behav.* 1985;22:5–13.

Jaiwal R, Chaturvedi CM. Elimination of testicular regression by 12-hr temporal relationship of serotonergic and dopaminergic activity in Indian palm squirrel, Funambulus pennanti. *J Neural Transm Gen Sect.* 1991; 84(1–2):45–52.

Jenck F, Moreau J, Mutel V, Martin J, Haefely W. Evidence for a role of 5-HTic receptors in the antiserotonergic properties of some antidepressant drugs. *Eur J Pharmacol.* 1993;231:223–229.

Johannes C, Araujo A, Feldman H, Derby C, Kleinman K, McKinlay JB. Incidence of erectile dysfunction in men 40 to 69 years old:longitudinal results from the Massachusetts male Aging Study. *J Urol.* 2000;163:460–463.

Johnston H, Payne A, Gilmore D, Wilson C. Neonatal serotonin reduction alters the adult feminine sexual behaviour of golden hamsters. *Pharmacol Biochem Behav.* 1990;35(3):571–575.

Jolicoeur FB, Gagne MA, Rivest R, Drumheller A, St-Pierre S. Atypical neuroleptic-like behavioral effects of neurotensin. *Brain Res Bull.* 1993;32:487–491.

Kakeyama M, Yamanouchi K. Lordosis in male rats: the facilitatory effect of mesencephalic dorsal raphe nucleus lesion. *Physiol Behav.* 1992;51(1):181–184.

Kaplan JM, Hao JX, Sodersten P. Apomorphine induces erection in chronic decerebrate rats. *Neurosci Lett.* 1991;129:205–208.

Kow LM, Tsai YF, Wang L, Pfaff DW. Electrophysiological analyses of serotonergic actions on neurons in hypothalamic ventromedial nucleus in vitro: receptor subtypes involved and implications for regulation of feeding and lordosis behaviors. *Chin J Physiol.* 1992;35(2):105–121.

Lindal E, Steffansson JG. The lifetime prevalence of psychosocial dysfunction among 55 to 57 year olds. *Soc Psychiatry Epidemiol.* 1993;28:91–95.

Lowy M. Erectile dysfunction in the Australian community. *Med J Aust.* 1999;171:342–343.

Linnankoski I, Gronrous M, Carlson S, Pertovaara A. Increased sexual behavior in male Macaca arctoides monkeys produced by atipamezole, a selective alpha 2-adrenoceptor antagonist. *Pharmacol Biochem Behav.* 1992;42(1):197–200.

Lorrain D, Matuszewitz L. Extracellular serotonin in the lateral hypothalamus is increased during the postejaculatory interval and impairs ejaculation in male rats. *J Neurosci.* 1997;17:936–937.

Luine V, Cowell J, Frankfurt M. GABAergic-serotonergic interactions in regulating lordosis. *Brain Res.* 1991;556(1):171–174.

Maeda N. Role of the dopaminergic , serotonergic, and cholinergic link in the expression of penile erection in rats. *Japanese J Pharmacol.* 1994a;66:59–66.

Maeda N. A screening concept based on a hypothesis led to a putative cognitive enhancer that stimulates penile erection. *Japanese J Pharmacol.* 1994b;64:147–153.

Maeda N. Involvement of raphe-hippocampal serotonergic and septo-hippocampal cholinerigc mechanisms in hte penile erection induced by FR121196, a putative cognitive enhancer. *Japanese J Pharmacol.* 1995;68:85–94.

Maeda N, Matsuoka N, Yamaguchi I. Possible involvement of the septo-hippocampal cholinergic and raphe-hippocampal serotonergic activation in the penile erection induced by fenfluramine. *Brain Res.* 1994a;652:181–190.

Maeda N, Matsuoka N, Yamaguchi I. Role of the dopaminergic, serotonergic, and cholinergic link in the expression of penile erection in rats. *Jpn J Pharmacol.* 1994b;66:59–66.

Marson L, McKenna KE. A role for 5-hydroxytryptamine in descending inhibition of spinal sexual reflexes. *Exp Brain Res.* 1992;88(2):313–320.

Mathias CJ, Bannister RB, Cortelli P. Clinical, autonomic and therapeutic observations in two siblings with postural hypotension and sympathetic failure due to an inability to synthesize noradrenaline from dopamine because of a deficiency of dopamine beta hydroxylase. *Q J Med.* 1990;75:517–533.

Matsuoka N. Brain somatostatin depletion by cysteamine attentuates the penile erection induced by serotonergic and dopaminergic but not cholinergic activation in rats. *Brain Res.* 1996;729:132–136.

McKenna K, Knight K, Mayers R. Modulation by peripheral serotonin of the threshold for sexual reflexes in female rats. *Pharmacol Biochem Behav.* 1991;40(1):151–156.

McKenna K. Central mechanisms in sexual function. *Sexual Dysfunction in Medicine.* 2001;2:40–47

McLean P. *Brain Mechanisms of Primal Sexual Functions and Related Behavior.* New York: Raven; 1975.

Mc Ginnis M, Williams W, Lumia A. Inhibition of male sexual behavior by androgen receptor blockade in preoptic area of hypothalamus, but not amygdala or septum. *Physiology & Behavior.* 1996;60:783–789.

Meinhardt W, Kropman R, Vermeij P, Nijeholt L, Zwartendijk J. The influence of medication on erectile function. *Int J Impotence Res.* 1997;9:17–26.

Marson L. Sexual reflexes in the female rat-evidence for spinal control. Paper presented at: Meeting of the Female Sexual Function Forum; 2001; Boston.

Melis M, Stancampiano R, Argiolas A. Effect of excitatory amino acid receptor antagonists on apomorphine-oxytocin-and ACTH-induced penile erection and yawning in male rats. *Eur J Pharmacol.* 1992;229:43–48.

Mendelson S, Gorzalka B. Sex differences in the effects of 1-(m-trifluoromethylphenyl) piperazine and 1-(m-chlorophenyl) piperazine on copulatory behavior in the rat. *Neuropharmacology.* 1990;29(8):783–786.

Mendelson SD. A review and reevaluation of the role of serotonin in the modulation of lordosis behavior in the female rat. *Neurosci Biobehav Rev.* 1992;16(3):309–350.

Minetti S, Fulginiti S. Sexual receptivity of adult female rats prenatally intoxicated with alcohol on gestational day 8. *Neurotoxicol Teratol.* 1991;13(5):531–534.

Mishra N, Tangri K, Bhargava K, Gupta M. Evidence for the inhibitory effect of 5-hydroxytryptamine at central and peripheral sites on ovulation in rabbits. *Clin Exp Pharmacol Physiol.* 1990;17(8):595–599.

Mos J, Vanlogten J, Bloetjes K. The effects of idazoxan and 8-OH-DPAT on sexual behaviour and associated ultrasonic vocalizations in the rat. *Neurosci Biobehav Rev.* 1991;15(4):505–515.

McKinlay J. The worldwide prevalence and epidemiology of erectile dysfunction. *Int J Impot Res.* 2000;12(suppl 4):6–11.

McKinlay JB, Digruttolo L, Glasser D, Sweeney M, Shirai M. International diferences in the epidemiology of male erectile dysfunction. *Int J Impot Res.* 1999;10(suppl):3–12

Meana M, Binik I, Khalife S, Cohen D. Affect and marital adjustment in women's ratings of dyspareunic pain. *Can J Psychiatry.* 1998;43:381–385.

Melman A, Gingell J. The epidemiology and pathophysiology of erectile dysfunction. *J Urology.* 1999;161:5–11.

Nusbaum M, Gamble G, Skinner B, Heiman J. The high prevalence of sexual concerns among women seeking routine gynecological care. *J of Fam Pract.* 2000;49:229–232.

Naganuma H, Egashira T, Fujii I. Neuroleptics induce penile erection in the rabbit. *Clin Exp Pharmacol Physiol.* 1993;20:177–183.

Nikulina E, Popova N. Serotonin's influence on predatory behavior of highly aggressive CBA and weakly aggressive DD strains of mice. *Aggess Behav.* 1986;12:277–283.

Penfield W, Rasmussen T. *The Cerebral Cortex of Man.* New York: Macmillan; 1950.

Pfaus J, Phillips A. Differential effects of dopamine receptor antagonists on the sexual behavior of male rats. *Psychopharmacology.* 1989;98:363–368.

Pomerantz SM. Quinelorane (LY163502), a D2 dopamine receptor agonist, acts centrally to facilitate penile erections of male rhesus monkeys. *Pharmacol Biochem Behav.* 1991;39(1):123–128.

Powers J, Schaumburg H. A fatal case of sexual inadequacy in men:adrenoleukodystrophy. *J Urol.* 1980;124:583–585.

Protias P, Windsor M, Mocaer E, Comoy E. Post-synaptic 5ht1a receptor involvement in yawning and penile erections induced by apomorphine, physostigmine and mCPP in rats. *Psychopharmacol.* 1995;120:376–383.

Protias P, Windsor M, Mocaer E, Comoy E. Post-synaptic 5ht1a receptor involvement in yawning and penile erections induced by apomorphine, physostigmine and mCPP in rats. *Psychopharmacol.* 1995;120:376–383.

Pinnock C, Stapleton A, Marshall V. Erectile dysfunction in the community:a prevalence study. *Med J Aust.* 1999;171:353–357.

Rago L, Saano V, Tupala E, Nieminen, SA, Airaksinen MM. 3H-atipamezole binding sites in mouse cerebral cortex:possible involvement of alpha 2 adrenoceptors in sexual behavior. *Methods Find Exp Clin Pharmacol.* 1992;14:23–71.

Randeva H, Davison R, Bouloux P. Endocrinlogy. In Carson C, Kirby R, Goldstein I, eds. *Textbook of Erectile Dysfunction.* Oxford U.K.: Isis; 1999:89–104.

Raynaud F, Pevet P. Effect of different photoperiods on the diurnal rhythm of 5-methoxytryptamine in the pineal gland of golden hamsters (Mesocricetus auratus). *J Neural Transm Gen Sect.* 1991;83(3):235–242.

Rehman J, Christ G, Alyskewyck M, Kerr E, Melman A. Experimental hyper-prolactinemia in a rat model: alteration in centrally mediated neuroerectile mechanisms. *Int J Impot Res.* 2000;12:23–32.

Retana-Marquez S, Salazer ED, Velazquez-Moctezuma J. Muscarinic and nicotinic influences on masculine sexual behavior in rats: effects of oxotremorine, scopolamine, and nicotine. *Pharmacol Biochem Behav.* 1993;44(4):913–917.

Retana-Marquez S, Velazquez-Moctezuma J. Evidence that the M1 muscarinic receptor subtype mediates the effects of oxotremorine on masculine sexual behavior. *Neuropsychopharmacology.* 1993;9(4):267–270.

Rodriguez-Manzo G, Fernandez-Guasti A. Reversal of sexual exhaustion by serotonergic and noradrenergic agents. *Behav Brain Res.* 1994;62(2):127–134.

Saenz de Tajada I. Pathophysiology of erectile dysfunction:the contribution of trabecular strcuture to function and the role of functional antagonism. *Int J Impot Res.* 2000;12(suppl 4):39–46.

Scimonelli T, Medina F, Wilson C, Celis M. Interaction of alpha-melanotropin (a-MSH) and noradrenaline in the median eminence in the control of female sexual behavior. *Peptides.* 2000;21:219–223.

Schwarcz G. Case report of inhibition of ejacualtion and retrograde ejacualtion as side effects of amoxapine. *Am J Psychaitry.* 1982;139:233–235.

Schreiner-Engel P, Schiavi R, White D, Ghizzanni A. Low sexual desire in women:the role of reproductive hormones. *Horm Behav.* 1989;23:221–234.

Shirai M, Marui E, Hayashi K, Ishii N, Abe T. Prevalence and correlates of erectile dysfunction in Japan. *Int J Impot Res.* 1999;102:36.

Segarra A, Luine V, Strand F. Sexual behavior of male rats is differentially affected by timing of perinatal ACTH administration. *Physiol Behav.* 1991;50(4):689–697.

Sietnieks A. Involvement of 5-HTsub 2 receptors in the LSD- and L-5-HTP-induced suppression of lordotic behavior in the female rat. *J. NEURAL TRANSM.* 1985;61(1-2):65–80.

Simon P, Guardiola B, Bizot-Espiard J, Schiavi P, Costentin J. 5-HT1A receptor agonist prevent in rats the yawning and penile erections induced by direct dopamine agonists. *Psychopharmacology.* 1992;108:47–50.

Simon P, Bertrand J, Costentin J. 5-Ht1A receptor blockade inreases penile erections induced by indirect serotonin agonists. *Neuroreport.* 1993;13(5):229–230.

Simon P, Guardiola B, Bizot-Espiard J, Schiavi P, Costenin J. 5-HT1a receptor agonists prevent in rats the yawning and penile erections induced by direct dopamine agonists. *Psychopharmacology.* 1992;108:47–50.

Sirinathsinghji D. Intrahypothalamic infusions of a synthetic heroin substitute, N-methyl-4-phenyl-1,2,3,6-tetrahydropyridine, potentiate mating behaviour in the female rat. *Brain Res.* 1985;346:130–135.

Sirinathsinghji DJS, Whittington PE, Audsley AR. Regulation of mating behaviour in the female rat by gonadotropin-releasing hormone in the ventral tegmental area: effects of selective destruction of the A10 dopamine neurones. *BRAIN RES.* 1986;374(1):167–173.

Smith B, Khatri A. Cortical localization of sexual feelings. *Psychosomatics.* 1979;20:771–776.

Smith ER, Maurice J, Richardson R, Walter T, Davidson JM. Effects of four beta-adrenergic receptor antagonists on male sexual behavior. *Pharmacol Biochem Behav.* 1990;36:713–717.

Stancampiano R, Melis MP, Argiolas A. Penile erection and yawning induced by 5ht1c receptor agonists in male rats: relationship with dopaminergic and oxytocinerfgic transmission. *Eur J Pharmacol.* 1994;261:149–155.

Stoleru S, Gregoire M, Gerard D, Decety J, Lafarge E, Cinotti L, Lavenne F, Le Bars D, Veret-maury E, Rada H, Collet C, Mazoyer B, Forest M, MAgnin F, Spira A, Comar D. Neuroanatomical correaltes of visually evoked sexual arousal in human males. *Arch Sex Behav.* 1999;28:1–21.

Umans JG, Lindheimer MD, Barron WM. Pressor effect of endothelium-derived relaxing factor inhibition in conscious virgin and gravid rats. *Am J Physiol.* 1990;259(2, pt 2):F293–296.

Uphouse L, Caldarola-Pastuszka M, Moore N. Inhibitory effects of the 5-HT1A agonists, 5-hydroxy- and 5-methoxy-(3-di-n-propylamino)chroman), on female lordosis behavior. *Neuropharmacology.* 1993;32(7):641–651.

Vachon P, Simmerman N, Zahran A, Carrier S. Increases in clitoral and vaginal blood flow following clitoral and pelvic plexus nerve stimualtions in the feamle rat. *Int J Impot Res.* 2000;12:53–57.

Varrin S, Heaton JP. Age-related changes in apomorphine-induced erections. *Neurobiol Aging.* 1992;13:175–177.

Verma K, Khaitan B, Singh O. The frequency of sexual dysfunction in patients attending a sex therapy clinic in North India. *Arch Sex Behav.* 1998;27:309–314.

Velazquez-Moctezuma J, Aguilar-Garcia A, Diaz-Ruiz O. Behavioral effects of neonatal treatment with clomipramine, scopolamine, and idazoxan in male rats. *Pharmacol Biochem Behav.* 1993;46(1):215–217.

Warner R, Thompson JT, Markowski VP, Loucks JA, Bazzatt JT, Eaton RC, Hull EM. Microinjection of the dopamine antagonist cis-flupenthixol into the MPOA impairs copulation, penile reflexes, and sexual motivation in male rats. *Brain Res.* 1991;540:177–182.

Watson N, Gorzalka B. Concurrent wet dog shaking and inhibition of male rat copulation after ventromedial brainstem injection of the 5-HT2 agonist DOI. *Neurosci Lett.* 1992;141(1):25–29.

Weidner W, Zoller G, Saverwein D. A modified technique for nerve-sparing retroperitoneal lymph node dissection in stage II nonseminomatous germ cell tumors using intraoperative measurement of bladder neck pressure alterations following sympathetic nerve fiber electrostimulation. *Eur Urol.* 1994;26(1):67–70.

Weiss RJ. Effects of antihypertensive agents on sexual function. *Am Fam Physician.* 1991;44(6):2075–2082.

Winn P. Cholinergic stimulation of substantia nigra: effects on feeding, drinking and sexual behaviour in the male rat. *Psychopharmacology* (Berl). 1991;104(2):208–214.

Xin Z. Penile sensitivity in aptients with primary premature ejaculation. *J Urol.* 1996;156:979–981.

Yamanouchi K, Kakeyama M. Effect of medullary raphe lesions on sexual behavior in male rats with or without treatments of p-chlorophenylalanine. *Physiol Behav.* 1992;51(3):575–579.

Yonezawa A, Kawamura S, Ando R. Chronic clonidine treatment and its termination: effects on penile erection and ejaculation in the dog. *Life Sci.* 1992;51(25):1999–2007.

Zarrindast MR, Mamandush SM, Rashidy-Pour A. Morphine inhibits dopaminergic and cholinergic induced ejaculation in rats. *Gen Pharmacol.* 1994;25(4):803–808.

Zarrindast MR, Shokravi S, Samini M. Opposite influences of dopaminergic receptor subtypes on penile erection. *Gen Pharmac.* 1992;23:671–675.

2. Sexual Side Effects of Antipsychotic Drugs

INTRODUCTION

Antipsychotic drugs are used to treat various forms of psychosis including schizophrenia, schizoaffective disorder, mood disorders, and psychotic disorders due to general medical conditions. They are also used as adjunctive medication in the treatment of mood disorders without psychosis and in the management of agitation in patients with medical disorders. Antipsychotic drugs are the primary therapy for people who have schizophrenia, a disabling psychotic disorder characterized by delusions and hallucinations. The treatment of schizophrenia is complicated by the severity and chronicity of the disorder, frequent drug noncompliance, and by disabling drug side effects such as acute dystonias, akathisia, parkinsonism, and tardive dyskinesia.

A number of methodological issues make the determination of the incidence of sexual dysfunction in people on antipsychotic drugs difficult. First, the population of patients taking antipsychotic drugs generally has a low baseline of sexual activity. Unless the psychotic disorder is under good control, it can be extremely difficult to obtain an accurate sexual history from the person. The patient's major sexual outlet may be masturbatory, and the patient may be uncomfortable providing this information. In view of the seriousness of the illnesses for which antipsychotic drugs are prescribed, the presence of sexual side effects has received minimal attention by most clinicians.

Case reports beginning in 1961 established the likelihood that antipsychotic drug use might be associated with sexual side effects. (Table 2.1

**Table 2.1   Sexual problems associated
with antipsychotics**

Delayed ejaculation
Decreased libido
Erectile dysfunction
Retrograde ejaculation
Painful ejaculation
Priapism
Deleyed orgasm
Amenorrhea
Galactorrhea

summarizes the sexual problems associated with antipsychotics.)
Some clinical series even suggested that approximately 50% of patients
on traditional antipsychotic drugs might have drug-induced sexual
dysfunction. With the introduction of newer agents, called atypical
antipsychotics, clinicians and patients have become more interested
in quality-of-life issues such as sexual function while receiving antipsychotic agents. Atypicals treat both negative symptoms (e.g., lack
of motivation and social withdrawal) as well as positive symptoms
(e.g., hallucinations, delusions).

Unfortunately, most psychiatric texts have minimal information concerning sexual dysfunction in people on antipsychotic agents. The
Physicians' Desk Reference (PDR) primarily consists of information
obtained in clinical trials, in which there was no direct questioning
about sexual function. As noted, few patients volunteer such information, so information in the *PDR* underestimates the frequency of
sexual side effects associated with drug treatment. Clinicians and patients have to depend on other sources of information. This chapter
summarizes the information currently available. It is important to realize that the major part of this information has been obtained from
clinical series and case reports.

TRADITIONAL OR TYPICAL ANTIPSYCHOTIC DRUGS

Traditional antipsychotics were discovered in the 1950s. These drugs
are also sometimes referred to as neuroleptics or typical antipsychotics to differentiate them from atypical antipsychotics such as
clozapine, olanzapine, risperidone, quetiapine and ziprasidone. All of
the typical antipsychotics bind to the dopamine D2 receptor, which
appears to be a necessary first step in their mechanism of action. It
is assumed that blockade of the D2 receptor in the mesolimbic cortical dopamine pathway is necessary for their antipsychotic activity,

and that the dopamine blockade in other pathways is responsible for the side effects of hyperprolatinemia and extrapyramidal side effects. The typical antipsychotics cause prolactin elevation, which has been posited to cause sexual dysfunction. Prolactin is tonically inhibited by dopamine, and dopamine blockade in the tuberoinfundibular pathway causes prolactin elevation. Most of the typical antipsychotics also have alpha-adrenergic blockade and antimuscarinic properties as side effects. Antiadrenergic activity is hypothesized to be a mechanism by which typical antipsychotics inhibit ejaculation and orgasm. Alpha-adrenergic blockade also may explain the propensity of these drugs to cause priapism or the safe enhancement of erectile function in a small number of patients.

Almost all classes of traditional antipsychotic drugs have been associated with sexual dysfunction in case reports. Although problems with erection and libido have been reported, the most common sexual side effect appears to be problems with ejaculation. Most traditional antipsychotics probably cause ejaculatory difficulties in approximately 19% of patients. It is unclear how often reports of absent ejaculation (failure of external emission) are actually due to retrograde ejaculation.

The few studies that have included female patients have found a similar incidence of problems with orgasm. In a 1976 study measuring the incidence of sexual problems in a group of patients taking thioridazine, 60% experienced sexual impairment, 44% had trouble with ejaculation, and 35% had difficulty maintaining erections. The senior author of that study was skeptical about this finding, so he took a dose of thioridazine and attempted to masturbate 4 hours later; he was unable to ejaculate. Of the typical antipsychotics, there have been more case reports of ejaculatory problems with thioridazine than any other agent. Even extremely small, presumably subtherapeutic, doses such as 30 mg have been reported to cause problems with ejaculation. Some clinicians have reported success using thioridazine to successfully treat premature ejaculation and troublesome nocturnal emissions. Painful ejaculation has been reported with a number of agents, including thioridazine, trifluoperazine, and haloperidol.

In isolated cases, improved erectile function has been reported with thioridazine, trifluoperazine, thiothixine, and mesoridazine; however, these appear to be infrequent occurrences. Fluphenazine and other antispychotics have been used to treat sexual offenders because of their antilibidinal properties. Of the older antipsychotics, molindone and loxapine were thought to have a low incidence of sexual dysfunction. However, recent data suggest that loxapine may have a

Table 2.2 Case reports of sexual dysfunction on traditional antipsychotics

Drug	Ejaculatory	Erectile	Female SD
Aliphatic phenothiazines			
Chlorpromazine (Thorazine)	Probable	Possible	Probable orgasm delay
Piperidine phenothiazines			
Thioridazine (Mellaril)	49–60%	44%	Probable orgasm delay
Mesoridazine (Serentil)	Probable	Possible	Probable orgasm delay
Piperazine phenothiazines			
Trifluoperazine (Stelazine)	80%	Possible	Probable orgasm delay
Fluphenazine (Prolixin)	75%	Possible	Probable orgasm delay
Perphenazine (Trilafon)	64%	Possible	Probable orgasm delay
Prochlorperazine (Compazine)	Probable	Possible	Probable orgasm delay
Thioxanthenes			
Chlorprothixene (Taractan)	Probable	Possible	Probable orgasm delay
Thiothixene (Navane)	Probable	Possible	Probable orgasm delay
Butyrophenones			
Haloperidal (Haldol)	25%	Unknown	Unknown
Diphenylbutylpiperidine			
Pimozide (Orap)	40%	Unknown	Probable orgasm delay
Dibenzazepine			
Loxapine (Loxitane)	30%	36%	Probable orgasm delay
Dihydroindolone			
Molindone (Moban)	Unknown	Unknown	Unknown

relatively high incidence of sexual dysfunction associated with its use.

Table 2.2 summarizes data on sexual dysfunction associated with traditional antipsychotics.

ATYPICAL ANTIPSYCHOTICS

Clozapine was the first atypical antipsychotic drug introduced in the United States. It had a major impact in the treatment of schizophrenia because of its effect on negative (social withdrawal and anhedonia) as well as positive (hallucinations and delusions) symptoms of schizophrenia. Added advantages of clozapine are that it causes minimal extrapyramidal side effects and minimal prolactin elevation. Other atypical antipsychotics include risperidone, olanzapine, and quetiapine. All but risperidone have been labeled as "prolactin sparing" because they have minimal effects on prolactin. However, these drugs all induce an alpha-adrenergic blockade as part of their pharmacologic profile. The mechanism of action for the atypical antipsychotics is unknown. These drugs have effects on multiple dopamine receptors as well as on serotonin receptors, especially 5HT2a and 5HT2c.

Recent data suggest that the so-called prolactin sparing antipsychotics (i.e., olanzapine, clozapine, and quietiapine) may have lower rates of sexual dysfunction than the traditional antipsychotics. Of the newer antipsychotics, risperidone appears to have the highest rate of sexual dysfunction. The incidence of sexual dysfunction on risperidone appears to be both dose-related and related to the degree of prolactin elevation. There have been isolated case reports of ejaculatory delay associated with risperidone, clozapine, and olanzapine. Risperidone has repeatedly been shown to cause more sexual side effects than olanzapine. A multicenter study found that the following incidence of sexual dysfunction: haloperidal, 25%; risperidone, 8%; olanzapine, 2%; clozapine, 0%. Not all clinical series have found that the incidence of sexual side effects on atypical antipsychotics is this much lower than conventional antipsychotics.

A study in Austria reported that haloperidol and clozapine had the same incidence of sexual dysfunction initially, but that tolerance developed to side effects on both drugs. There is some evidence of tolerance developing after 3–4 months of continued therapy.

All of the antipsychotic agents may have adverse effects on libido. Because of preexisting problems with libido, problems in reporting, and lack of precise definitions of libido, it is difficult to determine which drugs have a higher incidence of libido disturbances. Priapism has been reported with all of the newer agents as well as with most of the tradtional antipsychotic drugs.

Some authors have suggested that prolactin elevation is the mechanism by which antipsychotic drugs influence erectile capacity. Prolactinemia has been reported to interfere with neurotransmitter production and secretion. However, both hyperprolactinemia and sexual dysfunction could both be signs of a dopamine blockade. The ejaculatory disturbance associated with many antipsychotic drugs has been hypothesized to be either the result of alpha-adrenergic blockade or of dopamine blockade.

Table 2.3 Case reports of sexual dysfunction on atypical antipsychotics

Drug	Ejaculatory	Erectile	Female SD
Dibenzodiazpine			
Clozapine (Clozaril)	Transient?	Transient?	Unknown
Benzisoxazole			
Risperidone (Risperidal)	20–30%	15%	20%
Dibenzazepine			
Olanzapine (Zyprexa)	5%	5%	No effect
Quetiapine (Seroquel)	Possible ejaculatory delay	Unknown	Unknown
Ziprazodone (Geodon)	Unknown	Unknown	Unknown

The atypical antipsychotics may have lower incidence of sexual dysfunction for one or more of the following reasons:

1. lower elevation of prolactin

2. more 5HT2 activity than D2 blockade

3. more activity at other dopamine receptors than D2

4. greater mesolimbic specificity

Table 2.3 summarizes data on sexual dysfunction associated with atypical antipsychotics.

TREATMENT OF ANTIPSYCHOTIC-INDUCED SEXUAL DYSFUNCTION

There is some evidence in the literature to suggest that switching to a prolactin-sparing antipsychotic such as olanzapine (or *quetiapine*) may relieve sexual dysfunction induced by other drugs. Clinical series suggest that sildenafil reverses sexual dysfunction induced by antipsychotic drugs. Other clinicians have reported success with bromocriptine initiated at 2.5mg/day and titrated up to 25mg/day; or by using cabergoline, a longer-acting dopamine agonist, starting at .25mg twice

Table 2.4 Antidotes for antipsychotic-induced sexual dysfunction

25–50 mg imipramine for thioridazine
50–100 mg sildenafil
2.5–25 mg bromocriptine
.50–1 mg cabergoline

Table 2.5   Medical management of sexual side effects

1. Wait for tolerance to develop. This strategy should be reserved for patients who indicate that temporary cessation of sexual activities is not problematic. It should not be employed with patients who have a history of drug noncompliance of unexplained etiology.

2. Attempt dose reduction. This strategy might be attempted with patients who are treatment compliant, have a clear prodromal syndrome, and good social support.

3. If the problem is ejaculatory or orgasmic dysfunction, switch to an antipsychotic with less alpha-adrenergic blockade, such as olanzapine or haloperidol. Consider a trial of sildenafil.

4. If the patient is on risperidone and has ejaculatory problems, lower the dose or switch to olanzapine or quetiapine.

5. If the problem is low libido or erectile failure, switch to an atypical antipsychotic.

6. If the patient cannot be switched to an atypical antipsychotic, try adding bromocriptine 2.5 mg/day and increasing the dose by 2.5 mg/day, or cabergoline 2.5 mg twice a week increasing by .25 mg/week.

a week and increasing to .5 mg twice a week. Bromocriptine should be used with caution, as it has been reported to precipitate psychotic episodes. A report from Israel found that thioridazine-induced anorgasmia could be reversed by the addition of 25–50 mg of imipramine. The mechanism for this is unclear.

Table 2.4 summarizes antidotes for sexual dysfunction, and Table 2.5 summarizes the medical management of sexual side effects.

Priapism

Priapism is a prolonged, usually painful and persistent erection. Twenty-eight per cent of reported priapism cases were associated with oral medication involving psychiatric drugs, especially antipsychotics and trazodone. Priapism is a medical emergency warranting urological consultation if the erection persists more than 4–6 hours. Priapism can result in endothelial and trabecular necrosis, as well as widespread smooth muscle destruction (drug-induced). Priapism is felt to be the result of alpha-adrenergic antagonism. Other hypotheses concerning the mechanism of priapism involve adrenergic/cholinergic imbalance and hypersensitization of beta adrenergic receptors. Most episodes of priapism occur early in the morning. Approximately 50% result in permanent erectile failure. If urological consultation is unavailable, the usual treatment is corporeal aspiration with a large bore butterfly needle. After 20–50 ml of venous blood are withdrawn, the patient will usually experience reduction in pain. If the first intervention is ineffective or if the erection recurs after aspiration, the treatment of choice is irrigation of the corpus cavernosum with phenylephrine 100–200 μg, which can be repeated every 5 minutes.

Table 2.6 summarizes the treatment of priapism.

A
N
T
I
P
S
Y
C
H
O
T
I
C

D
R
U
G
S

Table 2.6 Treatment of priapism

Urology consult
Corporeal aspiration of 20–50 ml venous blood using large bore butterfly needle
Irrigation with 100–200 μg phenylephrine q 5 minutes

REFERENCES

Aizenberg D, Dorfman-Etrog P, Weizman A. Sexual dysfunction in male schizophrenic patients. *J Clin Psychiatry.* 1995;65:137–141.

Alcantara A, Nieto J. Spontaneous orgasms during risperidone treatment in a schizophrenic patients: a case report. *Hum Psychopharmacol.* 1998;13:135–136.

Arato M, Polgar M. Endocrinological changes in patients with sexual dysfunction under long-term neuroleptic treatment. *Pharmacopsychiatry.* 1979;14:425–431.

Asnis G, Sachar E, Langer G, Tabrizi M, Nathan R, Halpern F. Prolactin responses to haloperidal in normal young women. *Psychoneuroendocrinology.* 1988;13:515–520.

Baldwin D, Birtwistle J. Schizophrenia, antipsychotic drugs and sexual function. *Primary Care Psychiatry.* 1997;3:115–123.

Bartholomew A. A long acting phenothiazine as a possible agent to control deviant sexual behavior. *Am J Psychiatry.* 1968;124:917–923.

Berger S. Trifluoperazine and haloperidal: sources of ejaculatory pain? *Am J Psychiatry.* 1979;136:359.

Berlin R. Metoclopromide-induced reversible impotence. *West J Med.* 1986;144:359–361.

Blair J. Effects of antipsychotic drugs on reproductive function. *Dis Nerv Syst.* 1966;27:645–647.

Brambilla F, Guerrini A. Neuroendocrine effects of haloperidal therapy in chronic schizophrenia. *Psychopharmacology.* 1974;44:17–22.

Canuso C, Hnau M, Jhamb K, Green A. Olanzapine use in women with antipsychotic-induced hyperprolactinemia. *Am J Psychiatry.* 1998;155:1458.

Collins A, Kellner R. Neuroleptics and sexual function. *Integ Psychiatry.* 1986;4:96–108.

Compton M, Saldivia A, Berry S. Recurrent priapism during treatment with clozapine and olanzapine. *Am J Psychiatry.* 2000;157:659.

Conley R. Risperidone side effects. *J Clin Psychiatry.* 2000;61(Suppl 8):20–23.

Covington L, Cola P. Clozapine versus haloperidal: antipsychotic effects on sexual function in schizophrenia. *Sexuality and Disabilty.* 2000;18:41–48.

Crawford A, Beasley C, Tollefson G. The acute and long-term effect of olanzapine compared with placebo and haloperidal on serum plasma concentrations. *Schizophr Res.* 1997;26:41–54.

Daniels G, Goff D, Hayden D, Kearns A. Risperidone-associated hyperprolactinemia. *Endocr Pract.* 2000;6:425–429.

David S, Taylor C, Kinin B, Breier A. The effects of olanzapine, risperidone, and haloperidal on plasma prolactin levels in patients with schizophrenia. *Clin Ther.* 2000;22:1085–1096.

Deirmenjian J, Erhart S, Wirshing D, Spellberg B, Wirshing W. Olanzapine reversible priapism: a case report. *J Clin Psychopharmacol.* 1998;18:351–353.

Demyttenaere K, Fruyt J, Sienaert P. Psychotropics and sexuality. *Int Clin Psychopharmacol.* 1998;13(Suppl 6):35–41.

Dickson R, Glazer W. Hyperprolactinemia and male sexual dysfunction. *J Clin Psychiatry.* 1999a;60:125.

Dickson R, Glazer W. Neuroleptic-induced hyperprolactinemia. *Schizophrenia Bulletin.* 1999b;35:75–86.

Dickson R, Seeman M, Corenblum B. Hormonal side effects in women: typical versus atypical antipsychotic treatment. *J Clin Psychiatry.* 2000;61:10–15.

Emes C. Risperidone induced priapism. *Canad J Psychiatry.* 1994;39:96–108.

Fabian J. Psychotropic medications and priapism. *Am J Psychiatry.* 1993;150:349–350.

Fleischhacker W, Hummer M. Drug treatment of schizophrenia. *Drugs.* 1997;53:915–929.

Gazzola L, Opler L. Return of menstruation after switching from risperidone to olanzapine. *J Clin Psychopharmacol.* 1998;18:486–487.

Ghadirian A, Choviard G. Sexual dysfunction and plasma prolactin levels in treated schizophrenic outpatients. *J Nerv Ment Dis.* 1982;10:463–473.

Gold D, Justino F. Bicycle kickstand phenomena: prolonged erections associated with antipsychotic agents. *South Med J.* 1988;81:792–794.

Gordon M, DeGroot C. Olanzapine induced priapism. *J Clin Psychopharmacol.* 1999;19:192.

Gutierrez M, Stimmel G. Management of and counseling for psychotropic drug-induced sexual dysfunction. *Pharmacotherapy.* 1999;19:823–831.

Hammer M, Arana G. Hyperprolactinemia in antipsychotic-treated patients. *CNS Drugs.* 1998;10:209–222.

Hansen T, Casey D, Hoffman W. Neuroleptic intolerance. *Schizophr Bull.* 1997;23:567–582.

Hummer M, Kemmler G. Sexual disturbances during clozapine and haloperidal treatment for schizophrenia. *Am J Psychiatry.* 1999;56:631–633.

Jackson S, Walker, J. Self-administered intraurethral chlorpromazine: an unusual cause of priapism. *Am J Emergency Medicine.* 1991;9:171–175.

Kearns A, Goff D, Hayden D, Daniels G. Risperidone-associated hyperprolactinemia. *Endocrine Practice.* 2000;6:425–429.

Keene L, Davies P. Drug-related erectile dysfunction. *Adverse Drug React Toxicol Rev.* 1999;18:5–24.

Kotin J, Wilbert, D. Thioridazine and sexual dysfunction. *Am J Psychiatry.* 1976;133:82–85.

Marder S, Meibach, R. Risperidone in the treatment of schizophrenia. *Am J Psychiatry.* 1994;151:825–835.

Marken P, Hyakal R, Rfisher J. Management of psychotropic-induced hyperprolactinemia. *Clin Pharmacy.* 1992;11:851–856.

Markianos M, Hatzimanolis J, Lykouras L. Gonadal axis hormones in male schizophrenic patients during treatment with haloperidal and after switch to risperidone. *Psychopharmacology.* 1999;143:270–272.

Moinfar N, Goad S, Brink D, Klinger R. Clozapine-related priapism. *Hosp Community Psychiatry.* 1994;45:1044.

Montejo-Gonzalez A, Llorca G. New antipsychotic-induced sexual dysfunction: comparative incidence with risperidone and olanzapine using a questionnaire. *APA NR*. 1998;181–182.

Mutlu N, Ozkurkcugil C, Culha M, Turkan S, Gokalp A. Priapism induced by chlorpromazine. *Int J Clin Practice*. 1999;53:152–153.

Nicolson R, McCurley R. Risperidone-associated priapism. *J Clin Psychopharmacol*. 1997;17:133–134.

Petty R. Prolactin and antipsychotic medications: mechanism of action. *Schizophr Res*. 1999;35:67–73.

Raja M. Risperidone-induced absence of ejaculation. *Int Clin Psychopharmacol*. 1999;14:317–319.

Richter M, Crimson M. Pharmacology of sexual offenders. *Ann Pharmacol*. 1993;27:316–320.

Rosen R, Hanno P. Clozapine-induced priapism. *J of Urology*. 1992;148:876–877.

Salerian A, Deiber W, Vittone B, et al. Sildenafil for psychotropic-induced sexual dysfunction in 31 women and 61 men. *J Sex Marital Ther*. 2000;26:133–140.

Santoni J, Saubadu S. Adverse events associated with neuroleptic drugs: focus on neuroendocrine reactions. *Acta Ther*. 1995;21:193–204.

Seftel A, Saenz de Tejada I, Szetela B, Cole J, Goldstein I. Clozapine-associated priapism: a case report. *J of Urology*. 1992;147:146–148.

Shen WW, Park S. Thioridazine-induced inhibition of female orgasm. *Psychiatry J Univ. Ottawa*. 1982;7:249–251.

Shiwach R, Carmody T. Prolactogenic effects of risperidone in male patients: a preliminary study. *Acta Psychiatr Scand*. 1998;98:81–83.

Sirota P, Bogdanov I. Priapism associated with risperidone treatment. *Int J Psychiatry in Clin Practice*. 2000;4:237–239.

Stanniland C, Taylor D. Tolerabilty of atypical antipsychotics. *Drug Safety*. 2000;22:195–214.

Sullivan G, Lukoff D. Sexual side effects of antipsychotic medication: evaluation and interventions. *Hosp Community Psychiatry*. 1990;41:1238–1241.

Tejera C, Lorenzi J. Priapism in a patient receiving perphenazine. *J Clin Psychopharmacol*. 1992;12:448–449.

Tekell J, Smith E, Silva J. Prolonged erection associated with risperidone treatment. *Am J Psychiatry*. 1995;152:1097.

Thompson J, Ware M, Blashfield R. Psychotropic medication and priapism: a comprehensive review. *J Clin Psychiatry*. 1990;51:430–433.

Tollin S. Use of the dopamine agonists bromocriptine and cabergoline in the management of risperidone-induced hyperprolactinemia in patients with psychotic disorders. *J Endocrinol Invest*. 2000;23:765–770.

Tran P, Dellva M, Tollefson G, Beasley C, Potvin J, Kiesler G. Extrapyramidal symptoms and tolerability of olanzapine versus haloperidal in the acute treatment of schizophrenia. *J Clin Psychiatry*. 1997;58:205–211.

Valevski A, Modai I, Zharski E, Zemishlany Z, Weizman A. Effect of amantadine on sexual dysfunction in neuroleptic-treated male schizophrenic patients. *Clin Neuropharmacol*. 1998;21:355–357.

Zeigler J, Behav D. Clozapine-induced priapism. *Am J Psychiatry*. 1992;149:272–273.

3. Antianxiety Drugs and Sexual Dysfunction

Investigating the effects of antianxiety drugs on sexual function is complicated by the fact that both anxiety disorders and their treatment may be associated with sexual dysfunction. Patients with anxiety disorders have been found to have a high incidence of sexual disorders prior to pharmacotherapy. Recent studies in the Netherlands have found that women with panic disorder and obsessive–compulsive disorder have a high prevalence of hypoactive sexual desire disorder. It is assumed but unproven that similar relationships between anxiety disorders and male sexual dysfunction exist.

Many of the agents used to treat anxiety disorders may cause sexual dysfunction. Although selective serotonin reuptake inhibitors (SSRIs) are increasingly used to treat anxiety disorders, benzodiazepines are still commonly prescribed for this population. Beta-blockers and buspirone also are utilized, though to a lesser extent. All of the commonly prescribed benzodiazepines have been reported to be associated with sexual dysfunction. A double-blind placebo-controlled study has demonstrated a dose–response relationship between escalating doses of diazepam and orgasm delay in females. Case reports have suggested that low doses of lorazepam can be used to delay orgasm in the male with premature ejaculation. Table 3.1 summarizes the sexual side effects associated with benzodiazepines.

Most of the benzodiazepines appear to have a dose–response relationship between drug dose and sexual inhibition. A retrospective chart review of male veterans with posttraumatic stress disorder (PTSD) found that patients on clonazepam (average dose 3.4 mg) had a higher incidence of sexual dysfunction (primarily erectile problems) than patients on alprazolam (average dose 5 mg) and diazepam (average

Table 3.1 Sexual side effects associated with benzodiazepines

Drug	Impotence	Delayed Ejaculation	Female Sexual Dysfunction
Alprazolam (Xanax)	Probable	Yes	Female Sexual Dysfunction Orgasm Delay Probable
Chlordiazepoxide (Librium)	Unknown	Yes	Orgasm Delay Probable
Clonazepam (Klonopin)	Probable	Yes	Orgasm Delay Probable
Chlorazepate (Tranxene)	Unknown	Yes	Orgasm Delay Probable
Diazepam (Valium)	Probable	Yes	Yes
Lorazepam (Ativan)	Unknown	Yes	Probable
Buspirone (BuSpar)	No	No	
Propranolol (Inderal)	Yes	No	

dose 50 mg) or lorazepam (average dose 4 mg). In this study, switching the patients from clonazepam to either diazepam or lorazepam resolved the difficulty.

Another clinical series using sexual questionnaires with patients of both sexes on alprazolam found that 50% reported decreased libido as compared to pretreatment libido levels. Some patients reported difficulty with orgasm, and some men reported erectile difficulties. Reducing the dose or changing medication reversed sexual symptoms in most patients.

Other authors have reported that switching from diazepam to clonazepam resulted in the resolution of erectile dysfunction. Low-dose alprazolam has been reported to cause delayed ejaculation and loss of libido. Lorazepam also has been used successfully to delay ejaculation in men with rapid ejaculation. It is probable that many of the benzodiazepines marketed as sedative hypnotics interfere with the ability to reach orgasm, although this has not been reported. For example, one might expect delayed ejaculation and orgasm in patients who attempt to have sex in the morning after taking a long-acting benzodiazepine, such as flurazepam. Benzodiazepines are highly lipid soluble; this solubility is associated with their rapid passage into the brain. Because they can accumulate in fatty tissue, their activity may be prolonged in patients who are overweight.

It is of note that several case reports suggest that benzodiazepine use may be associated with sexual disinhibition. A possible animal model for this effect is the study of anxiolytics in subordinate male mice. Normally, subordinate male mice show impairment of their sexual performance in the presence of the male antagonist. Benzodiazepines improve the performance of subordinate mice toward female mice, as

Table 3.2   Recommendations for medical management

1. Reduce dose—most benzodiazepines cause sexual problems at higher doses.
2. Switch to a different benzodiazepine.
3. Consider a trial of sildenafil.
4. Consider use of an SSRI that has a low frequency of sexual side effects, such as citalopram.
5. Consider use of buspirone (warning: few patients find buspirone acceptable after prior exposure to benzodiazepines).

measured by proximal behavior, anogenital sniffing, and social grooming. It is probable that low doses of benzodiazepines may faciltiate sexual behavior in anxious individuals, whereas higher doses are inhibitory.

In contrast to studies of other species, human studies suggest that benzodiazepines may suppress both erectile and ejaculatory behavior. Studies in rats, stallions, and other animals have found that benzodiazepines facilitate erections and lordosis but inhibit ejaculation. Almost all benzodiazepines are sedating and have anticonvulsant, antianxiety, and muscle-relaxing properties.

This group of drugs is believed to work by potentiating gamma-aminobutyric acid (GABA) neuronal networks. GABA-nergic neurons form one of the brain's major inhibitory pathways. Benzodiazepines may exert some of their influence on sexual behavior through gamma-aminobutyric acid receptors in the midbrain central gray or ventral tegmental area. Although all benzodiazepines bind to GABA-A, there are some differences in affinities for receptors in different areas of the brain.

Buspirone does not appear to affect orgasm or erection, and it has been found to alleviate sexual problems in patients with generalized anxiety disorder. Buspirone acts as a partial 5HT1 a agonist, a different mechanism of action from the benzodiazepines. A large double-blind study demonstrated that buspirone 30–60 mg/day can successfully reverse SSRI-induced sexual dysfunction, usually after 1 week. Buspirone also has been reported to be associated with priapism.

A number of studies have suggested that propranolol may cause problems with erection, but it is not associated with ejaculatory problems. Table 3.2 contains recommendations for medical management.

REFERENCES

Agmo A, Fernandez H. Benzodiazepine receptor ligands and sexual behavior in the male rat: the role of GABAnergic mechanisms. *Pharmacol Biochem Behav.* 1991;38:871–878.

Balon R, Ramesh C, Pohl R. Sexual dysfunction associated with diazepam and not clonazepam. *Canad J Psychiatry.* 1989;34:947–948.

Brahams D. Benzodiazepines and sexual assault, Canada. *Lancet.* 1991;337:291–292.

Brock G, Lue T. Drug-induced male sexual dysfunction: an update. *Drug Safety.* 1993;8:414–426.

D'Amato FR, Pavone F. Role of anxiety in subordiante male mice sexual behavior. *Pharmacol Biochem Behav.* 1992;43:181–185.

Demyttenaere K, DeFruyt J, Sienaert P. Psychotropics and sexuality. *Int Clin Psychopharmacol.* 1998;13(Suppl 6):35–41.

Duncan L, Bateman D. Sexual function in women. *Drug Safety,* 8:225–234.

Dundee JW. Advantages and problems with benzodiazepine sedation. *Anesthesia Progress.* 1992;39:132–137.

Fava M, Borofsky GF. Sexual disinhibition during treatment with a benzodiazepine: a case report. *Int J Psychiatry in Medicine,* 21, 99–104.

Fernandez-Guasti A, Roldan-Roldan G, Larsson K. Anxiolytics reverse the acceleration of ejacaltion resulting from enforced intercopulatory intervals in rats. *Behav Neurosci.* 1991;105:230–240.

Fossey MD, Hammer MB. Clonazepam-related sexual dysfunction in male veterans with PTSD. *Anxiety.* 1994–5;1:233–236.

Frye CA, DeBold JF. 3 alpha-OH-DHP and 5-alpha-THDOC implants to the ventral tegmental area facilitate sexual receptivity in hamsters after progesterone priming to the ventral medial hypothalamus. *Brain Res.* 1993;28:130–137.

Frye CA, Vongher JM. Progestins' rapid facilitation of lordosis when applied to the ventral tegmentum corresponds to efficacy at enhancing gaba A receptor activity. *J Neuroendocrinology.* 1999;11:829–837.

Gao B, Cutler MG. Effects of chlordiazepoxide, buspirone and the 5-HT3 receptor antagonist, BRL 46470, on the behavior of oestrous and dioestrous female mice when encountering male partners. *Neuropharmacology.* 1993;32:969–975.

Ghadirian A, Annable L. Lithium, benzodiazepines, and sexual function in bipolar patients. *Am J Psychiatry.* 1992;149:841–849.

Gutierrez M, Stimmel G. Management of and counseling for psychotropic drug-induced sexual dysfunction. *Pharmacotherapy.* 1999;19:823–831.

Keene, L., & Davies, P. Drug-related erectile dysfunction. *Adverse Drug React Toxicol Rev.* 1999;18:5–24.

Kubacki A. Sexual disinhibition on clonazepam. *Can J Psychaitry.* 1987; 7:643–645.

Lydiard R, Howell E, Laraia M, Ballenger J. Sexual side effects of alprazolam. *Am J Psychiatry.* 1987;144:254–255.

McCarthy MM, Felzenberg E, Robbins A, Pfaff DW, Schwartz-Giblin N. Infusions of diazepam and allopregnanolone into the midbrain central gray facilitate open-field behavior and sexual receptivity in female rats. *Horm Behav.* 1995;29:279–295.

McDonnell SM, Garcia MC, Kenney RM. Pharmacological manipulation of sexual behavior in stallions. *J Reproduction and Fertility.* 1987;35, Suppl:45–49.

McDonnell SM, Kenney RM, Meckley PE, Garcia MC. Novel environmental suppression of stallion sexual behavior and effects of diazepam. *Physiology & Behavior*. 1986;37:503–505.

Meston, C., & Gorzalka, B. Psychoactive drugs and human sexual behavior. *J Psychoactive Drugs*. 1992;24:1–40.

Metz ME, Pryor JL, Nesvacil LJ, Aqbuzzahab F, Koznar J. Premature ejaculation a psychophysiological review. *J Sex & Marital Therapy*. 1997;23:3–23.

Munjack DJ & Crocker B. Alprazolam-induced ejaculatory inhibition. *J Clin Psychopharmacol*. 1986;6:57–58.

Nutt, D., & Hackman, A. Increased sexual function in benzodiazepine withdrawal. *Lancet*. 1986;2:1101–1102.

Riley, A., & Riley, E. The effect of single dose diazepam on female sexual response induced by masturbation. *Sexual and Marital Therapy*. 1986;1:49–53.

Sangal, R. Inhibited female orgasm as a side effect of alprazolam. *Am J Psychiatry*. 1985;142:1223–1224.

Segraves, R. Treatment of premature ejaculation with lorazepam. *Am J Psychiatry*. 1987;144:1240.

Virag R. Latrogenic priapism. *Lancet*. 1991;38:886.

4. Antidepressant Drugs and Sexual Dysfunction

INTRODUCTION

Antidepressants are used by millions of people. They are a "big" business—over 12 billion dollars are spent on antidepressants in the United States a year. Antidepressants are used not only for the treatment of depression but also for the treatment of anxiety disorders, premature ejaculation (see Chapter 20), paraphilias (see Chapter 21), and numerous other mental disorders and other conditions, such as diabetic neuropathy and various pain syndromes. Older antidepressants—heterocyclics and monoamine oxidase inhibitors—have been known as effective but at times troublesome drugs with various side effects, including the sexual ones. These shortcomings spurned the development of newer classes and types of antidepressants, such as the selective serotonin reuptake inhibitors (SSRIs), bupropion, mirtazapine, nefazodone, and venlafaxine. The introduction of new antidepressants with increased tolerability led to their use for indications not frequently if ever treated with antidepressants. These new drugs are generally considered equally effective (but not by everybody and not always) but better tolerated than the older antidepressants, though they are not totally free of side effects. Actually, use of newer antidepressants in less severe or serious conditions may have led, paradoxically, to a greater attention to their side effects. As is the case with the older drugs, some of the newer antidepressants are associated with sexual dysfunction. The character and frequency of the sexual dysfunction associated with different subgroups of antidepressants seem to vary somewhat. For example, predominantly serotonergic antidepressants (selective serotonin reuptake inhibitors [SSRIs] and the tricyclic antidepressant clomipramine) seem to be associated more frequently with delayed orgasm or anorgasmia than the other antidepressants.

45

Table 4.1   Causes of sexual dysfunction in depressed patients

- Part of depressive symptomatology
- Concomitant medical illness (e.g., diabetes mellitus)
- Primary sexual problem (e.g., dyspareunia)
- Side effects of antidepressant medication
- Side effects of other medications
- Effects of substance abuse
- Combination of some or all these factors

The management of the sexual dysfunction associated with antidepressants emerged as a challenging and complex clinical problem during the last decade or two. The complexity of the sexual dysfunction associated with antidepressants is increased by the fact that depression itself has been found to be associated with impairment of various aspects of sexual functioning. In addition, given that depression does not exist in a vacuum and frequently coexists with various medical conditions, these conditions and the medications used for their treatment also may contribute to sexual dysfunction. Table 4.1 summarizes the possible causes of sexual dysfunction in depressed patients.

Sexual dysfunction associated with antidepressants may have a profound effect on the quality of life of depressed patients and their subsequent compliance with treatment. Furthermore, this additional stressor could possibly lead to a worsening of the depressive symptomatology as a result of medication noncompliance or cognitive misinterpretation.

This chapter focuses on:

- Depression, anxiety, and sexual function
- Sexual dysfunction associated with antidepressants (heterocyclics, monoamine oxidase inhibitors, SSRIs and newer antidepressants), its description, epidemiology, types and mechanism of action, and diagnosis
- Management of sexual dysfunction associated with various antidepressants

As noted, antidepressants may be useful in some sexual disorders (premature ejaculation, paraphilias), and their use in these disorders is reviewed in other chapters of this book. Antidepressants and other agents discussed in this chapter are listed in Table 4.2.

Sexuality, Depression, and Anxiety

Unwanted changes in sexual functioning are a frequent symptom of depressive disorders. Decreased libido is the most common complaint from depressed patients, but other phases of the sexual cycle

Table 4.2 Pharmacological agents discussed in this chapter

Generic Name	Brand Name	Forms and Doses (mg)
ANTIDEPRESSANTS		
Heterocyclic Antidepressants		
amitriptyline	Elavil	t: 10, 25, 50, 75, 100, 150
		inj: 10/mL
amoxapine		t: 25, 50, 100, 150
clomipramine	Anafranil	c: 25, 50, 75
desipramine	Norpramin	t: 10, 20, 50, 75, 100, 150
doxepin	Sinequan	c: 10, 25, 50, 75, 100, 150
		o: 10/mL
imipramine	Tofranil PM	c: 150, 300, 600
	generic	t: 10, 25, 50
maprotiline		t: 25, 50, 75
nortriptyline	Pamelor (also generic)	t: 10, 25, 50, 75
		o: 2/mL
protriptyline	Vivactil	t: 10
trazodone	Desyrel	t: 50, 100, 150, 300
trimipramine	Surmontil	c: 25, 50, 100
Monoamine Oxidase Inhibitors (MAOIs)		
moclobemide***		
phenelzine	Nardil	t: 15
tranylcypromine	Parnate	t: 10
Newer, Miscellaneous Antidepressants		
bupropion	Wellbutrin	t: 75
	Wellbutrin SR	txr: 100, 150
	Zyban*	txr: 150
mirtazapine	Remeron	t: 15, 30, 45
	Remeron Sol Tab	tod: 15, 30, 45
mianserin***		
nefazodone	Serzone	t: 50, 10, 150, 200, 250
reboxetine***		
venlafaxine	Effexor	t: 25, 37.5, 50, 75, 100
	Effexor XR	c: 37.5, 75, 150
Selective Serotonin Reuptake Inhibitors (SSRIs)		
citalopram	Celexa	t: 20, 40
		o: 2/mL
escitalopram	Lexapro	t: 10, 20
fluoxetine	Prozac	pulv: 10, 20, 40
		t: 10
		o: 4/mL
	Sarafem	pulv: 10, 20
fluvoxamine	Luvox	t: 25, 50, 100
paroxetine	Paxil	t: 10, 20, 30, 40
		o: 20/mL
	Paxil CR	txr: 12.5, 25
sertraline	Zoloft	t: 25, 50, 100
		o: 20/mL
ANXIOLYTICS		
buspirone	Buspar	t: 5, 7.5, 10, 15, 30
chlordiazepoxide	Librium	c: 5, 10, 25
		inj: 20/mL

ANTIDEPRESSANT DRUGS

Table 4.2 (*Cont.*)

Generic Name	Brand Name	Forms and Doses (mg)
STIMULANTS		
dextroamphetamine	Adderal	t: 5, 7.5, 10, 12.5, 20, 30
	Adderal XR	c: 5, 10, 15, 20, 25, 30
	Dexedrine	t: 5
		c: 5, 10, 15
	Dextrostat	t: 5, 10
methylphenidate	Concerta	tex: 18, 36
	Metadate ER	tex: 10, 20
	Methylin	t: 5, 10, 20
	Ritalin	t: 5, 10, 20
	Ritalin SR	txr: 20
pemoline	Cylert	t: 18.75, 37.5, 75
		tc: 37.5
ANTIDOTES		
amantadine	Symmetrel	t: 100
		o: 10/mL
apomorphine***		
bethanechol	Urecholine	t: 5, 10, 25, 50
		inj: 5.15/mL
bromocriptine	generic	t: 2.5
		c: 5
cyproheptadine	Periactin	t: 4
	generic	t: 4
ginkgo biloba**		
granisetron	Kytril	t: 1
		inj: 1/mL
loratadine	Claritin	t: 10
		trd: 10
		o: 1/mL
neostigmine	Prostigmin	t: 15
		inj: .25/mL, .5/mL, 1/mL
	generic	inj: .5/mL, 1/mL
phentolamine***		
yohimbine	Aphrodyne	cap: 5.4
	generic	t: 5.4
ORAL VASOACTIVE AND OTHER AGENTS		
alprostadil	Caverject	pw: 5, 10, 20, 40 mcg/vial
	MUSE	supp: 125, 250, 500, 1000 mcg/supp
apomorphine***		
phentolamine***		
sildenafil	Viagra	t: 25, 50, 100

c = capsules; cap = caplets; inj = injection; o = oral concentrate; pulv = pulvules; pw = powder; supp = suppository; t = tablets; tc: chewable tablets; tex = extended-release tablets; tod = tablets orally disintegrated; trd: tablets rapidly disintegrating; txr = slow-release tablets or controlled-release tablets.
   * Used for smoking cessation.
   ** Various over-the-counter preparations.
   *** Not available in the United States.

(arousal, orgasm) also may be affected by depression. In earlier studies, the overall incidence of decreased libido was as high as 70–80%. In some studies, the decreased libido was associated with other symptoms of depression, such as weight loss, loss of energy, and disturbed sleep. Some researchers reported that not only the presence of depression but also its severity influenced the degree of sexual dysfunction associated with depression. The increase in severity of depression and anxiety was associated with greater loss of libido. Interestingly, increased libido and hypersexuality have been reported in depressed patients occasionally; however, this effect is a rather rare phenomenon. The evaluation of decreased libido in depression may be complicated by the overall anhedonia of the depressed state; however, most patients are clearly able to differentiate the loss of libido and the loss of interest in other activities.

Loss or decrease of libido is not the only impairment of sexual functioning associated with depression. Erectile dysfunction, arousal impairment, delayed ejaculation/orgasm, and anorgasmia have all been reported in depressed patients, though less frequently than loss of libido. Several research studies found impaired erectile capacity in depressed men. One study reported decreased nocturnal tumescence in depressed men when compared to healthy controls. Some researchers even consider depression to be a significant risk factor for development of erectile dysfunction.

However, the existence of sexual dysfunction associated with depression does not mean that depressed patients do not want to have good sexual functioning. Researchers in one poll found that depressed patients cited having a good sexual life as important to them at least as frequently as people in the general population. Interestingly, only a few depressed and nondepressed persons (2–3%) felt that the loss of sexual interest would prompt them to visit a physician.

As noted, antidepressants, especially SSRIs, are also frequently used in the treatment of various anxiety disorders. Several studies demonstrated that untreated patients with anxiety disorders report sexual dysfunction more frequently than normal controls. It also seems that among patients with anxiety disorders, sexual dysfunction is more common in patients with panic disorder and social phobia than in those with generalized anxiety disorder.

The occurrence of sexual dysfunction in association with depression and anxiety disorders, together with the fact that patients frequently would not spontaneously seek help for sexual dysfunction underscore the importance of instigating proactive baseline evaluation of sexual functioning prior to treatment with antidepressants.

Table 4.3   Antidepressants reported to cause sexual dysfunction (cited in studies and case reports)

Heterocyclics	MAOIs	SSRIs	Other
amitriptyline	isocarboxazid	citalopram	bupropion
amoxapine	phenelzine	escitalopram	mirtazapine
clomipramine	tranylcypromine	fluoxetine	nefazodone
desipramine		fluvoxamine	reboxetine*
doxepin		paroxetine	venlafaxine
imipramine		sertraline	
nortriptyline			
protriptyline			
trimipramine			
trazodone			

* Not available in the United States at present.

SEXUAL DYSFUNCTION AND ANTIDEPRESSANTS

Sexual dysfunction has been reported in case reports, case series, and studies involving almost all antidepressants (see Table 4.3).

However, some antidepressants have been found to have a lower frequency of associated sexual dysfunction than others (see Table 4.4).

Antidepressants can have an impact on any part of the sexual cycle. The various changes in sexual functioning associated with antidepressants that have been reported in numerous case reports and studies are listed in Table 4.5.

Table 4.4   Antidepressants with reportedly lower frequency of sexual dysfunction

Bupropion*
Mirtazapine
Moclobemide*,∞
Nefazodone
Reboxetine∞

* Some have claimed that bupropion and moclobemide have prosexual effects ("hyperorgasmia" with moclobemide?).
∞ Not available in the United States at present; moclobemide available in Canada.

Table 4.5   Antidepressant-induced types of sexual dysfunction

- Changes in libido (mostly decreased)
- Impaired erectile capacity, erectile dysfunction
- Priapism
- Changes in lubrication
- Clitoral engorgement
- Delayed ejaculation/orgasm
- Painful ejaculation
- Partial or complete anorgasmia
- Penile or vaginal anesthesia

Table 4.6   Varying estimates of sexual dysfunction associated with antidepressants

Source	Percentage	Antidepressants
Physicians' Desk Reference	1.9	fluoxetine
Zajecka et al., 1991	7.8	fluoxetine
Herman et al.	8.9	fluoxetine
Jacobsen	34	fluoxetine
Harrison et al.	30	imipramine
	40	phenelzine
Balon et al.	43.3	various
Couper-Smartt & Rodham	71	various
Patterson	75	fluoxetine
Monteiro et al.	92	clomipramine

Most of the early reports on antidepressant-associated sexual dysfunction were either anecdotal or nonsystematic, and the estimates of the incidence of sexual dysfunction associated with antidepressants varied widely. An example of various estimates of the frequency of sexual dysfunction associated with antidepressants is shown in Table 4.6.

Studies in Table 4.6 were noncomparative. Although these studies do not clarify the frequency of sexual dysfunction associated with antidepressants, they illustrate the confusion in the field. The incidence of sexual dysfunction associated with fluoxetine cited in the *Physicians' Desk Reference (PDR)* is quite low. It is known that the studies submitted for FDA approval usually quote only spontaneously reported side effects, including those reflecting sexual dysfunction. The estimate in the *PDR* is based on spontaneous reporting and not on proactive evaluation of sexual dysfunction. The percentage—1.9%—fairly well corresponds with the 2% of depressed people who would be prompted to visit their physician because of sexual dysfunction in the above-mentioned opinion poll.

Since the early noncomparative studies, numerous comparative studies have reported sexual dysfunction associated with antidepressants (for an excellent summary, see article by Montgomery and colleagues 2002). Most of these studies were not focused on sexual dysfunction as their primary research interest. The methodology and instruments used in these studies differ widely, and the frequency of sexual dysfunction varies widely, with numbers parallel to those cited in noncomparative studies. Most clinicians agree that the frequency of sexual dysfunction associated with antidepressants is probably between 30% and 50%. There is insufficient evidence to support a claim of drug–class differences in the frequency of sexual dysfunction. However, most reports and clinicians are in agreement that the incidence of sexual dysfunction with bupropion, mirtazapine, moclobemide, nefazodone, and maybe reboxetine is lower than with other drugs. Most researchers and clinicians also would agree that there are probably differences in the types of sexual dysfunction associated with different classes of antidepressants. For example, it seems that strongly serotonergic drugs cause delayed ejaculation/orgasm more frequently than other antidepressants, and heterocyclics are probably more frequently associated with erectile dysfunction. The evidence of prolonged ejaculation with SSRIs has been demonstrated by several excellent clinical and laboratory studies by researchers in the Netherlands (Waldinger and colleagues). For simplifying the issues, in this chapter we refer to studies of sexual dysfunction associated with antidepressants used in various mood and anxiety disorders. Interestingly, antidepressants have been shown to cause sexual dysfunction in healthy, nondepressed subjects, indicating that antidepressants may indeed be the cause of sexual dysfunction in depressed patients.

Changes in sexual function reported with various classes of antidepressants are summarized in Tables 4.7–4.10.

The possible differences in types of sexual dysfunction associated with different classes of antidepressants point indirectly to the

---

Table 4.7   Heterocyclic antidepressants and sexual dysfunction

- Decreased libido
- Erectile dysfunction (most frequent)
- Painful ejaculation
- Clomipramine—delayed ejaculation
- trazodone—priapism (1 in 5,000–6,000 cases)

Table 4.8   Monoamine oxidase inhibitors and sexual dysfunction

- Decreased libido
- Erectile dysfunction
- Delayed or absent ejaculation/orgasm
- Little or no dysfunction with moclobemide*

* Not available in the United States.

Table 4.9   Selective serotonin reuptake inhibitors and sexual dysfunction

- Decreased libido
- Erectile dysfunction
- Mostly delayed or absent ejaculation/orgasm
- Ejaculation delayed most with paroxetine

Table 4.10   Newer antidepressants and sexual dysfunction

- Bupropion
    Low frequency of sexual dysfunction/prosexual effects; used in treatment of
        sexual dysfunction in nondepressed subjects—role of dopamine
- Mirtazapine, mianserin*
    Lower frequency of sexual dysfunction—role of 5HT2 and 5HT3?
- Nefazodone
    Lower frequency of sexual dysfunction—role of 5HT2?
- Reboxetine*
    Lack of data; possibly lower frequency of sexual dysfunction
- Venlafaxine
    Delayed or absent ejaculation/orgasm

* Not available in the United States.

theoretical explanations of the mechanism of action associated with antidepressants.

Regulation of sexual functioning is a very complex and not fully under-stood process. It involves input from the central and peripheral ner-vous systems and interaction of multiple neurotransmitter systems, including the adrenergic, dopaminergic, muscarinic, and serotonergic ones. Other substances, such as vasoactive intestinal polypeptide and nitric oxide, seem to be involved in this process, too. In addition, vas-cular and muscle systems and various hormones play a very important role in the regulation of sexual functioning. For instance, an increase in testosterone levels increases sexual desire and arousal.

Libido, or sexual desire, is influenced by both physiological and attitu-dinal factors; it seems to be mediated by the limbic system and mod-ulated by dopamine, norepinephrine, and serotonin. Sexual arousal regulation also involves various neurotransmitter systems. Increases in dopamine and norepinephrine increase arousal, whereas central serotonergic activity usually leads to arousal inhibition. In males regulation of erection involves the cholinergic system, nitric oxide, the vascular system, and other substances such as cyclic guanosine monophosphate (cGMP) and phosphodiesterase 5 (which metabo-lizes cGMP). Finally, serotonin has a major central inhibitory effect on orgasm, whereas dopamine may have a stimulating effect on orgasm. The regulation of the entire process is much more complex.

This simplistic summary of the possible involvement of various neuro-transmitters only suggests that neurotransmitter systems affect var-ious aspects of sexual functioning but does not present definitive explanations or evidence. Furthermore, male sexual functioning has been studied more extensively than female sexual functioning. Al-though neural and neurotransmitter control of sexual functioning in both sexes seems to be analogous, our understanding of the regulation

Table 4.11 Neurotransmitters and sexual functioning*

Neurotransmitter Changes	Changes in Sexual Functioning
Acetylcholine increases	Increase in sexual arousal and orgasm in males; no data for females
Adrenaline increases	Increase in sexual arousal in both sexes; may also decrease arousal in both sexes when heightened nervous system arousal
Dopamine increases	Increase in sexual desire in both sexes; increase in sexual arousal in males (no data for females); may decrease orgasm in both sexes
Histamine increases/ decreases	Increase in arousal in males, no data for females Decrease in sexual desire in both sexes; decreased arousal in males
Norepinephrine increases	Increase in sexual arousal and orgasm in both sexes
Serotonin increases/ decreases	Increase in sexual arousal in males; decreased orgasm in males Decrease in sexual arousal in both sexes; decreased orgasm in both sexes

* Adapted from Meston & Frohlich, 2000.

of female sexual functioning is even poorer. Table 4.11 summarizes the available data on the putative effects of various neurotransmitters on sexual functioning.

On a superficial level, drugs with an exerting effect on the dopaminergic such as bupropion, have a positive effect on libido. Drugs serotonergic have a negative effect on sexual functioning, some decreasing libido and mainly delaying or suppressing orgasm. Drugs alpha- and beta-adrenergic receptors (such as some heterocyclics and MAOIs) frequently have an impact on erectile functioning. The effects of drugs are usually more complex, as many of them have dose-dependent biphasic effects. Some inhibit one component while enhancing another component of sexual function/behavior. The complicated interplay among medications, some neurotransmitter systems, and sexual functioning is reflected in the evidence summarized in Tables 4.12–4.15.

Diagnosing sexual dysfunction associated with antidepressants may be a complicated issue. As noted, various causative factors may contribute to sexual dysfunction in depressed patients, such as the

Table 4.12 Dopamine, sexual functioning, and medications

- Dopaminergic blockade (e.g., haloperidol infusion) of nucleus accumbens results in inhibition of sexual appetite.
- Dopamine antagonism diminishes sexual appetitive behavior without impairing ability to copulate.
- Dopamine agonist apomorphine induces erection (blocked by haloperidol).
- Low doses of D2 agonist induce intense erections.
- High doses of D2 agonist facilitate seminal emission and inhibit erection.
- Antipsychotics disrupt limbic–striatal interaction, cause decrease in sexual appetite.
- Bupropion may increase sexual appetite.

Table 4.13   Norepinephrine, sexual functioning, and medications

- Activation of peripheral adrenoreceptors in penis (cavernosal and vascular smooth muscles) maintains tonic muscular contraction.
- Priapism results from blockade of peripheral alpha-adrenoreceptors.
- Heterocyclics and MAOIs cause erectile dysfunction.

Table 4.14   Serotonin, sexual functioning, and medications

- Inhibition of serotonin synthesis in rats increases sexual activity.
- Drugs with central serotonergic activity reduce sexual activity.
- SSRIs and strongly serotonergic drugs cause anorgasmia and delayed ejaculation.
- Ecstasy, a serotonin agonist, causes enhancement of sensuous aspects of sex but inhibits ejaculation/orgasm.

Table 4.15   Gamma-aminobutyric acid (GABA), sexual functioning, and medications

- Stimulation of GABA receptors in lumbosacral spinal cord inhibits erectile reflexes in rats.
- Chlordiazepoxide experimentally enhances penile spinal reflexes.
- Chlordiazepoxide also can inhibit erection via action in hypothalamus.
- Benzodiazepines occasionally cause impaired sexual appetite and erection.
- Buspirone increased sexual desire in some patients.

depression itself, medical illness(es), antidepressants, other medications, herbal preparations used for the treatment of depression (St. John's wort), and substances of abuse. The effect of medication on sexual functioning may be difficult to differentiate from the other factors. Depending on patient memory may not be the most reliable approach either (given possible cognitive misinterpretation or pseudodementia in depressed patients). Thus a baseline evaluation of sexual functioning prior to starting the antidepressant medication is absolutely necessary. Without a baseline evaluation, it may be impossible to differentiate sexual dysfunction associated with medication from sexual dysfunction due to other factors, including depression. Diagnostic criteria are summarized in Table 4.16.

The baseline evaluation does not need to be a complicated one. However, it should include more than a casual question such as, "How is your sex life?" Specific questions about libido, arousal/lubrication/erection, orgasm, interpersonal relationships, and medications should be asked and answers documented. The same or similar questions should be asked later during the treatment with an antidepressant. Only in this way will the physician be able to assume, with some degree of certainty, that any subsequent sexual dysfunction is due to the antidepressant.

Table 4.16   Diagnostic criteria for sexual dysfunction associated with antidepressants*

A. Clinically significant sexual dysfunction that results in marked distress or interpersonal difficulty predominates in the clinical picture.

B. There is evidence from the history, physical examination, or laboratory findings that the sexual dysfunction is fully explained by antidepressant(s) use as manifested by the fact that the symptoms in Criterion A developed during, or within a month of, starting antidepressant administration (or substantial increase in dose).

C. The disturbance is not better accounted for by a sexual dysfunction that is not substance-induced. Evidence that the symptoms are better accounted for by a sexual dysfunction that is not substance-induced might include the following: The symptoms precede the onset of antidepressant administration; the symptoms persist for a substantial period of time (e.g., about a month) after antidepressant discontinuation, or are substantially in excess of what would be expected given the type or amount of the antidepressant used or the duration of use; or there is other evidence that suggests the existence of an independent non-antidepressant to induced sexual dysfunction (e.g., a history of recurrent nonsubstance-related episodes).

Specify if:
  with impaired desire
  with impaired arousal
  with impaired orgasm
  with sexual pain

* Adapted from *DSM-IV*, APA, 1994.

MANAGEMENT OF SEXUAL DYSFUNCTION ASSOCIATED WITH ANTIDEPRESSANTS

Management of sexual dysfunction associated with antidepressants starts with a baseline assessment of sexual functioning, which is a prerequisite for diagnosing sexual dysfunction as related to medications. Patients should be educated about the possibility of sexual dysfunction associated with antidepressants. Although opinions differ about the advisability of discussing sexual dysfunction prior to starting an antidepressant (some feel that it may encourage noncompliance), we feel that, in this modern era of mega-information, it is better to discuss this issue openly. The patient should be informed that there are various management strategies available, should the dysfunction occur, and that the dysfunction does not occur in all patients.

Given that some of the antidepressants (bupropion, mirtazapine, nefazodone) are known to have a lower frequency of reported sexual dysfunction, one might consider "preventing" the occurrence of sexual dysfunction associated with antidepressants by selecting one of these agents in the first case. However, this strategy should also encompass the specifics of each clinical situation (e.g., bupropion would probably not be used in anxiety disorders).

Several management strategies for handling sexual dysfunction associated with antidepressants are summarized in Table 4.17. (It is

Table 4.17   Management strategies for sexual dysfunction associated with antidepressants

1. Waiting for spontaneous remission/accommodation
2. Reduction to minimal effective dose
3. Scheduling sexual activity around the dose
4. Switching to another antidepressant with a lower frequency of sexual dysfunction
5. Prescribing drug holidays
6. Addition of antidotes
7. Use of other agents (e.g., sildenafil)

important to note that there is no FDA (Food and Drug Administration) approved agent for sexual dysfunction associated with antidepressants.)

Numerous case reports and case series report success in the management of sexual dysfunction associated with antidepressants. However, there are only a few good studies, and there are no data supporting the reliability and prevalent efficacy of one or another approach.

1. *Waiting for spontaneous remission/accommodation.* This is a rarely used approach because its effectiveness is usually low, and it may also require a long waiting period that may not be acceptable to many patients. Table 4.18 summarizes the evidence regarding this strategy.

2. *Reduction to minimal effective dose.* This is probably a more acceptable approach, even though it has its risks. The main problem here is finding the balance between the minimally effective dose and the subtherapeutic dose. Frequently the dose at which the alleviation of sexual dysfunction appears is also the dose at which depression or anxiety reappears. (See Table 4.19.)

Table 4.18   Waiting for spontaneous remission/accommodation

- Questionable approach.
- Spontaneous remission may occur from time to time (reported, e.g., with phenelzine, sertraline).
- Usually not effective with TCA-induced anorgasmia.
- In one study abnormal ejaculation/anorgasmia with fluoxetine did not remit after 6 months.
- Requires good doctor–patient relationship.
- May be acceptable for patients with a low frequency of sexual activity.

Table 4.19   Reduction to minimal effective dose

- May help occasionally
- Difficult balance between minimal therapeutic and subtherapeutic doses
- Frequently suggested approach in erectile dysfunction
- Dose-dependent effect demonstrated in one study with fluoxetine
- Worked with other SSRIs (e.g., paroxetine)

ANTIDEPRESSANT DRUGS

3. *Scheduling sexual activity around the dose.* Scheduling sexual activity around the dose has been suggested by some clinicians. It means administering the entire daily dose of the antidepressant just after sexual activity (e.g., often just before sleep). This strategy may work occasionally with some antidepressants that have short half-lives.

4. *Switching to another antidepressant with a lower frequency of sexual dysfunction.* This strategy has been described frequently as one of the more successful management approaches. Bupropion has a very low frequency of sexual dysfunction and has been described as having prosexual effects. Several studies described successful experiences of switching patients suffering from sexual dysfunction on SSRIs to bupropion. The switch led to alleviation of sexual dysfunction. Similarly, patients could be switched to mirtazapine or nefazodone (both found successful by some authors).

5. *Prescribing drug holidays.* Drug holidays, or even partial drug holidays (a variant of decreasing the dose) were explored in one small study. The antidepressant was stopped for a period of a few days and sexual activity recommended at the end of this period, just before the antidepressant therapy resumed. Partial drug holidays use only decreased dosage for a few days instead of a complete discontinuation. Drug holidays may be effective with short half-life drugs (e.g., paroxetine, sertraline), whereas they are not successful with long half-life drugs such as fluoxetine. We feel that this approach is probably not clinically suitable for several resons: (1) Encouraging the patient to stop and start medication frequently may encourage noncompliance. (2) Discontinuation of drugs with shorter half-life may occasionally cause withdrawal effects at the end of the drug holiday. (3) The long-term effects of this approach are unknown (stop and start—kindling?).

6. *Addition of antidotes.* Addition of antidotes may be the most frequently reported strategy. Various antidotes were introduced to "counteract" the effect of antidepressants on different neurotransmitters. Some of the effects were discovered accidentally.

Table 4.20 lists antidotes that have been used successfully (mostly in a single case or a few cases) for management of sexual dysfunction associated with antidepressants.

Paraphrasing Sir William Osler, when too many treatments (agents) for sexual dysfunction are available, none is effective all the time and in all cases, nor is any curative. Several open studies or case series demonstrated efficacy of some antidotes (e.g., buspirone, bupropion, yohimbine). One double-blind placebo-controlled study

Table 4.20 Antidotes and other agents used for management of sexual dysfunction

Amantadine	Methylphenidate
Bethanechol	Mirtazapine
Bromocriptine	Mianserin*
Bupropion	Neostigmine
Buspirone	Nefazodone
Cyproheptadine	Pemoline
Dextroamphetamine	Sildenafil
Ginkgo biloba	Trazodone
Granisetron	Yohimbine
Loratadine	

* Not available in the United States.

did not find differences between amantadine, buspirone, and placebo in the management of sexual dysfunction associated with fluoxetine. However, this study used doses—amantadine 100 mg/day or buspirone 20–30 mg/day—lower than those advocated by clinicians and in case reports (amantadine could be titrated to several hundred mg/day, buspirone 30 mg or more/day).

The effectiveness of some antidotes came into a question even in the open studies. For instance, some clinicians did not find ginkgo biloba useful in management of sexual dysfunction. Table 4.21 lists additional information on the more frequently used antidotes.

Table 4.21 Frequently used antidotes, their dosage and possible indications

Antidote	Dose	Sexual Dysfunction
Amantadine	100–600 mg/day in divided dose or prn	Anorgasmia; could be helpful for loss of desire or arousal
Bethanechol	prn 10–50 mg 1–2 hours before coitus	Dysfunction of arousal or orgasm
Bupropion (or bupropion SR)	prn 75–150 mg 1–2 hours before coitus, or daily 75–450 mg (mostly with SSRIs)	Dysfunction of desire, arousal, and orgasm
Buspirone	over 30 mg/day	Decreased desire; anorgasmia
Cyproheptadine*	prn 4–12 mg before coitus, or 4–16 mg/day	Anorgasmia
Dextroamphetamine	prn 5 mg 1–2 hours before coitus, or 5 mg or more/day	Dysfunction of desire, arousal, and orgasm
Methylphenidate	prn 5 mg or more, or 5–20 mg/day	Dysfunction of desire, arousal, and orgasm
Mirtazapine	15–45 mg/day	Impaired orgasm
Nefazodone	50 mg/day or more	Impaired orgasm
Neostigmine	prn 7.5–15 mg 1–2 hours before coitus, or 50–200 mg/day in divided doses	Dysfunction of arousal
Yohimbine**	prn 5.4–10.8 mg 1–2 hours before coitus, or 5.4 mg/day	Dysfunction of desire, arousal, and orgasm

* Cyproheptadine may cause severe sedation and possibly depression.
** Yohimbine may induce anxiety, especially in panic disorder patients.

A
N
T
I
D
E
P
R
E
S
S
A
N
T

D
R
U
G
S

Table 4.22 Sildenafil in antidepressant-associated sexual dysfunction

---

- Indicated in erectile dysfunction with various etiologies (60–80% success rate)
- Several studies and case reports on using sildenafil in sexual dysfunction associated with antidepressants
- Questionable effectiveness in females with antidepressant-associated sexual dysfunction
- Used with various antidepressants (SSRIs, mirtazapine, nefazodone, phenelzine)
- Frequently used as a first-line therapy
- Effective dose: 50–100 mg about an hour prior to intercourse
- Most frequently used dose in sexual dysfunction associated with antidepressants: 50 mg
- Lowest dose used: 25 mg (phenelzine)
- Infrequent, mild side effects (headaches, flushing, nasal congestion, changed vision)
- Not approved by the FDA for this indication

---

7. *Use of other agents, e.g., sildenafil.* Agents such as sildenafil may be used, based on their effectiveness in alleviating sexual dysfunction not associated with antidepressants. Sildenafil has been used for antidepressant-associated dysfunction (see Table 4.22), though it is not approved in this indication. Other theoretically useful agents may be apomorphine, phentolamine (both presently not available in the United States), and prostaglandine E1.

Mechanical devices (vacuum pump, penile rings) and intracorporeal injections of various agents mentioned in the chapter on treatment of erectile dysfunction should also be theoretically useful in antidepressant-associated sexual dysfunction. Tables 4.23–4.25 summarize suggestions for managing specific sexual dysfunctions. Note that all these approaches are suggested but not proven in solid studies (many of them reported as single cases).

As indicated in the above tables, some antidotes have been used more frequently with certain classes of antidepressants, either because of a

---

Table 4.23 Decreased libido

- Try to decrease dose
- Drug holidays (rather not)
- Small dose of neostigmine (7.5–15 mg) 30 min. before coitus
- Add dopaminergic agents (e.g., bupropion 150 mg/day or more; dextroamphetamine, methylphenidate, pemoline [starting with low dose, e.g., 5 mg of methylphenidate, and titrate up])
- Switch to another antidepressant (bupropion, nefazodone, trazodone—caution in males: priapism possible, though rare, with trazodone)

Table 4.24 Erectile dysfunction

- Try to decrease dose
- Drug holidays(?)
- Add antidotes (e.g., bethanechol 30 mg 1–2 hours prior to coitus)
- Add sildenafil (25–100 mg about an hour prior to coitus)
- Switch to another antidepressant (buspirone, mirtazapine, nefazodone, trazodone—caution in males: priapism possible, though rare, with trazodone)

Table 4.25 Ejaculatory/orgasmic dysfunction

- Wait for spontaneous remission/accommodation (rare)
- Decrease dose or try drug holidays (?)
- Add antidotes:
    amantadine 100–600 mg/day or prn (SSRIs)
    bethanechol 10–20 mg 1–2 hours before coitus (heterocyclics)
    bupropion 75 mg/day or more (SSRIs)
    buspirone 30 mg/day or more (SSRIs)
    cyproheptadine* 4–12 mg 1–2 hours before coitus (heterocyclics)
    yohimbine**5.4 mg T.I.D. or 5.4 mg or more prn 2–4 hours prior to coitus (SSRIs)
- Switch to another antidepressant (bupropion, mirtazapine, nefazodone; among heterocyclics, e.g., from imipramine or clomipramine to desipramine)

---

* Cyproheptadine may cause severe sedation and possibly depression.
** Yohimbine may induce anxiety, especially in panic disorder patients.

theoretical speculation that they may more likely to be helpful, or because of their availability and frequent use at that time. For example, bethanechol and cyproheptadine have been used more frequently for sexual dysfunction associated with heterocyclic antidepressants. These two substances have been also used for sexual dysfunction associated with MAOIs. Bupropion, buspirone, stimulants mirtazapine, nefazodone, and some other antidotes have been predominantly used for sexual dysfunction associated with SSRIs, and some of them for sexual dysfunction associated with venlafaxine.

Management of sexual dysfunction associated with antidepressants is a creative process that may be frequently based on clinical experience and intuition more than the data (when scarce). Switching to another antidepressant with a lower frequency of sexual dysfunction, use of various antidotes and other pharmacological agents (namely, sildenafil), and reducing the dose of antidepressant are the most frequently used and probably most prudent approaches. The selection of a particular strategy may depend on the clinical situation. It is probably easier to switch antidepressants in a patient who reports sexual dysfunction during a trial with a first-time antidepressant. However, it may be not possible to switch antidepressants in a treatment-resistant case where the clinician and patient finally arrived at an efficacious agent, but the efficacy is complicated by sexual dysfunction. In such a case, the use of antidotes or other agents may be more suitable.

CONCLUSIONS

Sexual dysfunction associated with antidepressants is a serious, complicated, and challenging clinical problem. Impairment of sexual functioning in depressed and anxious patients could have various causes, such as the depression or anxiety itself, medical illness, antidepressant medication, other medications, and substances of abuse. The

Table 4.26 General approach to sexual dysfunction associated with antidepressants

- Evaluate patient's sexual functioning prior to treatment.
- Exclude other possible causes of sexual dysfunction, such as medical illness or substance abuse.
- Discuss with the patient the possibility of sexual dysfunction associated with antidepressant.
- Educate patient about possible management strategies.
- Consider initiating an antidepressant with a low frequency of sexual dysfunction.
- Select appropriate management strategy, tailor it based on the character of dysfunction, type of medication, evidence in literature, clinical situation (first-time use of antidepressant vs. treatment resistance), convenience, and patient's special needs.
- Reevaluate dysfunction and effectiveness of management strategy periodically.

frequency of sexual dysfunction associated with various antidepressants is usually in the range of 30–50%, but could be even higher. Some antidepressants, such as bupropion, mirtazapine, moclobemide, and nefazodone, have a lower frequency of sexual dysfunction. The management of sexual dysfunction associated with antidepressants should start with a baseline evaluation of the patient's sexual functioning and should include a discussion of possible sexual dysfunction with the patient as well as education regarding possible management strategies, should the need arise. Management of sexual dysfunction itself is a complicated process which could encompass a variety of strategies. These strategies include waiting for remission, reduction of the antidepressant dose, scheduling sexual activity around the dose, switching to an antidepressant with a lower frequency of sexual dysfunction, and the use of various antidotes and vasoactive pharmacological agents. The most frequently used strategies are switching to another antidepressant, using the antidotes and other agents, and dose reduction. One might also consider starting the patient on an antidepressant with a lower frequency of sexual dysfunction. Table 4.26 summarizes the approach to sexual dysfunction associated with antidepressants.

REFERENCES

Aizenberg D, Gur S, Zemishlany Z, Granek M, Jacksmian P, Weizman A. Mianserin, a 5-HT $_{2a/2c}$ and α_2 antagonist, in the treatment of sexual dysfunction induced by serotonin reuptake inhibitors. *Clin Neuropharmacol.* 1997;10:210–215.

Aizenberg D, Shiloh R, Zemishlany Z, Weizman A. Low-dose imipramine for thioridazine-induced anorgasmia. *J Sex & Marital Ther.* 1996;22:225–229.

Aizenberg D, Zemishlany Z, Hermesh H, Karp L, Weizman A. Painful ejaculation associated with antidepressants in four patients. *J Clin Psychiatry.* 1991;52:461–463.

Aizenberg D, Zemishlany Z, Weizman A. Cyproheptadine treatment of sexual dysfunction induced by serotonin reuptake inhibitors. *Clin Neuropharmacol.* 1995;18:320–324.

Aldrich AP, Cook MD, Pedersen LR. Retrospective review of selective serotonin reuptake inhibitor-induced libido disturbance in women. *Clin Drug Invest.* 1996;11:353–359.

American Psychiatric Association. *Diagnostic and Statistical Manual of Mental Disorders* 4th ed. Washington DC: American Psychiatric Association;1994.

Arnott S, Nutt D. Successful treatment of fluvoxamine-induced anorgasmia by cyproheptadine. *Br J Psychiatry.* 1994;164:838–839.

Ashton, AK, Ahrens K, Gupta S, Masand PS. Antidepressant-induced sexual dysfunction and ginkgo biloba. *Am J Psychiatry.* 2000;157:836–837.

Ashton AK, Hamer T, Rosen RC. Serotonin reuptake inhibitor-induced sexual dysfunction and its treatment: a large-scale retrospective study of 596 outpatients. *J Sex & Marital Ther.* 1997;23:165–176.

Ashton AK, Rosen RC. Bupropion as an antidote for serotonin reuptake-induced sexual dysfunction. *J Clin Psychiatry.* 1998a;59:112–115.

Ashton AK, Rosen RC. Accommodation to serotonin reuptake inhibitor-induced sexual dysfunction. *J Sex & Marital Ther.* 1998b;24:191–192.

Assalian P. Sildenafil for St. John Wort-induced sexual dysfunction. *J Sex & Marital Ther.* 2000;26:357–358.

Assalian P, Margolese HC. Treatment of antidepressant-induced sexual side effects. *J Sex & Marital Ther.* 1996;22:218–223.

Azadzoi KM, Payton T, Krane RJ, Goldstein I. Effects of intracavernosal trazodone hydrochloride: animal and human studies. *J Urol.* 1990;144:1277–1282.

Baldwin DS. Psychotropic drugs and sexual dysfunction. *Int Rev Psychiatry.* 1995;7:261–273.

Baldwin DS. Depression and sexual function. *J Psychopharmacol.* 1996;10(Suppl 1):30–34.

Balogh S, Hendricks SE, Kang J. Treatment of fluoxertine-induced anorgasmia with amantadine. *J Clin Psychiatry.* 53:212–213.

Balon R. The effects of antidepressants on human sexuality: diagnosis and management. *Primary Psychiatry.* 1995;2:46–51.

Balon R. Intermittent amantadine for fluoxetine-induced anorgasmia. *J Sex & Marital Ther.* 1996;22:290–292.

Balon R. Fluvoxamine-induced erectile dysfunction responding to sildenafil. *J Sex & Marital Ther.* 1998;24:313–317.

Balon R, Yeragani VK, Pohl R, Ramesh C. Sexual dysfunction during antidepressant therapy. *J Clin Psychiatry.* 1993;54:209–212.

Bartlik BD, Kaplan P, Kaplan HS. Psychostimulants apparently reverse sexual dysfunction secondary to selective serotonin re-uptake inhibitors. *J Sex & Marital Ther.* 1995;21:262–268.

Barton JL. Orgasmic inhibition by phenelzine. *Am J Psychiatry.* 1974;136: 1616–1617.

Beasley CM, Nilsson ME, Koke SC, Gonzales JS. Efficacy, adverse events, and treatment discontinuations in fluoxetine clinical studies of major depression: a meta-analysis of the 20-mg/day dose. *J Clin Psychiatry.* 2000;61:722–728.

Beaumont G. Sexual side-side effects of clomipramine. *J Int Med Res.* 1977;51:37–44.

ANTIDEPRESSANT DRUGS

Benazzi F, Mazzoli M. Fluoxetine-induced sexual dysfunction: a dose-dependent effect? *Pharmacopsychiatry.* 1994;27:246.

Berk M, Acton M. Citalopram-associated clitoral priapism: a case series. *Int Clin Psychopharmacol.* 1997;12:121–122.

Bhopal JS. St John's wort-induced sexual dysfunction. *Can J Psychiatry.* 2001;46:456–457.

Bodkin JA, Lasser RA, Wines JD, Jr, Gardner DM, Baldessarini RJ. Combining serotonin reuptake inhibitors and bupropion in partial responders to antidepressant monotherapy. *J Clin Psychiatry.* 1997;58:137–145.

Brubaker RV. Fluoxetine-induced sexual dysfunction reversed by loratadine. *J Clin Psychiatry.* 2002;63:534.

Burke WJ. Gergel I, Bose J. Fixed-dose trial of the single isomer SSRI escitalopram in depressed outpatients. *J Clin Psychiatry.* 2002;63:331–336.

Casper RC, Redmond DE, Jr, Katz MM, Schaffer CB, Davis JM, Koslow SH. Somatic symptoms in primary affective disorder: Presence and relationship to the classification of depression. *Arch Gen Psychiatry.* 1985;42:1098–1104.

Clayton AH. Recognition and assessment of sexual dysfunction associated with depression. *J Clin Psychiatry.* 2001;62(Suppl 3):5–9.

Clayton AH, McGarvey EL, Abouesh AI, Pinkerton RC. Substitution of an SSRI with bupropion sustained-release following SSRI-induced sexual dysfunction. *J Clin Psychiatry.* 2001;62:185–190.

Clayton AH, Owens JE, McGarvey EL. Assessment of paroxetine-induced sexual dysfunction using the Changes in Sexual Functioning Questionnaire. *Psychopharmacol Bull.* 1995;31:397–406.

Clayton AH, Pradko JF, Croft HA, Montano CB, Leadbetter RA, Bolden-Watson C, Bass KI, Donahue RMJ, Jamerson BD, Metz A. Prevalence of sexual dysfunction among newer antidepressants. *J Clin Psychiatry.* 2002;63:357–366.

Cohen AJ. Fluoxetine-induced yawning and anorgasmia reversed by cyproheptadine treatment. *J Clin Psychiatry.* 1992;53:174.

Coleman CC, King BR, Bolden-Watson C, Book MJ, Segraves RT, Richard N, Ascher J, Batey S, Jamerson B, Metz A. A placebo-controlled comparison of the effects on sexual functioning of bupropion sustained-release and fluoxetine. *Clin Ther.* 2001;23:1040–1058.

Couper-Smartt JD, Rodham R. A technique for surveying side effects of tricyclic drugs with reference to reported sexual effects. *J Int Med Res.* 1973;1:473–476.

Croft H, Settle E, Jr, Houser T, Batey SR, Donahue RM, Asher JA. A placebo-controlled comparison of the antidepressant efficacy and effects on sexual functioning of sustained-release bupropion and sertraline. *Clin Ther.* 1996;21:643–658.

Davidson JTR. Sexual dysfunction and antidepressants. *Depression.* 1995;2:233–240.

DeCastro RM. Reversal of MAOI-induced anorgasmia with cyproheptadine. *J Clin Psychopharmacol.* 1985;4:169.

Dorevich A, Davis H. Fluvoxamine-associated sexual dysfunction. *Ann Pharmacother.* 1994;28:872–874.

Ekselius L, Von Knorring L. Effect on sexual function of long-term treatment with selective serotonin reuptake inhibitors in depressed patients treated in primary care. *J Clin Psychopharmacol.* 2001;21:154–160.

Ellison JM. Exercise-induced orgasms associated with fluoxetine treatment of depression. *J Clin Psychiatry.* 1996;57:596–597.

Ellison JM. Antidepressant-induced sexual dysfunction: review, classification, and suggestions for treatment. *Harv Rev Psychiatry.* 1998;6:177–189.

Ellison JM, DeLuca P. Fluoxetine-induced genital anesthesia relieved by ginkgo biloba. *J Clin Psychiatry.* 1998;59:199–200.

Elmore JL, Quattlebaum JT. Female sexual stimulation during antidepressant treatment. *Pharmacotherapy.* 1997;17:612–616.

Fava M, Rankin M. Sexual functioning and SSRIs. *J Clin Psychiatry.* 2002;63(Suppl 5):13–16.

Feiger A, Kiev A, Shrivastava RK, Wisselink PG, Wilcox CS. Nefazodone versus sertraline in outpatients with major depression: focus on efficacy, tolerability, and effects on sexual function and satisfaction. *J Clin Psychiatry.* 1996;57(Suppl 2):53–62.

Ferguson JM. The effects of antidepressants on sexual functioning in depressed patients: a review. *J Clin Psychiatry.* 2001;62(Suppl 3):22–34.

Ferguson JM, Shrivastava RK, Stahl SM, Hartford JT, Borian F, leni J, McQuade RD, Jody D. Reemergence of sexual dysfunction in patients with major depressive disorder: double-blind comparison of nefazodone and sertraline. *J Clin Psychiatry.* 2001;62:24–29.

Figueira I, Possidente E, Marques C, Hayes K. Sexual dysfunction: a neglected complication of panic disorder and social phobia. *Arch Sex Behav.* 2001;30:369–377.

Fishbain DA. Impact of sildenafil on male erectile disorder due to psychological factors. *Can J Psychiatry.* 2000;45:85–86.

Gardner EA, Johnston JA. Bupropion—an antidepressant without sexual physiological action. *J Clin Psychopharmacol.* 1985;5:24–29.

Gartrell N. Increased libido in women receiving trazodone. *Am J Psychiatry.* 1986;143:781–782.

Gelenberg AJ, Laukes C, McGahuey C, Okayli G, Moreno F, Zentner L, Delgado P. Mirtazapine substitution in SSRI-induced sexual dysfunction. *J Clin Psychiatry.* 2000;61:356–360.

Gilaberte I, Montejo AL, De La Gandara J, Perez-Sola V, Bernardo M, Massana J, Martin-Santos R, Santiso A, Noguera R, Casais L, Perez-Camo V, Arias M, Judge R. Fluoxetine in the prevention of depressive recurrences: a double-blind study. *J Clin Psychopharmacol.* 2001;21:417–424.

Gitlin MJ. Psychotropic medications and their effects on sexual function: diagnosis, biology, and treatment approaches. *J Clin Psychiatry.* 1994;55:406–413.

Gitlin MJ. Treatment of sexual side effects with dopaminergic agents. *J Clin Psychiatry.* 1995;56:124.

Gitlin MJ, Suri R, Altshuler L, Zuckerbrow-Miller J, Fairbanks L. Bupropion-sustained release as a treatment for SSRI-induced sexual side effects. *J Sex & Marital Ther.* 2002;38:131–138.

ANTIDEPRESSANT DRUGS

Goldbloom DS, Kennedy SH. Adverse interaction of fluoxetine and cyproheptadine in two patients with bulimia nervosa. *J Clin Psychiatry*. 1991;52:261–262.

Goldstein DJ, Mallinckrodt C, Lu Y, Demitrack MA. Duloxetine in the treatment of major depressive disorder: a double-blind clinical trial. *J Clin Psychiatry*. 2002;63:225–231.

Greenberg HR. Erectile impotence during the course of Tofranil therapy. *Am J Psychiatry*. 1965;121:1021.

Grimes JB, Labbate LA. Spontaneous orgasm with the combined use of bupropion and sertraline. *Biol Psychiatry*. 1996;40:1184–1186.

Gross MD. Reversal by bethanechol of sexual dysfunction caused by anticholinergic antidepressants. *Am J Psychiatry*. 1982;139:193–194.

Guelfi JD, Ansseau M, Timmerman L, Korsgaard S. Mirtazapine versus venlafaxine in hospitalized severely depressed patients with melancholic features. *J Clin Psychopharmacol*. 2001;21:425–431.

Harrison WM, Rabkin JG, Ehrhardt AA, Stewart JW, McGrath PJ, Ross D, Quitkin FM. Effects of antidepressant medication on sexual function: a controlled study. *J Clin Psychopharmacol*. 1986;6:144–149.

Harvey KV, Balon R. Clinical implications of antidepressant drug effects on sexual function. *Ann Clin Psychiatry*. 1995;7:189–201.

Hedges DW, Reimherr FW, Strong RE, Halls CH, Rust C. An open trial of nefazodone in adults outpatients with generalized anxiety disorder. *Psychopharmacol Bull*. 1996;32:671–676.

Herman JB, Brotman AW, Pollack MH, Falk WE, Biederman J, Rosenbaum JF. Fluoxetine-induced sexual dysfunction. *J Clin Psychiatry*. 1990;51:25–27.

Hollander E, McCarley A. Yohimbine treatment of sexual side effects induced by serotonin reuptake blockers. *J Clin Psychiatry*. 1992;53:207–209.

Hsu JH, Shen WW. Male sexual side effects associated with antidepressants: a descriptive clinical study of 32 patients. *Int J Psychiatry Med*. 1995;25:191–201.

Hypericum Depression Trial Study Group. Effect of Hypericum perforatum (St. John's wort) in major depressive disorder. A randomized controlled trial. *JAMA*. 2002;287:1807–1814.

Jacobsen FM. Fluoxetine-induced sexual dysfunction and an open trial of yohimbine. *J Clin Psychiatry*. 1992;53:119–122.

Jani NN, Wise TN. Antidepressants and inhibited female orgasm: a literature review. *J Sex & Marital Ther*. 1988;14:279–284.

Jones SD. Ejaculatory inhibition with trazodone. *J Clin Psychopharmacol*. 1984;4:279–281.

Karp JF, Frank E, Ritenour A, McEachran A, Kupfer DJ. Imipramine and sexual dysfunction during the long-term treatment of recurrent depression. *Neuropsychopharmacology*. 1994;11:21–27.

Kennedy SH, Eisfeld BS, Dickens SE, Bacchiochi JR, Bagby RM. Antidepressant-induced sexual dysfunction during treatment with moclobemide, paroxetine, sertraline, and venlafaxine. *J Clin Psychiatry*. 2000;61:276–281.

Kennedy SH, McCann SM, Masellis M, McIntyre RS, Raskin J, McKay G, Baker GB. Combining bupropion SR with venlafaxine, paroxetine, or fluoxetine:

a preliminary report on pharmacokinetic, therapeutic, and sexual dysfunction effects. *J Clin Psychiatry.* 2002;63:181–186.

Kiev A, Feiger A. A double-blind comparison of fluvoxamine and paroxetine in the treatment of depressed outpatients. *J Clin Psychiatry.* 1997;58:146–152.

Kotler M, Cohen H, Aizenberg D, Matar M, Loewenthal U, Kaplan Z, Miodownik H, Zemishlany Z. Sexual dysfunction in male posttraumatic stress disorder patients. *Psychother Psychosom.* 2000;69:309–315.

Kraupl Taylor F. Loss of libido in depression. *Br Med J.* 1972;1:105.

Labbate LA. Sexual dysfunction and antidepressants. *Primary Psychiatry.* 2001;8:65–68.

Labbate LA, Brodrick PS, Nelson RP, Lydiard RB, Arana GW. Effects of bupropion sustained-release on sexual functioning and nocturnal erections in healthy men. *J Clin Psychopharmacol.* 2001;21:99–103.

Labbate LA, Grimes JB, Arana GW. Serotonin reuptake antidepressant effects on sexual functioning in patients with anxiety disorders. *Biol Psychiatry.* 1998;43:904–907.

Labbate LA, Grimes JB, Hines A, Pollack MH. Bupropion treatment of serotonin reuptake antidepressant-associated sexual dysfunction. *Ann Clin Psychiatry.* 1997;9:241–245.

Labbate LA, Lare SB. Sexual dysfunction in male psychiatric outpatients: validity of the Massachusetts General Hospital Sexual Functioning Questionnaire. *Psychother Psychosom.* 2001;70:221–225.

Landen M, Eriksson E, Agren H, Fahlen T. Effects of buspirone on sexual dysfunction in depressed patients treated with selective serotonin reuptake inhibitors. *J Clin Psychopharmacol.* 1999;19:268–271.

Lane RM. A critical review of selective serotonin reuptake inhibitor-related sexual dysfunction; incidence, possible aetiology and implications for management. *J Psychopharmacol.* 1997;11:72–82.

Lauerma H. A case of moclobemide-induced hyperorgasmia. *Int Clin Psychopharmacol.* 1995;10:123–124.

Lesko LM, Stotland NL, Segraves RT. Three cases of female anorgasmia associated with MAOIs. *Am J Psychiatry.* 1982;139:1353–1354.

Levenson JL. Priapism associated with bupropion treatment. *Am J Psychiatry.* 1995;152:813.

Lue TF. Erectile dysfunction. *N Engl J Med.* 2000;342:1802–1813.

Margolese HC, Assalian P. Sexual side effects of antidepressants: a review. *J Sex & Marital Ther.* 1996;22:209–217.

Masand PS, Ashton AK, Gupta S, Frank B. Sustained-release bupropion for selective serotonin reuptake inhibitor-induced sexual dysfunction: a randomized, double-blind, placebo-controlled, parallel-group study. *Am J Psychiatry.* 2001;158:805–807.

Mathew RJ, Weinman ML. Sexual dysfunction in depression. *Arch Sex Behav.* 1982;11:323–325.

Mavissakalian M, Perel J, Guo S. Specific side effects of long-term imipramine management of panic disorder. *J Clin Psychopharmacol.* 2002;22:155–161.

McGahuey CA, Delgado PL, Geleberg AJ. Assessment of sexual dysfunction using the Arizona Sexual Experience Scale (ASEX) and implications for the treatment of depression. *Psychiatr Ann.* 1999;29:39–45.

McLean JD, Forsythe RG, Kapkin IA. Unusual side effects of clomipramine associated with yawning. *Can J Psychiatry.* 1983;28:569–570.

Meston CM, Frohlich PF. The neurobiology of sexual function. *Arch Gen Psychiatry.* 2000;57:1012–1030.

Meston CM, Gorzalka BB. Psychoactive drugs and human sexual behavior: the role of serotonin activity. *J Psychoactive Drugs.* 1992;24:1–40.

Michael A, Owen A. Venlafaxine-induced increased libido and spontaneous erection. *Br J Psychiatry.* 1997;170:193.

Michael A, Ramana R. Nefazodone-induced spontaneous ejaculation. *Br J Psychiatry.* 1996;169:672–673.

Michelson D, Schmidt M, Lee J, Tepner R. Changes in sexual function during acute and six-month fluoxetine therapy: a prospective assessment. *J Sex & Marital Ther.* 2001;27:289–302.

Modell JG. Repeated observations of yawning, clitoral engorgement, and orgasm associated with fluoxetine administration. *J Clin Psychopharmacol.* 1989;9:63–65.

Modell JG, Katholi CR, Modell JD, DePalma RL. Comparative sexual side effects of bupropion, fluoxetine, paroxetine, and sertraline. *Clin Pharmacol Ther.* 1997;61:476–487.

Modell JG, May RS, Katholi CR. Effect of bupropion-SR on orgasmic dysfunction in nondepressed subjects: a pilot study. *J Sex & Marital Ther.* 2000;26:231–240.

Monteiro WO, Noshirvani HF, Marks IM, Lelliot PT. Anorgasmia from clomipramine in obsessive–compulsive disorder: a controlled trial. *Br J Psychiatry.* 1987;151:107–112.

Montejo-Gonzales AL, Llorca G, Izquierdo JA, Ledesma A, Bousono M, Calcedo A, Carrasco JL, Ciudad J, Daniel E, De La Gandara J, Derecho J, Franco M, Gomez MJ, Macias JA, Martin T, Perez V, Sanchez JM, Sanchez S, Vicens E. SSRI-induced sexual dysfunction: fluoxetine, paroxetine, sertraline, and fluvoxamine in a prospective, multicenter, and descriptive clinical study of 344 patients. *J Sex & Marital Ther.* 1997;23:176–194.

Montejo-Gonzales AL, Llorca G, Izquierdo JA, Rico-Villademoros F. Incidence of sexual dysfunction associated with antidepressant agents: a prospective multicenter study of 1,022 outpatients. *J Clin Psychiatry.* 2001;62(Suppl 3):10–21.

Montgomery SA, Baldwin DS, Riley A. Antidepressant medications: a review of the evidence for drug-induced sexual dysfunction. *J Affect Disord.* 2002;69:119–140.

Nafziger AN, Bertino JS, Jr, Goss-Bley AI, Kashuba ADM. Incidence of sexual dysfunction in healthy volunteers on fluvoxamine therapy. *J Clin Psychiatry.* 1999;60:187–190.

Neil JR. Penile anesthesia associated with fluoxetine. *Am J Psychiatry.* 1991;148:1603.

Nelson EB, Shah VN, Welge JA, Keck PE, Jr, A placebo-controlled, crossover trial of granisetron in SRI-induced sexual dysfunction. *J Clin Psychiatry.* 2001;62:469–473.

Nemeroff CB, Ninan PT, Ballenger J, Lydiard RB, Feighner, J, Patterson WM, Greist JH. Double-blind multicenter comparison of fluvoxamine versus sertraline in the treatment of depressed outpatient. *Depression*. 1995;3:163–169.

Nininger JE Inhibition of ejaculation by amitriptyline. *Am J Psychiatry*. 1978;135:750–751.

Nofzinger EA, Thase ME, Reynolds CR III, Frank E, Jennings JR, Garamoni GL, Fasiczka AL, Kupfer DJ. Sexual dysfunction in depressed men: assessment by self-report, behavioral, and nocturnal penile tumescence measures before and after treatment with cognitive behavioral therapy. *Arch Gen Psychiatry*. 1993;50:24–30.

Norden M. Buspirone treatment of sexual dysfunction associated with selective serotonin re-uptake inhibitors. *Depression*. 1994;2:109–112.

Nurnberg HG, Hensley PL, Lauriello J, Bogenschutz MP. Sildenafil treatment of antidepressant-associated sexual dysfunction: a 12-case treatment replication in a naturalistic clinical setting. *Primary Psychiatry*. 2001;8:69–78.

Nurnberg HG, Levine PE. Spontaneous remission of MAOI-induced anorgasmia. *Am J Psychiatry*. 1987;144:805–807.

Othmer E, Othmer SC. Effect of buspirone on sexual function in patients with generalized anxiety disorder. *J Clin Psychiatry*. 1987;48:201–203.

Patterson WM. Fluoxetine-induced sexual dysfunction. *J Clin Psychiatry*. 1993;54:71.

Pecknold JC, Langer SF. Priapism: trazodone versus nefazodone. *J Clin Psychiatry*. 1996;57:547–548.

Pescatori ES, Engelman JC, Davis G, Goldstein I. Priapism of the clitoris: a case report following trazodone use. *J Urol*. 1993;149:1557–1559.

Pettinati HM, Volpicelli JR, Luck G, Kranzler HR, Rukstalis MR, Cnaan A. Double-blind clinical trial of sertraline treatment for alcohol dependence. *J Clin Psychopharmacol*. 2001;21:143–153.

Phillipp M, Kohnen R, Benkert O. A comparison study of moclobemide and doxepin in major depression with special reference to effects on sexual dysfunction. *Int Clin Psychopharmacol*. 1993;7:149–153.

Phillips RL, Jr, Slaughter JR. Depression and sexual desire. *Am Fam Physician*. 2000;62:782–786.

Physicians' Desk Reference (56th ed). Montvale, NJ: Medical Economics Company; 2002.

Pollack MH, Zaninelli R, Goddard A, McCafferty JP, Bellew KM, Burnham DB, Iyengar MK. Paroxetine in the treatment of generalized anxiety disorder: results of a placebo-controlled, flexible-dosage trial. *J Clin Psychiatry*. 2001;62:350–357.

Posternak MA, Zimmerman M. The effectiveness of switching antidepressants during remission: a case series of depressed patients who experienced intolerable side effects. *J Affect Disord*. 2002;69:237–240.

Power-Smith P. Beneficial sexual side-effects from fluoxetine. *Br J Psychiatry*. 1994;164:249–250.

Price J, Grunhaus LJ. Treatment of clomipramine-induced anorgasmia with yohimbine: a case report. *J Clin Psychiatry*. 1990;51:32–33.

Purcell P, Ghurye R. Trazodone and spontaneous orgasm in elderly postmenopausal woman: a case report. *J Clin Psychopharmacol*. 1995;15:293–295.

Quirk KC, Einarson TR. Sexual dysfunction and clomipramine. *Can J Psychiatry*. 1982;27:228–231.

Rabkin JG, Quitkin F, Harrison W, Tricamo E, McGrath P. Adverse reactions to monoamine oxidase inhibitors. I. A Comparative study. *J Clin Psychopharmacol*. 1984;4:270–278.

Rabkin JG, Quitkin FM, McGrath P, Harrison W, Tricamo R. Adverse reactions to monoamine oxidase inhibitors. II. Treatment correlates and clinical management. *J Clin Psychopharmacol*. 1985;5:2–9.

Rapp MS. Two cases of ejaculatory impairment related to phenelzine. *Am J Psychiatry*. 1979;136:1200–1201.

Ravindran AV, Guelfi JD, Lane RM, Cassano G. B. Treatment of dysthymia with sertraline: a double-blind, placebo-controlled trial in dysthymic patients without major depression. *J Clin Psychiatry*. 2000;61:821–827.

Reynolds RD. Sertraline-induced anorgasmia treated with intermittent nefazodone. *J Clin Psychiatry*. 1997;58:89.

Riley AJ, Riley EJ. Cyproheptadine and antidepressant-induced anorgasmia. *Br J Psychiatry*. 1986;148:217–218.

Rosenbaum JF, Pollack MH. Anhedonic ejaculation with desipramine. *Int J Psychiatry Med*. 1988;18:85–88.

Rothschild AJ. Selective serotonin reuptake inhibitor-induced sexual dysfunction: efficacy of a drug holiday. *Am J Psychiatry*. 1995;152:1514–1516.

Roy-Byrne PP, Pages KP, Russo JE, Jaffe C, Blume AW, Kingsley E, Cowley DS, Ries RK. Nefazodone treatment of major depression in alcohol dependent patients: a double-blind, placebo-controlled trial. *J Clin Psychopharmacol*. 2000;20:129–136.

Russell JM, Koran LM, Rush J, Hirschfeld RMA, Harrison W, Friedman ES, Davis S, Keller M. Effect of concurrent anxiety on response to sertraline and imipramine in patients with chronic depression. *Depress Anxiety*. 2001;13:18–27.

Segraves RT. Effects of psychotropic drugs on human erection and ejaculation. *Arch Gen Psychiatry*. 1989;46:275–284.

Segraves RT. Antidepressant-induced sexual dysfunction. *J Clin Psychiatry*. 1998;59(Suppl 4):48–54.

Segraves RT. Two additional uses for sildenafil in psychiatric patients. *J Sex & Marital Ther*. 1999;25:265–266.

Segraves RT, Croft H, Kavoussi R, Ascher JA, Batey SR, Foster VJ, Bolden-Watson C, Metz A. Bupropion sustained release (SR) for the treatment of hypoactive sexual desire disorder (HSDD) in nondepressed women. *J Sex & Marital Ther*. 2001;27:303–316.

Segraves RT, Kavoussi R, Hughes AR, Batey SR, Johnston JA, Donahue R, Ascher J. Evaluation of sexual functioning in depressed outpatients: a double-blind comparison of sustained-release bupropion and sertraline treatment. *J Clin Psychopharmacol*. 2000;20:122–128.

Seidman SN. Exploring the relationship between depression and erectile dysfunction in aging men. *J Clin Psychiatry*. 2002;63(Suppl 5):5–12.

Sovner R. Anorgasmia associated with imipramine but not desipramine: case report. *J Clin Psychiatry*. 1983;44:345–346.

Sovner R. Treatment of tricylic antidepressant-induced orgasmic inhibition with cyproheptadine. *J Clin Psychopharmacol*. 1984;4:169.

Steele TE, Howell EF. Cyproheptadine for imipramine-induced anorgasmia. *J Clin Psychopharmacol*. 1986;6:326–327.

Sullivan G. Increased libido in three men treated with trazodone. *J Clin Psychiatry*. 1988;49:202–203.

Thase ME, Reynolds CF III, Jennings JR, Frank E, Garamoni GL, Nofzinger EA, Fascizka AL, Kupfer DJ. Diminished noctural penile tumescence in depression: a replication study. *Biol Psychiatry*. 1992;31:1136–1142.

Thase ME, Reynolds CF III, Jennings JR, Frank E, Howell JR, Houck PR, Berman S, Kupfer DJ. Nocturnal penile tumescence is diminished in depressed men. *Biol Psychiatry*. 1988;24:33–46.

Yager J. Bethanechol chloride can reverse erectile and ejaculatory dysfunction induced by tricyclic antidepressants and mazindol. *J Clin Psychiatry*. 1986;47:210–211.

Waldinger MD, Hengeveld MW, Zwinderman AH. Ejaculation-retarding properties of paroxetine in patients with primary premature ejaculation: a double-blind, randomized, dose-response study. *Br J Urol*. 1997;79:592–595.

Waldinger MD, Hengeveld MW, Zwinderman AH, Olivier B. Effect of SSRI antidepressants on ejaculation: A double-blind, randomized, placebo-controlled study with fluoxetine, fluvoxamine, paroxetine, and sertraline. *J Clin Psychopharmacol*. 1998;18:274–281.

Waldinger MD, Olivier B. Sexual dysfunction and fluvoxamine therapy. *J Clin Psychiatry*. 2001;62:126–127.

Waldinger MD, Zwinderman AH, Olivier B. Antidepressants and ejaculation: A double-blind, randomized, placebo-controlled, fixed-dose study with paroxetine, sertraline, and nefazodone. *J Clin Psychopharmacol*. 2001a;21:283–297.

Waldinger MD, Zwinderman AH, Olivier B. SSRIs and ejaculation: A double-blind, randomized, fixed-dose study with paroxetine and citalopram. *J Clin Psychopharmacol*. 2001b;21:556–560.

Walker PW, Cole JO, Gardner EA, Hughes AR, Johnston JA, Bates SR, Lineberry CG. Improvement in fluoxetine associated sexual dysfunction in patients switched to bupropion. *J Clin Psychiatry*. 1993;54:459–465.

Ware MR, Emmanuel NP, Johnson MR, Brawman-Mintzer O, Knapp R, Crawford-Harrison M, Lydiard RB. Self-reported sexual dysfunction in anxiety disorder patients. *Psychopharmacol Bull*. 1996;32:530.

Warner MD, Peabody CA, Whiteford HA, Hollister LE. Trazodone and priapism. *J Clin Psychiatry*. 1981;48:244–245.

Yassa R. Sexual disorders in the course of clomipramine treatment: a case report of three cases. *Can J Psychiatry*. 1982;27:148–149.

Yeragani VK, Gershon S. Priapism related to phenelzine therapy. *N Engl J Med*. 1987;317:117–118.

Zajecka J. Strategies for the treatment of antidepressant-related sexual dysfunction. *J Clin Psychiatry*. 2001;62(Suppl 3):35–43.

Zajecka J, Amsterdam JD, Quitkin FM, Reimherr FW, Rosenbaum JF, Tamura RN, Sundell KL, Michelson D, Beasley CM, Jr. Changes in adverse events reported by patients during 6 months of fluoxetine therapy. *J Clin Psychiatry*. 1999;60:389–394.

Zajecka J, Dunner DL, Gelenberg AJ, Hirschfeld RMA, Kornstein SG, Ninan PT, Rush AJ, Thase ME, Trivedi MH, Arnow BA, Borian FE, Manber R,

Keller MB. Sexual function and satisfaction in the treatment of chronic major depression with nefazodone, psychotherapy, and their combination. *J Clin Psychiatry.* 2002;63:709–716.

Zajecka J, Fawcett J, Schaff M, Jeffries H, Guy C. The role of serotonin in sexual function: fluoxetine-associated orgasm dysfunction. *J Clin Psychiatry.* 1991;52:66–68.

Zajecka J, Mitchell S, Fawcett J. Treatment-emergent changes in sexual function with selective serotonin reuptake inhibitors as measured with the Rush Sexual Inventory. *Psychopharmacol Bull.* 1997;33:755–760.

5. Mood Stabilizers

INTRODUCTION

This chapter focuses on the assessment and management of sexual dysfunction associated with drugs used for stabilizing mood (i.e., lithium and anticonvulsants), but not on sexual dysfunction associated with some drugs (i.e., antipsychotic and antianxiety drugs) used to treat acute mania. These antipsychotic and antianxiety drugs are mentioned in this chapter, but the sexual dysfunction associated with these two drug classes is reviewed in Chapters 2 and 3. In addition to long-term mood stabilization, some of the mood stabilizers are used to treat acute mania, mainly in combination with antipsychotics (typical and atypical), but even alone, when some patients undergo loading with mood stabilizers. Table 5.1 lists mood stabilizers available in the United States.

Assessing sexual dysfunction in patients treated for a bipolar illness is a complicated matter. Given that several drugs are usually used in the management of bipolar patients, changes in sexual function may be due the illness itself, to mood stabilizing drugs, or to other drugs (not necessarily psychotropic ones). These changes in sexual functioning associated with bipolar disorders usually include decreased sexual interest and desire during the depressive phase and excessive involvement in pleasurable activities—sexual indiscretions, among others—with a high potential for painful consequences during manic phases.

It is important to emphasize that most of the so-called mood stabilizers have not been approved by the Food and Drug Administration (FDA) for treatment of mood disorders. In fact, only lithium is approved for treatment of the manic episode of a bipolar disorder. Anticonvulsants are approved for the treatment of various forms

Table 5.1 Mood stabilizers available in the United States

Generic Name	Brand Name	Forms and Doses (mg)*
carbamazepine	Tegretol	tc: 100
		t: 200
		txr: 100/200/400
		o: 20/mL
	Carbatrol	cer: 200/300
clonazepam	Klonopin	t: 0.5/1/2
divalproex sodium	Depakote sprinkle	c: 125
	Depakote tablets	t: 125/250/500
	Depakote ER	t: 500
gabapentin	Neurontin	t: 600/800
		c: 100/300/400
		o: 50/mL
haloperidol	Haldol	t: 0.5/1/2/5/10/20
		o: 2/mL
		p: 5/mL
	Haloperidol decanoate	pl: 50/mL; 100/mL
lamotrigine	Lamictal	t: 25/100/150/200
		tc: 2/5/25
lithium carbonate	Eskalith	c: 300
	Eskalith CR	cr: 450
	Lithobid	txr: 300
lithium citrate	Lithium citrate	s: 8 mEq/5 mL
lorazepam	Ativan	t: 0.5/1/2
		p: 2/mL; 4/mL
nipodipine	Nimotop	c: 30
olanzapine	Zyprexa	t: 2.5/5/7.5/10
	Zyprexa.Zydis	tod: 5/10/15/20
oxcarbazepine	Trileptal	t: 150/300/600
		o: 60/mL
risperidone	Risperdal	t: 0.25/0.5/1/2/3/4
		o: 1/mL
tiagabine hydrochloride	Gabitril	t: 2/4/12/16/20
topiramate	Topamax	t: 25/100/200
		c: 15/25
valproate sodium	Depacon injection	p: 100/mL
valproic acid	Depakene	c: 250
		s: 50/mL
verapamil hydrochloride	Calan	t: 40/80/120
		txr: 120/180/240
	Covera HS	txr: 180/240
	Isoptin SR	txr: 120/180/240
	Verelan	c: 120/180/240/360
	Verelan PM	cer: 100/200/300
	Verapamil hydrochloride	t: 40/80/120/180/240
		c: 120/180/240

* c = capsules; cer = extended release capsules; cr = controlled release; o = oral concentrate; p = parenteral concentrate; pl = parenteral concentrate, long acting; s = syrup; t = tablet; tc = chewable tablets; tod = orally disintegrated tablets; tsd = single-dose tablets (slow release); txr = slow release tablets.

of epilepsy only. However, some of them have been widely used for treatment of bipolar disorders. None of the mentioned antidotes has been approved by the FDA for the treatment of sexual dysfunction.

SEXUAL DYSFUNCTION IN PATIENTS WITH MOOD DISORDERS

As already noted, changes in sexual functioning may be associated with either depression (decreased desire or libido) or mania (increased involvement in sexual activity). Changes in sexual desire, thought, and behavior during depression and mania were observed centuries ago. All phases of the sexual cycle can be affected during depression, but decreased libido is the most frequent complaint. The incidence of reduced sexual desire in clinically depressed patients varied in several studies from 31% to 62% to even 77% (bipolar depressed patients). It is not only the presence of depression itself, but also its severity that is associated with various degrees of sexual dysfunction. Increasing severity of depression and anxiety was associated with greater loss of libido. Cognitive impairment also showed strong correlation with loss of sexual interest (among other variables). Erectile dysfunction, arousal impairment, delayed ejaculation or orgasm, and partial or complete anorgasmia occur less frequently than decreased libido in depressed patients. Several studies found changes in erectile capacity in depressed men. Men with a depressive disorder also have significantly diminished nocturnal penile tumescence time and rigidity: 40% of 34 depressed men had decreased nocturnal penile tumescence, compared to 15% of 28 healthy controls. Decreased nocturnal penile tumescence in depressed men is estimated to be as frequent as 57%. The average reduction in erection time in one study was 30%, and the average decrease in penile rigidity was 15–25%. Interestingly, nocturnal penile tumescence disturbances did not improve early during remission of clinical depression. Remitted patients in this study were also more satisfied with their sex lives after treatment, despite the relative absence of change in level of daily sexual activity. The researchers felt that this increased satisfaction reflected the depressed patients' cognitive appraisal of sexual function as less satisfying and pleasurable. Some authors consider depression a significant risk for the development of erectile dysfunction. However, increased libido and hypersexuality also have been reported in depressed patients. It has been hypothesized that hypersexuality in depressed patients may serve as a compensation for their lack of sexual gratification or as a means of denying that any sexual dysfunction exists.

The manic phase of a bipolar disorder is frequently associated with hypersexuality: 30–65% of manic patients manifest hypersexuality, whereas only about 15% experience diminished libido. In a summary of the relatively limited data on changes in sexual behavior during different phases of bipolar illness, hypersexuality was reported in 57%

Table 5.2 Sexual dysfunctions associated with mood disorders

Depressed mood (either in major depression or depressive phase of bipolar disorder)	Mania, hypomania
Frequent	**Frequent**
Decreased libido (interest, desire) Erectile dysfunction (manifested by diminished nocturnal penile tumescence)	Increased libido Hypersexuality Promiscuity, extramarital affairs Increased sexual intensity
Less Frequent	**Less Frequent**
Inadequate vaginal lubrication Delayed orgasm/ejaculation Partial or complete anorgasmia Dyspareunia Premature ejaculation Increased libido Hypersexuality	Nudity, sexual exposure

of manic patients, averaged across seven studies, with a range 25–80%. It was also noted that bipolar patients may have a decreased sexual drive. Interestingly, researchers observed that 40% of cyclothymic patients had episodic or unexplained promiscuity or extramarital affairs. Other researchers have noted the association between mania and increased sexual activity. However, it is not clear whether the hypersexuality is an intrinsic feature of mania, or whether it is secondary to symptoms such as grandiosity, impulsivity, and hyperactivity.

Obviously, changes in sexual function during depression and mania can influence any estimates of sexual dysfunction associated with medications used for treating depression and mania. It is also well known that depressed patients frequently do not spontaneously report their sexual dysfunction. All these factors need to be taken into account when evaluating and treating sexual dysfunction that is presumably associated with depression or mania. Table 5.2 summarizes the sexual dysfunctions associated with mood disorders.

SEXUAL DYSFUNCTION ASSOCIATED WITH MOOD STABILIZERS

The literature on sexual dysfunction associated with mood stabilizers is scarce, and the "data" are frequently limited to case reports or methodologically unsophisticated studies.

Lithium

Lithium is the oldest and most frequently used mood stabilizer. Its efficacy has been confirmed in numerous studies. Therapeutic use of lithium requires maintaining serum lithium levels of 0.6 to 1.5 mEq/L. Sexual responsiveness may be dampened by lithium. Several studies have found sexual dysfunction associated with lithium. In one study, half of the patients experienced troublesome decreses in sexual drive, decreases in frequency of sexual intercourse, and decreases in sexual intensity. However, patients did not experience diminishment in enjoyment of sex and orgasm once intercourse began. In early studies, other researchers observed that a small portion of their bipolar patients treated prophylactically with lithium reported impaired sexual functioning. (For instance, in a double-blind segment of a larger study, 3 of 10 bipolar patients reported impaired sexual functioning, two of them complaining of erectile dysfunction and one reporting decreased libido). In another fairly large survey, only one of 237 patients complained of loss of libido and potency during long-term lithium treatment. Several other research studies reported decreased libido and impaired erection. Interestingly, in one research study lithium frequently decreased sperm motility and caused other changes in spermiogram.

More recent small studies suggested that the frequency of sexual dysfunction associated with lithium might be higher than previously thought. One study reported that 4 of 25 men (16%) suffered from sexual dysfunction associated with lithium, three from decreased libido and one from erectile dysfunction. In another small and restrospective study, 3 of 10 female patients (30%) and 5 of 14 male patients (36%) reported lithium to be associated sexual dysfunction. However, control subjects in this same study, who were not taking lithium, reported similar frequencies of sexual dysfunction (7 of 25 female controls and 5 of 17 male controls). Another group of researchers also reported sexual dysfunction associated with lithium in bipolar and schizoaffective disorder patients. In this study, reduction of sexual thoughts occured in 23% of participating men, loss of erection during coitus in 20% of participating men, and diminished frequency of waking erection in 14% of participating men. However, almost all the patients in this study were satisfied with their sexual performance and reported a maintence of the pleasure they experienced during sexual activity. Lithium-associated sexual dysfunction was not a source of distress and did not cause noncompliance with medication in this study.

In a multiple regression analysis of data from 104 patients treated with various medications for bipolar disorder, one group of researchers found that lithium, when given alone, was associated with sexual dysfunction in 17% patients. However, the combination of lithium and benzodiazepines was associated with sexual dysfunction in 49% patients, while the combination of lithium and other medications (tricyclic antidepressants, antipsychotics, carbamazepine) was associated with sexual dysfunction in only in 17% patients.

There does not seem to be a relationship between serum lithium level and sexual dysfunction, although one study reported an association between high lithium level and increased libido.

It is important to note that, in one study, lithium decreased self-rated "good sexual feelings" in healthy volunteers.

It is difficult to speculate on the mechanism of lithium-induced sexual dysfunction. However, it is possible that its enhancement of serotonergic transmission may play a role in the sexual dysfunction associated with this mood stabilizer.

In summary, evidence from the literature suggests that lithium may cause sexual dysfunction in a minority of patients treated for a bipolar disorder. The sexual dysfunction associated with lithium is limited mainly to decreased libido and erectile dysfunction. Table 5.3 summarizes the sexual dysfunctions associated with lithium.

Table 5.3   Sexual dysfunction associated with lithium[*]
(frequency is usually low, 20–30%; however, decreased libido up to 50%)

Decreased sexual drive
Decreased sexual frequency
Decreased sexual intensity
Erectile dysfunction

Rare findings (one study):
   Decreased sperm motility
   Various changes in spermiogram

[*] Note: Sexual dysfunction is higher when lithium is combined with benzodiazepines.
Unclear relationship between sexual dysfunction and lithium level—probably none.

Anticonvulsants

Anticonvulsants have become increasingly popular in the treatment of bipolar disorders. The anticonvulsants used in this context include carbamazepine, gabapentin, lamotrigine, oxcarbazepine, topiramate, valproate, and possibly tiagabine. Most of the reports on sexual dysfunction associated with anticonvulsants come from the epilepsy literature. (For details on anticonvulsant-associated sexual dysfunction and changes in sex hormone levels associated with anticonvulsants, see Chapter 10.)

The literature on sexual dysfunction associated with anticonvulsants used in the treatment of bipolar disorders is scarce. In epilepsy patients, carbamazepine-associated sexual dysfunction was observed in 13% of patients. Valproic acid seemed to have the lowest frequency and the least effect on sex hormones in people with epilepsy.

Three case reports noted anorgasmia associated with gabapentin in men treated for bipolar disorder. In two cases, gabapentin-associated anorgasmia and lack of pleasure caused noncompliance, and sexual dysfunction returned to baseline after gabapentin was stopped. Other researchers switched the patient to valproic acid, which resolved the anorgasmia while still controlling the symptoms. The *Physicians' Desk Reference* (*PDR*) lists the incidence of sexual dysfunction associated with gabapentin as 1.5% (results from epilepsy treatment studies).

One group of researchers described the case of a female with schizoaffective disorder who was treated with lamotrigine and developed low libido and unpleasant sensations in her genitals and erogenous zones. In contrast, another group reported improved sexual function in three men after lamotrigine was added or substituted for their various anticonvulsant treatments for epilepsy.

To date, there are no reports on sexual dysfunction associated with other anticonvulsants in the treatment of bipolar disorders.

The specific mechanisms of action, whereby sexual dysfunction is associated with anticonvulsants, remain unclear. They are probably multifactorial, and different mechanisms of action are involved for different anticonvulsants. The anticonvulsant effect on sex hormones and sex hormone binding globulin should be considered one mechanism of action. Direct effect on various neurotransmitters (e.g., serotonin), both centrally and peripherally, is another possible explanation. Table 5.4 summarizes the sexual dysfunctions associated with anticonvulsants.

Table 5.4   Sexual dysfunction associated with anticonvulsants[*] in mood disorders

	Frequency	Type of Dysfunction
Carbamazepine	Unknown (13% in epilepsy)	No data in bipolar disorder (Changes of hormone levels in epilepsy) (Ejaculatory failure in trigeminal neuralgia-1 case)
Gabapentin	1.5% (?) (epilepsy data)	Anorgasmia and lack of pleasure
Lamotrigine	Unknown	Loss of libido (one case) Improvement of sexual dysfunction in epilepsy
Valproic acid	Unknown (Low in epilepsy)	No data (Least effect on hormones in epilepsy)

[*] No data on oxcarbazepine, topiramate, tiagabine.

Calcium Channel Blockers, Benzodiazepines, and Antipsychotics Used as Mood Stabilizers

Two calcium channel blockers, verapamil and nimodipine, occasionally have been used in the treatment of bipolar disorders. No sexual dysfunction associated with these two drugs during treatment of bipolar disorder has been reported. However, calcium channel blockers were associated with 1% incidence of sexual dysfunction in patients treated for hypertension. Sexual dysfunction associated with these drugs used to treat bipolar disorders could be fairly low, too.

Benzodiazepines such as clonazepam and lorazepam occasionally have been used to treat bipolar disorders. Clonazepam, according to the *PDR*, is associated with ejaculatory problems in 1–2% and impotence in 1–3% of male patients. Clonazepam also was associated with sexual dysfunction in veterans with posttraumatic stress disorder (PTSD). Finally, as noted, benzodiazepines (with clonazepam being the most frequently used, in 86% of patients) in combination with lithium were associated with sexual dysfunction in 49% of bipolar patients.

Sexual dysfunction is frequently associated with the antipsychotic medication used in the treatment of bipolar disorders. Antipsychotics may cause various sexual dysfunctions, including serious ones such as priapism, and changes in sex hormone (i.e., prolactin) levels. For details, see Chapter 2.

It is reasonable to assume that the combination of mood stabilizers with either antipsychotics or benzodiazepines may lead to a higher incidence of sexual dysfunction. Table 5.5 summarizes the sexual dysfunctions associated with additional drugs used as mood stabilizers.

Table 5.5   Sexual dysfunction associated with other medications used to treat mood disorders

	Frequency	Type of Dysfunction
Calcium channel blockers	Unknown (1% in hypertension)	No data
Benzodiazepines (alprazolam,chlordiazepoxide diazepam)*	Unknown (1–3% in other disorders)	No data (Delayed ejaculation, orgasm in other disorders, rarely impaired erection)
Antipsychotics	Unknown (Up to 50% in other disorders)	No data (Hyperprolactinemia, lower sexual desire, erectile dysfunction, priapism, retrograde ejaculation, delayed orgasm/anorgasmia, reproductive side effects in other disorders)

* Sexual dysfunction is higher when benzodiazepines are combined with lithium.

MANAGEMENT OF SEXUAL DYSFUNCTION ASSOCIATED WITH MOOD STABILIZERS

Literature on the management of sexual dysfunction associated with mood stabilizers is scarce. It is very important to establish whether the sexual dysfunction predated the use of the current medications. As noted, both depression and mania may be associated with changes in sexual functioning in some patients (no information is available on the frequency of sexual dysfunction during the euthymic mood, however). Thus establishing baseline sexual functioning of all patients prior to starting any treatment is extremely important.

There are several management approaches to dealing with medication associated with sexual dysfunction:

- Waiting for spontaneous remission of sexual dysfunction
- Reducing the dose
- Scheduling medication in relation to sexual activity
- Switching to medication with a lower frequency of sexual dysfunction
- Drug holidays
- Using antidotes, vacuum erectile devices, or prosthesis
- Selecting a primary treatment agent associated with a lower frequency of sexual dysfunction.

None of these approaches has been studied rigorously and only a few of them have been reported successful (case reports). Lowering the lithium dose was associated with improvement of sexual dysfunction in one case. In two cases of lithium-associated sexual dysfunction, sexual functioning returned to baseline levels whenever lithium was discontinued in one case (not always an option) and spontaneously remitted after two months of lithium therapy in the other. Repeated discontinuation of lithium led to repeated cessation of sexual dysfunction in one man in another study sample of 25 men.

The literature on management of sexual dysfunction associated with anticonvulsants used to treat bipolar disorders is similarly scarce. Both patients in two case reports returned to their usual orgasm and ejaculation abilities after gabapentin discontinuation. One of the patients reported resolution of gabapentin-associated sexual dysfunction after switching to valproic acid. Interestingly, as noted, in three men treated with anticonvulsants for epilepsy, sexual dysfunction improved after switching to, or adding, lamotrigine.

The management of antipsychotic-associated sexual dysfunction is reviewed in Chapter 2, and the management of anxiolytic-associated sexual dysfunction is reviewed in Chapter 3. Management strategies may include various approaches, even the use of sildenafil when

Table 5.6   Management options for mood stabilizers associated sexual dysfunction

Switching to another mood stabilizer (lamotrigine?, valproic acid?*)
Selecting a mood stabilizer with theoretically low frequency of sexual dysfunction (lamotrigine?, valproic acid?*)
Possible use of antidotes (e.g., sildenafil)—untested

* No data available.

erectile dysfunction occurs in response to antipsychotics. It has been suggested that the strategies employed to manage antipsychotic-associated sexual dysfunction in patients with bipolar disorders should include the elimination of other drugs that may cause sexual dysfunction (e.g., change from SSRIs to bupropion or nefazodone), reduction of the dose, and a change in the antipsychotic agent (e.g., consider olanzapine or quetiapine). The efficacy and safety of various antidotes in this population are unknown. There are no reports on management of sexual dysfunction in bipolar patients treated with calcium channel blockers.

Some of these general strategies used in the management of sexual dysfunction are not viable options (e.g., drug holidays) during treatment with mood stabilizers. Scheduling sexual activity around the dose of a mood stabilizer (i.e., just *prior* to taking the entire daily dose) may not be the best strategy either, due to the need to maintain steady levels of the medication. Spontaneous remission may occur occasionally, but its frequency is unknown. In summary, the most favorable management options are listed in Table 5.6.

Furthermore, when selecting additional medications for use in the depressive or manic phase of a bipolar disorder, the possible side effect of sexual dysfunction should be taken into account. Bupropion, mirtazapine, and nefazodone seem to have lower frequencies of sexual dysfunction than, for instance, SSRIs, and thus may be a more suitable option for some depressed bipolar patients. Similarly, some antipsychotics (older: loxapine, molindone; newer: olanzapine, quetiapine[?]) may have lower frequencies of sexual dysfunction and thus may be better tolerated by bipolar patients.

Monitoring and addressing sexual dysfunction during the treatment of bipolar disorders may help enhance compliance with the treatment regime. Psychotherapy, behavioral therapy, and sexual therapy also could be useful as adjunctive strategies in the management of sexual dysfunction. Creativity and caution remain the basic guiding strategies in the management of mood stabilizer-associated sexual dysfunction.

The general approach to assessing and managing possible sexual dysfunction associated with mood stabilizers is listed in Table 5.7.

Table 5.7   General strategies for management of sexual dysfunction associated with mood stabilizers

Physician	Patient
1. Establish baseline sexual functioning	1. Reduce psychosocial stressors
2. Help to eliminate other possible causes of sexual dysfunction (e.g., smoking, substance abuse)	2. Participate in psychoeducation
3. Initiate monotherapy whenever possible	3. Initiate exercise program and healthy lifestyle (smoking cessation, elimination of substance abuse)
4. Choose mood stabilizer with possible low incidence of sexual dysfunction	
5. Switch to mood stabilizer with possible lower incidence of sexual dysfunction	
6. Consider antidotes	
7. Use alternative treatment strategies (psychotherapy, sex therapy)	
8. Encourage patient with his/her tasks	

CONCLUSIONS

Sexual dysfunction occurs in a relatively low number of patients treated mood stabilizers for a bipolar illness. Because any sexual dysfunction could cause noncompliance and thus destabilize the patient, it is nonetheless important to consider it throughout the assessment process. However, this assessment process is complicated by the opposite changes in sexual functioning that occur during the depressive and manic phases. No information on sexual dysfunction in untreated euthymic patients with bipolar disorders exists. The exact frequency of sexual dysfunction associated with mood stabilizers and its mechanism of action are not known. Enhancement of serotonergic transmission has been suggested as an explanation for lithium-associated sexual dysfunction. Hormonal changes have been implicated in sexual dysfunction associated with older anticonvulsants, with the exception of valproic acid. The mechanism of action associated with newer anticonvulsants may be different. The mechanism of action in antipsychotic-associated sexual dysfunction is complex (see Chapter 2).

The management strategies of sexual dysfunction associated with mood stabilizers have not been properly studied. Using monotherapy, selecting mood stabilizers with a lower frequency of sexual dysfunction and/or hormonal changes, and using some antidotes seem to be the most prudent strategies at the present time. (Sildenafil, although untested, may be of help in erectile dysfunction; however, we suggest caution in using sildenafil in acutely manic patients.) Careful selection of an antidepressant with a lower frequency of sexual dysfunction for the depressive phase, and an antipsychotic agent with a lower frequency of sexual dysfunction for the manic phase, in addition to a mood stabilizer, should also be part of the management strategy.

REFERENCES

American Psychiatric Association. *Diagnostic and Statistical Manual of Mental Disorders.* 4th ed. Washington, DC: American Psychiatric Association; 1994.

Aizenberg D, Sigler M, Zemishlany Z, Weizman A. Lithium and male sexual function in affective patients. *Clin Neuropharmacol.* 1996;6:515–519.

Akiskal HS, Djenderedjian AH, Rosenthal RH, Khami MK. Cyclothymic disorder: validating criteria for inclusion in the bipolar affective group. *Am J Psychiatry.* 1977;134:1227–1233.

Akiskal HS, Pinto O. The evolving bipolar spectrum, prototypes I, II, III, and IV. *Psychiatr Clin North Am.* 1999;22:517–534.

Bergen D, Daugherty S, Eckenfels E. Reduction of sexual activities in females taking antiepileptic drugs. *Psychopathology.* 1992;25:1–4.

Blay SL, Ferraz MPT, Calil HM. Lithium-induced male sexual impairment: two case reports. *J Clin Psychiatry.* 1982;43:497–498.

Brannon GE, Rolland PD. Anorgasmia in a patient with bipolar disorder type 1 treated with gabapentin. *J Clin Psychopharmacol.* 2000;20:379–381.

Brunet M, Rodamilans M, Martinez-Osaba, et al. Effects of long-term antiepileptic therapy on the catabolism of testosterone. *Pharmacol Toxicol.* 1995;76:371–375.

Casper RC, Redmond Jr, DE, Katz MM, Schaffer CB, Davis JM, Koslow SH. Somatic symptoms in primary affective disorder: presence and relationship to the classification of depression. *Arch Gen Psychiatry.* 1985;42:1098–1104.

Compton MT, Miller AH. Priapism associated with conventional and atypical antipsychotic medications: a review. *J Clin Psychiatry.* 2001a;62:362–366.

Compton MT, Miller AH. Sexual side effects associated with conventional and atypical antipsychotics. *Psychopharmacol Bull.* 2001b;35:89–108.

Connell JMC, Rapeport WG, Beastall GH, Brodie JM. Changes of circulating androgens during short-term carbamazepine therapy. *Br J Clin Pharmac.* 1984;17:347–351.

Erfurth A, Amann B, Grunze H. Female genital disorder as adverse symptom of lamotrigine treatment. A serotoninergic effect? *Neuropsychobiology.* 1998;38:200–201.

Fossey MD, Hammer MB. Clonazepam-related sexual dysfunction in male veterans with PTSD. *Anxiety.* 1995;1:233–236.

Ghadirian A-M, Annable L, Belanger M-C. Lithium, benzodiazepines, and sexual function in bipolar patients. *Am J Psychiatry.* 1992;149:801–805.

Goodwin FK, Jamison KR. *Manic-Depressive Illness.* New York: Oxford University Press;1990:310–311.

Husain AM, Carwile ST, Miller PP, Radtke RA. Improved sexual function in three men taking lamotrigine for epilepsy. *South Med J.* 2000;93:335–336.

Judd LL, Hubbard B, Janowsky DS, Huey LY, Attewell PA. The effect of lithium carbonate on affect, mood, and personality of normal subjects. *Arch Gen Psychiatry.* 1977;34:346–351.

Kaneda Y. Risperidone-induced ejaculatory dysfunction: a case report. *Eur Psychiatry.* 2001;16:134–135.

Kivela SL, Pahkala K. Clinician-rated symptoms and signs of depression in aged Finns. *Int J Soc Psychiatry.* 1988;34:274–284.

Kolomaznik M, Švejnohová D, Janoušek I, Suva J. Lithium a mužská sexualita [Lithium and male sexuality.] *Čas Lék Čes.* 1980;119:521–526.

Kristensen E, Jorgensen P. Sexual function in lithium-treated manic–depressive patients. *Pharmacopsychiat.* 1987;20:165–167.

Kuperman JR, Asher I, Modai I. Olanzapine-associated priapism. *J Clin Psychopharmacol.* 2001;21:247.

Labbate LA, Rubey RN. Gabapentin-induced ejaculatory failure and anorgasmia. *Am J Psychiatry.* 1999;156:972.

Leigh H, Walsh T. Sexual dysfunction in psychiatric disorders. *Medical Aspects of Human Sexuality.* 1988;22(July):64–70.

Leris ACA, Stephens J, Hines JEW, McNicholas TA. Carbamazepine-related ejaculatory failure. *Br J Urol.* 1997;79:485.

Lorimy F, Loo H, Deniker P. Clinical effects of long-term lithium treatment on sleep, appetite and sexuality. *L'Encephale.* 1977;3:227–239.

Matthew RJ, Weinman M, Claghorn JL. Tricyclic side effects without tricyclics in depression. *Psychopharmacol Bull.* 1980;16:58–60.

Mattson RH, Cramer JA, Collins JF, et al. Comparison of carbamazepine, phenobarbital, phenytoin, and primidone in partial and secondarily generalized tonic–clonic seizures. *N Engl J Med.* 1985;313:145–151.

Montes JM, Ferrando L. Gabapentin-induced anorgasmia as a cause of noncompliance in a bipolar patient. *Bipolar Disord.* 2001;3:52.

Nofzinger EA, Thase ME, Reynolds III CR, et al. Sexual dysfunction in depressed men: assessment by self-report, behavioral, and nocturnal penile tumescence measures before and after treatment with cognitive behavioral therapy. *Arch Gen Psychiatry.* 1993;50:24–30.

Physicians' Desk Reference. 56th ed. Montvale, NJ: Medical Economics Company; 2002.

Raboch J, Smolík P, Souček K. Lithium a mužská sexualita [Lithium and male sexuality.] *Čs Psychiatry.* 1983;79:29–32.

Raspa RF, Wilson CC. Calcium channel blockers in the treatment of hypertension. *Am Fam Physician.* 1993;48:461–470.

Roose SP, Glassman AH, Walsh BT, Cullen T. Reversible loss of nocturnal penile tumescence during depression: a preliminary report. *Neuropsychobiology.* 1982;8:284–288.

Sangal R. Inhibited female orgasm as a side effect of alprazolam. *Am J Psychiatry.* 1985;142:1223–1224.

Seger A, Lamberti JS. Priapism associated with polypharmacy. *J Clin Psychiatry.* 2001;62:128.

Segraves RT. Overview of sexual dysfunction complicating the treatment of depression. *J Clin Psychiatry Monograph S.* 1992;10:4–10.

Segraves RT. Effects of antipsychotic, antianxiety, and mood-stabilizing agents on sexual function. *Primary Psychiatry.* 1999a;6:37–39.

Segraves RT. Two additional uses for sildenafil in psychiatric patients. *J Sex Marital Ther.* 1999b;25:265–266.

Strand J, Wise TN, Fagan PJ, Schmidt Jr CW. Erectile dysfunction and depression: category or dimension? *J Sex Marital Ther.* 2002;28:175–181.

Thase ME, Reynolds III CF, Jennings JR, et al. Nocturnal penile tumescence is diminished in depressed men. *Biol Psychiatry.* 1988;24:33–46.

Thase ME, Reynolds III CF, Jennings JR, et al. Diminished nocturnal penile tumescence in depression: a replication study. *Biol Psychiatry.* 1992;31:1136–1142.

Vestergaard P, Amdisen A, Schou M. Clinically significant side effects of lithium treatment. *Acta Psychiatr. Scand.* 1980;62:193–200.

Vinařová E, Uhlíř O, Štika L, Vinař O. Side effects of lithium administration. *Act Nerv Super (Praha).* 1972;14:105–107.

Wang PW, Ketter TA. Pharmacokinetics of mood stabilizers and new anticonvulsants. *Psychopharmacol Bull.* 2002;36:44–66.

Zarate CA. Antipsychotic drug side effect issues in bipolar manic patients. *J Clin Psychiatry.* 2000;61(Suppl 8):52–61.

6. Drugs Associated with Sexual Dysfunction Used in Gastrointestinal Practice

ANTIDIARRHETIC AGENTS

Diarrhea is an extremely common symptom. Clearly, a differential diagnosis is critical prior to symptomatic management. Common antidiarrhetic agents such as Lomotil (diphenoxlate and atropine), Motofen (difenoxine plus atropine), Donnatal (atropine, phenobarbital, hyoscyamine, and scolopine), and Levsin (hyoscyamine) are all anticholinergic agents. There have been no reports of these agents causing sexual problems. Many clinicians attribute erectile dysfunction on various agents as the result of anticholinergic side effects. However, the role of cholinergic stimulation in normal sexual function remains unclear. Erectile tissue is richly innervated with both cholinergic and adrenergic receptors. The role of the cholinergic receptors also remains unclear. Acetylcholine is not the principal neurotransmitter involved in penile erection. In laboratory students, atropine has not been found to have an effect on vaginal lubrication in response to sexual stimulation. It is possible that these agents may negatively impact erectile function as a side effect, but they are usually taken briefly, during a period of acute distress, when sexual activity is infrequently initiated. Imodium (loperamide), a peripheral opiate agonist, also has not been reported to cause sexual dysfunction.

ANTIEMETIC AGENTS

Many medical conditions, medications, and procedures induce nausea and vomiting. Antiemetic agents are most effective when given prophylactically. Uncontrolled nausea and vomiting can have severe adverse effects on quality of life, and protracted nausea and vomiting can result in dehydration, malnutrition, and metabolic disturbances. The pressure associated with severe vomiting can cause rupture of the esophagus or mucosal tears in the cardioesophageal area. Nausea and vomiting secondary to cancer chemotherapy are hypothesized to involve stimulation of the dopamine type 2 receptors and serotonin type 3 receptors. Both cancer chemotherapy and radiation release serotonin from the enterochromaffin cells of the gastrointestinal tract, and the serotonin binds to vagal 5HT3 receptors. The "vomiting center" consists of intertwined neural networks in the nucleus tractus solitaris of the medulla oblongata. The "chemoreceptor trigger zone" is located in the floor of the fourth ventricle and sends impulses to the vomiting center.

Drugs commonly used for nausea include *phenothiazines* such as prochlorperazine (Compazine), metoclopramide (Reglan), and promethazine (Phenergan), and *serotonergic 5HT3 blockers* such as ondansetron (Zofran), gransetron (Kytril), and dolasetron (Anzemet). Gransetron has been reported to reverse SSRI-induced anorgasmia, although this finding was not replicated in a double-blind controlled study. None of the 5HT3 blockers has been reported to be associated with sexual problems. Compazine (prochlorperazine) and Reglan (metoclopramide) are dopamine D2 blockers and have been associated with erectile dysfunction. It is important to point out that most individuals are not sexually active while experiencing severe diarrhea and nausea. This sexual side effects of anti-nausea and anti-diarrhea drugs could be overlooked.

ANTACID AGENTS

Acid indigestion may affect over 95 million Americans a month, and over $1 billion dollars of over-the-counter remedies are sold annually. The treatment of acid indigestion, peptic ulcer disease, and gastroesophageal reflux disease has advanced tremendously over the last few decades. Prior to the introduction of cimetidine (Tagamet), antacids and modification of diet were often the recommended treatments for "heartburn." After cimetidine, three more H2 blockers were introduced in the U.S. market: ranitidine (Zantac), Axid (nizatidine), and famotidine (Pepcid). Proton pump inhibitors such as omeprazole (Prilosec) and lansoprazole (Prevacid) provide more effective control of gastroesophageal reflux disease. Additional agents are expected to reach the U.S. market in the near future.

Cimetidine

Cimetidine, introduced in 1978, was subsequently reported to be related to decreased libido, erectile dysfunction, and gynecomastia. In various clinical series, gynecomastia and/or impotence on high-dose cimetidine has been reported to occur in 40–60% of male patients. In most cases, sexual dysfunction and gynecomastia disappeared when cimetidine was discontinued and ranitidine was started. Libido disturbances also have been noted in women on cimetidine. Cimetidine has even been reported to be effective in the treatment of hypersexuality; minor changes in testosterone, prolactin, and gonadotrophins have been reported, as have cases of hyperprolactinemia. Sexual side effects associated with cimetidine have been attributed to its (1) antiandrogenic and estrogenic properties, (2) ganglionic blocking effects, and (3) effects on central histaminic function. Elevated estrogen levels are not usually associated with conventional cimetidine doses. Sexual dysfunction appears to be dose-related, as high doses of this drug have been reported to have very high incidences of erectile dysfunction (i.e., 40–60%). Erectile tissue contains histaminic receptors, and histamine relaxes human corpus cavernosa strips in a dose-dependent fashion. This effect is inhibited by cimetidine and potentiated by the histamine-1 receptor antagonist, mepyramine. Intracorporeal injection of histamine induces penile erections. This histamine link could be a mechanism by which H2 blockers cause erectile problems. However, current evidence is unclear as to whether erectile function is mediated by H1, H2, or H3 receptors.

Other Antacid Agents

Ranitidine has been frequently advocated as a substitute drug for cimetidine-induced erectile dysfunction. However, erectile dysfunction and gynecomastia also have been reported with this drug. Rantidine has no interaction with the androgen receptor in vitro and appears not to influence reproductive hormone levels. There have been no reports of sexual problems with famotidine. One case report suggests a possible relationship between nizatidine (Axid) and erectile problems.

Gynecomastia and erectile problems have been reported with proton pump inhibitors such as omeprazole (Prilosec). The significance of these reports is difficult to evaluate. To date, there have minimal reports of sexual side effects with lansoprazole (Prevacid). Metoclopramide (Reglan), a dopamine agonist that is sometimes used to improve gastric emptying, has definitely been associated with erectile failure.

Table 6.1 The impact of common gastrointestinal drugs on sexual function

Drug	Erection	Ejaculation	Female SD
Axid (nizatidine)	Unknown	Unknown	Unknown
Compazine (prochlorperazine)	Yes	No	Decreased Llbido
Donnatal (atropine, phenobarbital, hyoscyamine, scolopine)	No	No	Unknown
Imodium (loperamide)	No	No	Unknown
Levsin (hyoscyamine)	No	No	Unknown
Lomotil (atropine plus diphenoxlate)	No	No	Unknown
Motofen (atropine plus difenoxin)	No	No	Unknown
Pepcid (famotidine)	Unknown	Unknown	Unknown
Prevacid (lansoprazole)	No	No	Unknown
Prilosec (omeprazole)	Unknown	No	Unknown
Reglan (metoclopramide)	Yes	No	Decreased Llbido
Tagamet (cimetidine)	Yes	No	Possible Libido Impairment
Xantac (ranitidine)	Yes?	No	Unknown
Zofran (ondansetron)	No	No	Unknown

Table 6.1 summarizes the impact of common gastrointestinal drugs on sexual function.

REFERENCES

Adakan P, Karim S. Male sexual dysfunction during treatment with cimetidine. *Br Med J*. 1979;1:1282–1283.

Beeley L. Drug-induced sexual dysfunction and infertility. *Adverse Drug React Acute Poisoning Rev*. 1984;3:23–42.

Bera F, Jonville-Bera A, Doustin P, Autret E. Impotence and gynecomastia secondary to hyperprolactinemia induced by rantidine. *Therapie*. 1994;49: 361–362.

Bias P, Milan G. Dysfunction of the hypothalamo–hypophyseal–gonadal axis induced by histamine H2 antagonists. *Minerva Med*. 1985;76:579–586.

Brock G, Lue T. Drug-induced male sexual dysfunction: an update. *Drug Safety*. 1993;8:414–426.

Cara AM, Lopes-Martin RA, Antunes E, Nahoun C, DeNucci G. The role of histamine in human penile erection. *Br J Urol*. 1995;75:220–224.

Carlson E, Ippoliti A. Cimetidine, an H2 antihistamine, stimulates prolactin secretion in man. *J Clin Endocrin Metab*. 1977;45:367–370.

Carvajal A, Arias L. Gynecomastia and sexual disorders after the administration of omeprazole. *Am J Gastroenterology*. 1995;90:1–2.

Collen M, Howard J, McArthur K, et al. Comparison of ranitidine and cimetidine in the treatment of gastric hypersecretion. *Ann Intern Med*. 1984;100:52–58.

Cooper JW, Wade WE. *Gastrointestinal Drug Therapy in the Elderly*. New York: Haworth Press; 1998.

DeVault KR. Overview of medical therapy for gastroesophageal reflux disease. *Gasteroenterol Clin*. 1999;24:1–16.

Dutertre J, Soutif D, Jonville A. Sexual disturbances during omeprazole therapy. *Lancet.* 1991;338:1022.

Gifford L, Aeugle M, Myerson R, Tannenbaum J. Cimetidine postmarket outpatient surveillance program. *JAMA.* 1980;243:1532–1535.

Gora-Harper M, Balmer C, Castellano F, et al. ASHP therapeutic guideines on the pharmacological management of nausea and vomiting in adult and pediatric patients receiving chemotherapy or radiation or undergoing surgery. *Am. J Health Syst Pharm.* 1999;56:1–76.

Gwee MC, Cheah L. Actions of cimetidine and rantidine at some cholinergic sites: implications in toxicology and anesthesia. *Life Sci.* 1986;4:383–388.

Gwee M, Cheah L, Lee S. Ganlion blocking activity of cimetidine in the anesthetized cat. *Clin Exp Pharamcol Physiol.* 1985;12:475–480.

Jensen R, Collen M, Pandol S. Cimetidine-induced impotence and breast changes in patients with gastric hypersecretory states. *N Eng J Med.* 1983;308:883–887.

Jensen R, Collen M, McArthur K, et al. Comparison of the effectiveness of ranitidine and cimetidine in inhibiting acid secretion in patients with gastric hypersecretory states. *Am J Med.* 1984;77(Suppl 5B):90–105.

Keene L, Davies P. Drug related erectile dysfunction. *Adverse Drug React Toxicol Rev.* 1999;18:5–24.

Lardinois C, Mezzaferri, E. Cimetidine blocks testosterone synthesis. *Arch Int Med.* 1985;145:920–922.

Long J, Smyth P, Culliton M, Cunningham S, et al. Prolactin and the hypothalamic–pituitary–testicular axis in cimetidine-treated men. *Ir J Med.* 1985;78:48–51.

Peden N, Cargill J, Browning M, Sanders J, Wormsley K. Male sexual dysfunction during treatment with cimetidine. *Br Med J.* 1978;1:659.

Perez EA. Use of dexamthasone with 5-HT3-receptor antagonists for chemotherapy-induced nausea and vomiting. *Cancer J Sci Am.* 1998;4:72–77.

Schiller LR. Diarrhea. *Med. Clin North Am.* 2000;84:1–15.

Tsai SJ. Metoclopramide-induced impotence and akathisia: a case report. [Chinese Medical Journal.] 1996;57:443–446.

Wiseman S, McAuley J, Freidenberg G, Friedman D. Hypersexuality in patients with dementia: possible response to cimetidine. *Amer Acad Neurol.* 2000;54:1–3.

Zimmerman T. Problems associated with medical treatment of peptic ulcer disease. *Am J Med.* 1984;77(5B):51–56.

7. Drugs Associated with Sexual Dysfunction Used in Urological Practice

Urologic drugs associated with sexual dysfunction include drugs used to treat incontinence, benign prostatic hypertrophy, metastatic prostate cancer, and other urological neoplasms.

INCONTINENCE

Urinary incontinence is a condition with significant social and economic effects (e.g., protective underwear, medications, surgery). Population surveys indicate that the median incontinence rates for women and men over 50 years old are 35% and 17%, respectively. For patients less than 50, women still had higher rates of incontinence than men, 28% versus 4%. Incontinence rates in men are clearly age-related.

Drugs commonly used to treat incontinence include: anticholinergic agents such as oxybutynin and tolterodine; imipramine, a tricyclic antidepressant; and chlorpheniramine, an antihistamine. A recent survey of patients in the Veterans Medical Centers found that the most commonly prescribed drugs were oxybutynin chloride, dicyclomine, and imipramine; the next most commonly prescribed drugs were propantheline and hyoscyamine. It is interesting to note that the majority of patients did not routinely fill their prescriptions.

Imipramine is a tricyclic antidepressant with antihistaminic, anticholinergic, serotonergic, and adrenergic properties. Imipramine is associated with difficulty reaching orgasm or ejaculatory difficulty in 30–40% of patients taking therapeutic levels for depression. The incidence of sexual problems on lower doses of imipramine, such as those used to

93

Table 7.1   The impact of drugs treating incontinence on sexual function

	Effect on Erection	Effect on Orgasm	Effect on Female Sexual Function
chlorpheniramine	Unknown	Unknown	Unknown
dicyclomine (Bentyl)	Unknown	Unknown	Unknown
hyoscyamine (Levsin)	Unknown	Unknown	Unknown
imipramine (Tofranil)	Unknown	30–40%	Probable orgasm delay
oxybutynin (Ditropan)	Unknown	No	Unknown
propantheline	Unknown	Unknown	Unknown
tolterodine (Detrol)	Unknown	No	Unknown

treat incontinence, is unknown. Imipramine has been noted in case reports to cause erectile problems. Imipramine may exert its effect on sexual function by its affinity for the 5HT1C receptor or by alpha-adrenergic blockade. Double-blind controlled studies of sexual side effects on imipramine have not been conducted.

Chlorpheniramine, an antihistaminic agent, and flavoxate, an antispasmotic agent, are also used to treat incontinence. Neither appears to be associated with sexual dysfunction. Chlorpheniramine is believed to work by blocking histaminic-mediated release of acetylcholine. There is minimal evidence that other drugs used to treat incontinence are associated with sexual dysfunction. Table 7.1 summarizes the impact of drugs treating incontinence on sexual function.

Many of the drugs used to treat incontinence have anticholinergic properties. However, it is unlikely that anticholinergic activity directly influences human sexual behavior.

As noted, the human corpus cavernosum is innervated by cholinergic nerves and contains cholinergic receptors. Administration of exogenous acetycholine chloride to precontracted corpus cavernosum tissue results in smooth muscle relaxation. However, atropine, a muscarinic antagonist, has little effect on human erectile function. Physiological studies implicate the parasympathetic nervous system in erection, whereas conflicting pharmacological data refute the concept that only acetylcholine works at neuroeffector junctions in the penis. Current conceptualizations suggest that acetylcholine probably works synergistically with other vasodilators released by nerves or contained in the vascular tissues. It is worth noting that cholinergic fibers also are present in organs mediating ejaculation and, presumably, female orgasm. Studies in the rat have convincingly demonstrated that stimulation of the cholinergic septohippocampal pathway is involved in penile erection. Although it has never been demonstrated, it is probable that cholinergic fibers exert a modulating effect on adrenergic fibers. Orgasm appears to be mediated by alpha-1 adrenergic fibers. There is no clear evidence, to date, that anticholinergic drugs directly interfere with sexual function in the human. Case reports that cholinergic agents sometimes reverse anorgasmia induced by serotonergic antidepressants suggest that acetylcholine exerts some action that modulates the activity of other neurotransmitter systems.

BENIGN PROSTATIC HYPERTROPHY

Approximately 40% of men over the age of 65 has lower urinary tract symptoms suggestive of benign prostatic hypertrophy. Symptomatic treatment of this condition is based on two components of the disease: (1) the static component caused by the physical mass of the prostate tissue; and (2) the dynamic component of urethral and prostatic muscle tone, which is mediated by alpha-1 adrenoceptors. Current medical treatment of benign prostatic hypertrophy includes the use of finasteride and alpha-adrenoceptor blockers such as phenoxybenzamine, prazosin, terazosin, doxazosin, and tamsulosin. A large number of studies has investigated the efficacy and side effects of these agents. Unfortunately, very few have employed direct questioning about sexual function. Table 7.2 summarizes the impact of drugs treating benign prostatic hypertrophy on sexual function.

Finasteride

Finasteride is a 5 alpha-reductase inhibitor that blocks the conversion of testosterone to dihydrotestosterone. Although it was originally felt to have a low incidence of sexual side effects, studies using

Table 7.2   The impact of drugs treating benign prostatic hypertrophy on sexual function

	Effect on Erection	Effect on Orgasm	Female Sexual Function
doxazosin (Cardura)	No	Yes	Unknown
finasteride (Proscar)	20%	Delayed	Unknown
prazosin (Minipress)	Unknown	20%	Unknown
tamsulosin (Flomax)	No	10–26%	Unknown
terazsin (Hytrin)	No	Yes	Unknown

direct inquiry have found problems with erection and/or ejaculation in 22–33% of patients. Although some clinicians reported that early sexual side effects with this drug dissipated with continued treatment, others have reported that the effect on sexual function appears to increase with duration of usage such that there is a higher incidence of sexual problems after 6 months of use than after 3 months. Decreased libido is a commonly noted side effect. Most patients report a decreased amount of ejaculate upon starting finasteride treatment. The decreased availability of dihydrotestosterone to androgen receptors in the central nervous system may be the explanation for the sexual side effects associated with this drug. Studies comparing finasteride with alpha-adrenergic blocking agents have reported more ejaculatory and erectile impairment on finasteride than alpha blockers.

Alpha-Adrenoceptor Blockers

Adrenergic alpha-1 blocking agents are often utilized to treat the symptoms of benign prostatic hypertrophy. Most of the alpha-adrenergic blockers have a tendency to improve erectile function but also may increase the risk of priapism. They also can cause ejaculatory delay or failure. Recent studies suggest that there may be at least three types of alpha-1 receptors with alpha-1a found predominantly in the prostate. Most of the alpha-1blockers used in the treatment of benign prostatic hypertrophy do not differentially affect one alpha-1 receptor type more than another. Tamsulosin affects alpha-1a adrenoceptors more than alpha-1b or alpha-1d. Some clinicians have reported that the alpha-blockers do not cause sexual problems, whereas closer reading of the data indicates that erectile function improved whereas ejaculatory function deteriorated. In addition, tolerance may develop to ejaculatory problems caused by alpha blockers.

When used as an antihypertensive agent, prazosin has a high incidence of ejaculatory failure and has even been studied for possible use as a male contraceptive. In female rats, prazosin injected into the ventral medial nucleus of the hypothalamus inhibits lordosis. The positive effect of prazosin on erectile function may be related to its inhibition of contraction in corpus cavernosum tissue. Relaxation of this tissue faciltates vasoperfusion and penile turgidity. The frequency with which prazosin causes ejaculatory problems in patients with prostatic hypertrophy symptoms is unknown.

Tamsulosin and alfuzosin cause ejaculatory impairment in 10–26% of patients. Double-blind trials of tamsulosin have reported problems with ejaculation in 10% of men at .4 mg/day and in 26% at .8 mg/day.

The frequency of ejaculatory problems on doxazosin is unknown but assumed to be similar to that of the other alpha-1 blockers.

PROSTATIC CANCER

Prostate cancer is the most common urological malignancy and the second most common malignancy in men. Many men with prostatic cancer have metastatic disease at the time of detection. It has been known since the 1940s that prostate cancer activity is dependent upon androgens and that surgical castration or estrogen administration produced disease regression and served as a palliative treatment. For these men, androgen ablation therapy remains the treatment of choice. Surgical or medical reduction of plasma testosterone to castrate levels results in delay of disease progression. Low-dose estrogen, luteinizing-hormone releasing hormone (LHRH) agonists, and orchiectomy have similar efficacy. These benefits are achieved at considerable psychosocial costs, however. It is also known that hypogonadal men usually have diminished sexual activity, a decrease in sexual interest, and a decrease in spontaneous erections. Estrogens act to decrease the production of testosterone by inhibiting the release of luteinizing hormone from the anterior pituitary.

Flutamide is a nonsteroidal derivative of toluidine that has been shown to interfere with the binding of testosterone and dihydrotestosterone to the androgen receptor. Its sexual side effects are less devastating than estrogen therapy and it has some efficacy in ameliorating advanced prostate cancer. It has been combined with LHRH therapy, but LHRH has a high frequency of sexual side effects. Flutamide also has been combined with finasteride, the rationale being that addition of a 5 alpha-reductase inhibitor would provide more complete intraprostatic androgen blockade. This particular strategy appears to have disasterous effects on sexual function, however. Approximatley 35% of men reported absent or delayed ejacualtion.

The majority of androgens is produced by the Leydig cells of the testes, which are under control of the hypothalamic axis by cyclic release of gonadotropic releasing hormone (GnRh) and luteinizing hormone (LH). Drugs used to treat metastatic cancer of the prostate include the LHRH agonists and the androgen receptor blockers. The LHRH agonists are synthetic analogues of LHRH. The drug initially stimulates LH secretion and androgen production but produces inhibitory effects on the pituitary and gonads, causing long-term profound suppression of testosterone. LHRH agonists such as nafarelin,

Table 7.3   The impact of LHRH agonists on sexual function

	Effect on Erection	Effect on Orgasm	Female SD
flutamide (Eulexin)	Yes	Yes	Probable
leuprolide (Lupron)	86%	Yes	Probable
nafarelin (Synaril)	Yes	Yes	Probable
nilutamide (Nilandron)	Yes	Yes	Probable

buserelin, goserelin, and leuprolide all block the pituitary release of gonadotropins and thus decrease the production of androgen, thereby reducing testosterone production to castrate levels. These drugs cause a marked decrease in libido and a decrease in ejaculatory demand. One study found that patients having coitus between 2–4 times monthly had a total cessation of sexual desire and sexual activity on leuprolide therapy. Nocturnal penile tumescence, the number of erectile episodes, maximum rigidity, and circumference also were diminished. Other studies indicate that LHRH agonists produce a decrease in libido, impotence, and breast swelling. It is assumed but unproven that the suppression of libido occurs via the central nervous system. Table 7.3 summarizes the impact of LHRH agonists on sexual function.

Bicalutamide, a nonsteroidal antiandrogen, may have fewer sexual side effects than flutamide and the GnRH agonists. The combination of flutamide and finasteride has been reported to cause gynecomastia and ejaculatory problems in 35% of patients, when direct inquiry of sexual behavior is utilized. Other androgen receptor antagonists include ketoconazole, and nilutamide. Cyproterone acetate is not available in the U. S. market. Table 7.4 summarizes the impact of antiandrogen drugs treating prostatic cancer.

Table 7.4   The impact of antiandrogens on sexual function

	Erection	Ejaculation	Female SD
Bicalutamide (Casodex)	Yes	Yes	Probable
Flutamide (Eulexin)	Yes	Yes	Probable
Ketoconazole (Nizoral)	Yes	Yes	Decreased libido
Nilutamide (Nilandron)	Yes	Yes	Probable

REFERENCES

Atala A, Amin M. Current concepts in the treatment of genitourinary tract disorders in the older individual. *Drugs Aging*. 1991;1:176–193.

Broderick G, Foreman M. Iatrogenic erectile dysfunction: pharmacological and surgical therapies that alter male sexual behavior and erectile performance. In Carson C, R Kirby, I Goldstein, editors. *Textbook of Erectile Dysfunction*. Oxford, U.K.:Isis, 1999:233–256.

Brufsky A, Fontaine-Rothe P, Berlane K, et al. Finasteride and flutamide as potency-sparing androgen: ablative therapy for advanced adenocarcinoma of the prostate. *Urol*. 1997;49:913–920.

Boccardo F, Rubagotti A, Barichello M, Battaglia M, et al. Bicalutamide monotherapy versus flutamide plus goserlin in prostate cancer patients: results of an italian prostate cancer project. *J Clin Oncol*. 1999;17:2027–2028.

Carraro J, Raynaud J, Koch G, et al. Comparison of phytotherpay (permixon) with finasteride in the treatment of benign prostate hyperplasia: a randomized international study of 1,098 patients. *Prostate*. 1996;29:231–240.

Chapple C, Baert L, Thind P, et al. Tamsulosin 0.4 mg once daily: tolerability in older and younger patients with lower urinary tract symptoms suggestive of benign prostatic obstruction. *Eur Urol*. 1997;32:462–470.

da Silva, FC, Fossa SD, Aaronson N, Serbouti S, et al. The quality of life in patients with newly diagnosed M1 prostate cancer. *Eur J Cancer*. 1996;32:72–77.

Debuyne FMJ, Jardin A, Colloi D, et al. Sustained-release alfuzosin, finaseride and the combination of both in the treatment of benign prostatic hyperplasia. *Eur Urol*. 1998;34:169–175.

Fitzpatrick J, Kirby R, Krane R, Adolfsson J, Newling D, Goldstein I. Sexual dysfunction associated with the management of prostate cancer. *Eur Urol*. 1998;33:513–522.

Girman CJ, Kolman C, Liss CL, Bolognese JA, Binkowitz BS, Stoner E. Effects of finasteride on health-related quality of life in men with symptomatic benign prostatic hypertrophy. *Prostate*. 1996;29:83–90.

Gormley G, Stoner E. The effect of finasteride in men with benign prostatic hypertrophy. *New Engl J Med*. 1992;327:1185–1191.

Hendry W, Althof S, Benson G, et al. Male orgasmic and ejaculatory disorders. In Jardin A, Wagner G, Khoury S, Giuliano F, Padma-Nathan H, Rosen R, editors. *Erectile Dysfunction*. Plymouth, U.K.:Health Publications;2000: 477–506.

Hofner K, Claes H, DeReijke TM, Folkestad B, Speakman MJ. Tamusulsin 0.4 mg once daily: effect on sexual function in patients with lower urinary tract symptoms suggestive of benign prostatic hypertrophy. *Eur Urol*. 1999;36:335–341.

Kirby R, Robertson C, Turkes A. Finasteride in association with either flutamide or gosserelin as combination hormonal therapy in patients with stage M1 carcinoma of the prostate gland. *Prostate*. 1999;40:105–114.

Lepor H. Long-term evaluation of tamsulosin in benign prostatic hyperplasia: placebo-controlled double-blind extension of phase III trial. *Urol*. 1998;51:901–906.

Malone DC, Okano GJ. Treatment of urge incontinence in Veterans Affairs Medical Centers. *Clin Therapeutics.* 1999;21:867–877.

Marumo K, Baba S, Murai M. Erectile function and nocturnal penile tumescence in patients with prostate cancer undergoing luteinizing hormone-releasing agonist therapy. *Int J Urol.* 1999;6:19–23.

Moinpour CM, Lovato LC, Thompson IM. Profile of men randomized to the prostate cancer prevention trial: baseline health-related quality of life, urinary, and health behaviors. *J Clin Oncol.* 2000;18:1942–1953.

Nichel J, Fradet Y. Efficay and safety of finasteride therapy for benign prostatic hypertrophy: results of a 2-year randomized controlled trial. *Canad Med Assoc J.* 1996;155:1251–1259.

Saenz de Tejada I, Cavidad N, Heaton J, et al. Anatomy, physiology and pathophysiology of erectile function. In Jardin A, Wagner G, Khoury S, Giuliano F, Padma-Nathan H, Rosen R, editors. *Erectile Dysfunction.* Plymouth, U.K., XX: Health Publications; 2000:65–102.

Sarosdy M, Schellhammer PF, Soloway M, Vogelzang N, Crawford ED, et al. Endocrine effects, efficacy and tolerability of a 10.8 mg depot formulation of gopserelin acetate administered every 13 weeks to patients with advanced prostate cancer. *BJU Int.* 1999;83:801–806.

Schou J, Holm NR, Meyhoff HH. Sexual function in patients with symptomatic benign prostatic hyperplasia. *Scand J Urol Nephrol.* 1996;30(Suppl);119–122.

Schroper FH, Collette L, de Reijke TM, Whean P. Prostate cancer treated by Anti-Androgens; is sexual function preserved? *BR J Cancer.* 2000;82:283–290.

Uygur M, Gur E. Erectile dysfunction following treatments of benign prostatic hyperplasia. *Andrologia.* 1998;30:5–10.

8. Cardiovascular Drugs

Cardiovascular diseases include a wide variety of conditions such as myocardial infarction, angina pectoris, coronary artery disease, arrhythmias and disturbances of conduction in general, hypertension, atherosclerosis, and others. Numerous drugs are used to treat various aspects of cardiovascular diseases, such as calcium channel blockers, antiarrhythmics, beta-blockers, coronary vasodilatators, peripheral vasodilatators, antilipidemic agents, and various antihypertensives (e.g., diuretics, angiotensin converting enzyme (ACE) inhibitors, combination agents). Sexual functioning in patients suffering from cardiovascular disease and the treatment for cardiovascular disease are areas clouded in numerous myths. For instance, many patients reduce or postpone resumption of sexual activity for a long time after suffering a myocardial infarction. Many are afraid of coital death. However, coital death is a rare event. On the other hand, resumption of sexual activity after a long abstinence may be very stressful and anxiety provoking. Many drugs used for the treatment of cardiovascular diseases are associated with sexual dysfunction. Nevertheless, the scope of sexual dysfunction associated with these drugs might be overstated (or, at least, solid evidence is lacking) and some of them occasionally could be found helpful. Many of them affect aspects of vascular functioning involved in the regulation of one phase of sexual functioning—arousal (erection in males, swelling response in females). The currently most well-known medication for treatment of erectile dysfunction, sildenafil, was originally studied as a potential agent for angina pectoris and hypertension.

As is the case with many medications and diseases, sexual function and dysfunction associated with both have not always been well studied. The reasons for the relative lack of studies on sexual functioning with cardiovascular agents are similar to the reasons for the lack of studies of sexual dysfunction associated with other medications—confounding variables of sexual dysfunction associated with cardiovascular diseases, lack of valid instruments to measure sexual dysfunction, patient fear and misconception, and lack of interest in these studies on the part of the pharmaceutical industry. In addition, cardiovascular risk factors, such as diabetes mellitus and smoking, also are risk factors for sexual dysfunction (namely, erectile disorder). For various reasons, sexual function/dysfunction in patients with cardiovascular disease and patients treated with cardiovascular drugs has been studied much more extensively in males, though some data from female patients are available.

Sexual dysfunction associated with cardiovascular agents can be a complicated and challenging issue requiring an active and creative approach by the treating physician. Sexual dysfunction associated with cardiovascular diseases and agents used to treat these diseases can have a significant effect on the patient's quality of life.

This chapter reviews several areas related to sexual dysfunction associated with cardiovascular agents:

- Cardiovascular changes during sexual activity and changes in sexuality associated with cardiovascular disease
- Sexual dysfunction associated with various cardiovascular agents, its description, epidemiology, types, mechanism of action, and diagnosis
- Management of sexual dysfunction associated with various cardiovascular agents

Cardiovascular agents available in the United States are listed in Table 8.1.

Table 8.1 Cardiovascular drugs available in the United States

Generic Name	Brand Name	Forms and Doses (mg)
ADRENERGIC BLOCKERS		
doxazosin mesylate	Cardura	t: 1, 2, 4, 8
phenoxybenzamine hydrochloride	Dibenzyline	c: 10
prazosin hydrochloride	Minipress	c: 1, 2, 5
reserpine	Serpasil	t: .1, .25
terazosin hydrochloride	Hytrin	c: 1, 2, 5, 10
ADRENERGIC STIMULANTS		
clonidine hydrochloride	Catapress	t: .1, .2, .3
	Catapress-TTS	td: .1, .2, 3

Table 8.1   (*Cont.*)

Generic Name	Brand Name	Forms and Doses (mg)
guanfacine hydrochloride	Tenex	t: 1, 2
methyldopa	Aldomet	t: 125, 250, 500

ALPHA/BETA ADRENERGIC BLOCKERS

carvedilol	Coreg	t: 3, 125, 6.25, 12.5, 25
labetalol hydrochloride	Normodyne	t: 100, 200, 300
		inj: 5/ml

ANGIOTENSIN CONVERTING ENZYME (ACE) INHIBITORS

benazepril hydrochloride	Lotensin	t: 5, 10, 20, 40
captopril	Capoten	t: 12.5, 25, 50, 100
enalapril maleate	Vasotec	t: 2.5, 5, 10, 20
enalaprilat	Vasotec IV	inj: 1.25/mL
fosinopril sodium	Monopril	t: 10, 20, 40
lisinopril	Prinivil	t: 2.5, 5, 10, 20, 40
	Zestril	t: 2.5, 5, 10, 20, 30, 40
moexipril	Univasc	t: 7.5, 15
perindopril erbumine	Aceon	t: 2, 4, 8
quinapril	Accupril	t: 5, 10, 20,40
ramipril	Altace	c: 1.25, 2.5, 5, 10
trandolapril	Mavik	t:1, 2, 4

ANGIOTENSIN-2 RECEPTOR ANTAGONISTS

candesartan cilexetil	Atacand	t: 4, 8, 16, 32
eprosartan mesylate	Teveten	t: 400, 600
Irbesartan	Avapro	t: 75, 150, 300
losartan potassium	Cozaar	t: 25, 50, 100
telmisartan	Micardis	t: 40, 80
valsartan	Diovan	c: 80, 160

ANTIARRHYTHMICS

Group 1

disopyramide phosphate	Norpace	c:100,150
		cex: 100, 150
flecainide acetate	Tambocor	t: 50, 100, 150
mexiletine hydrochloride	Mexitil	c: 150, 200, 250
procainamide hydrochloride	Procanbid	tex: 500, 1000
propafenone hydrochloride	Rythmol	t: 150, 225, 300
quinidine sulphate	Quinidex Extentabs	tex: 300
quinidine gluconate		inj: 80/mL
tocainide hydrochloride	Tonocard	t: 400, 600

Group 2

acebutolol hydrochloride	Sectral	c: 200, 400
esmolol hydrochloride	Brevibloc	inj: 10/mL, 250/mL
propranolol hydrochloride	Inderal	t: 10, 20, 40, 60, 80
		inj: 1/mL
	Inderal LA	lat: 60, 80, 120, 160
sotalol hydrochloride	Betapace	t: 80, 120, 160, 240
	Betapace AF	t: 80, 120, 160

Group 3

amiodarone hydrochloride	Cordarone	t: 200
		inj: 50/mL
	Pacerone	t: 200
dofetilide	Tikosyn	t: 125, 250, 500
ibutilide fumarate	Corvert	inj: .1/mL
sotalol hydrochloride	Betapace	t: 80, 120, 160, 240
	Betapace AF	t: 80, 120, 160

CARDIOVASCULAR DRUGS

Table 8.1 (*Cont.*)

Generic Name	Brand Name	Forms and Doses (mg)
Group 4		
diltiazem hydrochloride	Cardizem CD	c: 120, 180, 240, 300
	Cardizem	inj: 5/mL
	Cardizem Lyo-Ject	25 mg/syringe
	Cardizem Monovial	100 mg/infusion
verapamil hydrochloride	Calan	t: 40, 80, 120
	Calan SR	cp: 120, 180, 240
Miscellaneous Antiarrhythmics		
adenosine	Adenocard	inj: 3/mL
digoxin	Lanoxicaps	c: .05, .1, .2
	Lanoxin	t: .125, .25
	Lanoxin Elixir	O: .05/mL
	Lanoxin Injection	inj: .1/mL, .25/mL
ANTILIPIDEMICS		
atorvastatin calcium	Lipitor	t: 10, 20, 40
cerivastatin sodium	Baycol	t: .2, .3, .4, .8
cholestyramine	Questran	powder: 4g/9g
	Prevalite	can: 231g
clofibrate	Atromid-S	c:500
colesevelam hydrochloride	WelChol	t:625
colestipol hydrochloride	Colestid	t: 1000
fenofibrate	Tricor	c: 67, 134, 200
fluvastatin sodium	Lescol	c:20, 40
gemfibrozil	Lopid	t: 600
lovastatin	Mevacor	t: 10, 20, 40
niacin	Niaspan	tex: 500, 750, 1000
pravastatin sodium	Pravachol	t: 10, 20, 40
simvastatin	Zocor	t: 40, 80
BETA-BLOCKERS		
acebutolol hydrochloride	Sectral	c: 200, 400
atenolol	Tenormin	t:25, 50, 100
		inj: .5/mL
betaxolol hydrochloride	Kerlone	t: 10
bisoprolol fumarate	Zebeta	t: 5, 10
carteolol hydrochloride	Cartrol	t:2.5, 5
esmolol hydrochloride	Brevibloc	inj: 10/mL, 250/mL
metoprolol succinate	Toprol-XL	tex: 50, 100, 200
nadolol		t: 20, 40, 80
penbutolol	Levatol	t: 20
pindolol	Visken	t:5, 10
propranolol hydrochloride	Inderal	t: 10, 20, 40, 60, 80
		inj: 1/mL
	Inderal LA	lat: 60, 80, 120, 160
sotalol hydrochloride	Betapace	t: 80, 120, 160, 240
	Betapace AF	t: 80, 120, 160
timolol maleate	Blocadren	t: 5, 10, 20
CALCIUM CHANNEL BLOCKERS		
amlodipine besylate	Norvasc	t: 2.5, 5, 10
bepridil hydrochloride	Vascor	t:200, 300
diltiazem hydrochloride	Cardizem CD	c: 120, 180, 240, 300
	Cardizem	inj: 5/mL
	Cardizem Lyo-Ject	25 mg/syringe
	Cardizem Monovial	100 mg/infusion
	Tiazac	cex: 120, 180, 240, 360, 420
felodipine	Plendil	tex: 2.5, 5, 10

Table 8.1   *(Cont.)*

Generic Name	Brand Name	Forms and Doses (mg)
isradipine	DynaCirc	c: 2.5, 5
	DynaCirc CR	tex: 5, 10
nicarpidine hydrochloride	Cardene IV	inj: 2.5/mL
nifedipine	Adalat	c: 10, 20
	Adalat CC	t: 30, 60, 90
	Procardia	c: 10, 20
	Procardia XL	tex: 30, 60, 90
nimodipine	Nimotop	c: 30
nisoldipine	Sular	t: 10, 20, 30, 40
verapamil hydrochloride	Calan	t: 40, 80, 120
	Calan SR	cp: 120, 180, 240
	Covera-HS	t: 180, 240
	Isoptin-SR	tex: 120, 180, 240
	Veralan	cex: 120, 180, 240, 360
	Veralan PM	cex: 100, 200, 300

COMBINATION PREPARATIONS

amiloride/hydrochlorothiazide	Moduretic	t:5/50
amlodipine/benazepril hydrochloride	Lotrel	c: 2.5/10, 5/10, 5/20
atenolol/chlorthalidone	Tenoretic	t: 50/25, 100/25
benazepril hydrochloride hydrochlorothiazide	Lotensin HCT	t: 5/6.25, 10/12.5, 20/12.5, 20/25
bisoprolol fumarate/hydrochlorothiazide	Ziac	t: 2.5/6.25, 5/6.25, 10/6.25
clonidine hydrochloride/chlorthalidone	Clorpres	t: 0.1/15, 0.2/15, 0.3/15
	Combipres	
enalapril maleate	Lexxel	t: 5/2.5, 5/5
felodipine		
enalapril maleate/hydrochlorothiazide	Vaseretic	t: 5/12.5, 10/25
hydrochlorothiazide/triameterene	Dyazide	c: 25/37.5
ibesartan/hydrochlorothiazide	Avalide	t: 150/12.5, 300/12.5
lisinopril/hydrochlorothiazide	Prinzide	t: 10/12.5, 20/12.5, 20/25
	Zestoretic	t: 10/12.5, 20/12.5, 20/25
losartan potassium hydrochlorothiazide	Hyzaar	t: 50/12.5, 10/12.5
methyldopa/chlorothiazide	Aldoclor	t: 250/250
methyldopa/hydrochlorothiazide	Aldoril	t: 250/15, 250/25, 500/30, 500/50
moexipril hydrochloride/ hydrochlorothiazide	Uniretic	t: 7.5/12.5, 12.5/25
nadolol/bendroflumethiazide	Corzide	t: 40/5, 80/5
prazosin hydrochloride/polythiazide	Minizide	c: 1/05, 2/05, 5/05
propranolol/hydrochlorothiazide	Inderide	t: 40/25, 80/25
	Inderide LA	c: 160/50, 120/50, 80/50
quinapril hydrochloride/ hydrochlorothiazide	Accuretic	t: 10/12.5, 20/12.5, 20/25
spironolactone/hydrochlorothiazide	Aldactazide	t: 25/25, 50/50
timolol maleate/hydrochlorothiazide	Timolide	t: 10/25
trandolapril/verapamil hydrochloride	Tarka	t: 2/180, 1/240, 2/240, 4/240
triamterene/hydrochlorothiazide	Maxzide	t: 75/50
	Maxzide-25mg	t: 37.5/25
valsartan/hydrochlorothiazide	Diovan HCT	c: 80/12.5, 160/12.5

DIURETICS

acetazolamide	Diamox	t: 125, 250
amiloride hydrochloride	Midamor	t: 5
bumetamide	Bumex, Burimex	t: .5, 1, 2
		inj; .25/mL
chlorothiazide	Diuril	t: 250, 500
		O: 50/mL
		v (inj): 500 (powder)

Table 8.1   (*Cont.*)

Generic Name	Brand Name	Forms and Doses (mg)
chlorthalidone	Thalitone	t: 15
dichlorphenamide	Daranide	t: 50
ethacrynate sodium	Sodium Edecrin	v (inj): 50 (powder)
ethacrynic acid	Edecrin	t: 25, 50
furosemide	Lasix	t: 20, 40, 80
hydrochlorothiazide	HydroDiuril	t: 25, 50
	Microzide	c: 12.5
hydroflumethiazide	Diucardin	t: 50
indapamide		t: 1.25, 2.5
methyclothiazide	Enduron	t: 2.5, 5
metolazone	Mykrox	t: .5
	Zaroxolyn	t: 2.5, 5, 10
polythiazide	Renese	t: 1, 2, 4
spironolactone	Aldactone	t: 25, 50, 100
torsemide	Demadex	t: 5, 10, 20, 100
		inj: 10/mL
triamterene	Dyrenium	c: 50, 100

INOTROPIC AGENTS

digoxin	Digitek	t: .125, .25
	Lanoxicaps	c: .05, .1, .2
	Lanoxin	t: .125, .25
	Lanoxin Elixir	o: .05/mL
	Lanoxin Injection	inj: .1/mL, .25m/L
dobutamine	Dobutrex Solution	inj: 12.5/mL
ephedrine	Pressor	c: 25, 50
milrinone lactate	Primacor	inj: 200μg/mL

MISCELLANEOUS

abciximab	ReoPro	inj: 2/mL
alteplase, recombinant	Activase	inj: 29 millU/50 mL, 58 millU/100 mL
epinephrine injection	Adrenaline Chloride Sol.	inj: 1/mL
hydralazine	Apresoline	t: 10, 25, 50, 100
mecamylamine hydrochloride	Inversine	t: 2.5
metyrosine	Demser	c: 250
minoxidil	Loniten	t: 2.5, 10
reteplase recombinant	Retavase	inj: 10.4 U/vial
streptokinase	Streptase	inj: 250,000 IU/vial, 750,000 IU/vial, 1,5000,000 IU/vial
tenecteplase	TNKase	inj: 50 mg/vial

VASODILATATORS

Coronary

isosorbide dinitrate	Isordil Sublingual	t: 2.5, 5, 10
	Isordil Titradose	t: 5, 10, 20, 30, 40
	Sorbitrate Oral Tbl	t: 5, 10, 20, 40
	Chewable Sorbitrate Tbl	tc: 10, 20, 30, 40
isosorbide mononitrate	Imdur	t: 30, 60, 120
	Ismo	t: 20
nitroglycerin	Nitro Dur	td: .1/hr, .2/hr, .3/hr, .4/hr, .6/hr, .8/hr
	Nitrolingual Pumpspray	s: .4/per dose
	Nitrostat	ts: .3, .4, .6

Peripheral

epoprostenol sodium	Flolan	inj: .5/17 mL, 1.5/17 mL
fenoldopam mesylate	Corlopam	inj: 10/mL
milrinone lactate	Primacor	inj: 1/mL in vial, 200 μg/mL in bag

Table 8.1 (*Cont.*)

Generic Name	Brand Name	Forms and Doses (mg)
VASOPRESSORS		
epinephrine	EpiPen	inj: .15 mg/autoinjector, .3 mg/autoinjector
metaraminol bitartrate	Aramine	inj: 10/mL
midodrine hydrochloride	ProAmatine	t: 2.5, 5

c = capsules; can = can; cex = extended-release capsules; cp = caplets; inj = injections; lat = long-acting tablets; o = oral suspension; s = spray; t = tablets; tc = chewable tablets; td = transdermal system (patch); tex = extended-release tablets; ts = sublingual tablets; v = vials.

SEXUALITY, CARDIOVASCULAR FUNCTIONING, AND CARDIOVASCULAR DISEASE

Various cardiovascular changes during sexual activity have been described in normal volunteers and in patients with various cardiovascular diseases. These changes are summarized in Table 8.2. For more detailed information the reader is also referred to a review article by Rerkpattanapipat, Stanek, and Kotler (2001).

The effort required by sexual activity is usually lower than believed by many patients and physicians; it is mild to moderate and comparable to daily activities. Several studies found the increase of heart rate and blood pressure during sexual activity to be lower than, for instance, during a stair-climbing test, or comparable to walking and other activities of daily life. Some suggested that the stair-climbing test might be an adequate test of physiological responses comparable to sexual activity in most patients. In some studies, even the peak heart rate during sexual activity in patients with stable coronary artery disease was comparable to peak heart rate during fairly routine daily activities. Interestingly, several research studies addressed the question of whether some healthy male positions during sexual activity involve different cardiovascular changes. In two studies, there were

CARDIOVASCULAR DRUGS

Table 8.2 Cardiovascular changes during sexual activity

- Increase in resting heart rate (higher during orgasm than during intromission; mean peak heart rate about 100–140 beats/min.)
- Increase in both systolic and diastolic blood pressure
  —systolic: by 40—100 mmHg
  —diastolic by 20—55 mmHg
- Ventricular ectopic activity (most sex-related arrhythmias are simple ectopic beats similar to patterns during regular daily activity)
- Increased energy expenditure in cardiovascular system

no significant differences in the heart rate or blood pressure responses during sexual activity between male-on-top and male-underneath positions. However, in one of these studies, the male-on-top position required more metabolic expenditure than the other position.

However, one small study with hypertensive patients found a very wide fluctuation of both heart rate and blood pressure during coitus, with occasional brief episodes (several seconds) of extremely high blood pressure (mean coital levels for eight hypertensive males: 238/138 mmHg, and heart rate 131/min.; mean levels for three hypertensive females: 216/127 mmHg and heart rate 96/min.; peak value blood pressure in one subject with baseline blood pressure of 204/123 mmHg: 300/175 mmHg). Nevertheless, these subjects did not report any complications.

Some cardiovascular diseases may be accompanied by changes in vascular functioning and thus also by sexual dysfunction associated with vascular damage. Vascular disease is actually one of the most common organic factors in the etiology erectile dysfunction. Thus risk factors for vascular disease are also risk factors for sexual dysfunction in the form of erectile dysfunction. Hypertension is a well-known risk factor for vascular disease and also for erectile dysfunction. Several studies found higher rates of erectile problems among newly diagnosed untreated hypertensive males when compared to normotensive controls. Nonmedicated hypertensive males with erectile problems had reduced nocturnal penile tumescence and abnormal penile pulsatile flow (both indicating hemodynamic impairment) compared to normotensive controls in one study. The estimates of erectile failure incidence among untreated hypertensive patients vary between 8% and 20% and increase with age. The estimates of ejaculatory disturbance in these patients vary between 7% and 10% (compared to 4% in the so-called normal population). Some of the common risk of cardiovascular disease and sexual dysfunction are listed in Table 8.3.

Myocardial infarction and coital death are frequent concerns of patients with cardiovascular disease. However, the risk of both these

Table 8.3   Common preventable/treatable risks for cardiovascular changes and sexual dysfunction

- Diabetes mellitus
- Smoking
- Obesity
- Sleep apnea
- Hypertension
- Chronic obstructive pulmonary disease (COPD)

Table 8.4 Physician's role in addressing sexual functioning/dysfunctioning in patients with cardiovascular disease

- Actively discuss sexual functioning with the patient.
- Obtain history of sexual functioning prior to cardiovascular disease/event.
- Evaluate general health.
- Evaluate cardiac status.
- Evaluate exercise tolerance.
- Evaluate psychological status (level of depression, anxiety).
- Involve spouse in the discussion of sexual activity.
- Provide practical advice regarding sexual activity.
- Recommend physical fitness program.
- Provide medications to relieve symptoms of cardiac disease during sexual activity (e.g., beta-blockers or nitroglycerine—but nitrates are contraindicated in patients using sildenafil, and vice versa)

adverse events is relatively low. In one study, coital deaths accounted for only .6% of sudden deaths, most of them occurring during extramarital affairs and in hotels. In another study, sexual activity was considered a contributor to the development of myocardial infarction in .9% cases, and the risk among coronary artery disease patients was not higher than in the general population. Nevertheless, many patients with cardiovascular diseases, particularly myocardial infarction, report decreased sexual activity (between 22% and 75% in postmyocardial infarction patients). There are numerous reasons for the decreased sexual activity, including fear of death, depression, and physical symptoms such as chest pain.

Although sexual functioning and possible sexual dysfunction associated with the disease and/or medication could be a frequent concern of patients with untreated and/or treated cardiovascular disease, neither patients nor physicians typically address these issues. The physician's role in addressing patients' sexual functioning/dysfunction and some practical advice for the patient are summarized in Tables 8.4 and 8.5. (Both tables are adapted from the text in the article by Rerkpattanapipat et al. 1999.)

Table 8.5 Practical tips regarding sexual activity for patients with cardiovascular disease (especially postmyocardial infarction)

- Discuss your concerns about sexual functioning openly with your physician.
- Resume sexual activity as soon as you desire.
- Avoid sex after meals (wait 3 hours) or after alcohol consumption.
- Avoid sex in extreme temperatures.
- Avoid sex when tired, fatigued.
- Avoid sex during periods of extreme stress.
- Report unusual symptoms during or after sexual activity to your physician (e.g., chest pain, long palpitations, marked fatigue, sleeplessness).

CARDIOVASCULAR DRUGS

All these issues underscore the importance of obtaining a baseline evaluation of sexual functioning prior to starting pharmacological treatment of cardiovascular diseases.

SEXUAL DYSFUNCTION AND CARDIOVASCULAR DRUGS

Sexual dysfunction associated with various cardiovascular drugs has been a well-known fact for a long time. Numerous case reports, case series, and studies have described sexual dysfunction associated with cardiovascular drugs. Antihypertensives and diuretics have been associated with sexual dysfunction most frequently. As with other conditions and medication-associated sexual dysfunction, one might ask whether the sexual dysfunction is due to the condition, and whether the medication causes the sexual dysfunction at all. Not all cardiovascular agents have been studied in relation to sexual function in normal volunteers. However, some data suggest that beta-blockers, especially propranolol, may cause sexual dysfunction in healthy males. As noted, baseline evaluation of sexual functioning prior to starting the medication would help to elucidate the relationship between the medication and any subsequent sexual dysfunction.

The various changes in sexual functioning reported with cardiovascular drugs are summarized in Tables 8.6 and 8.7.

Sexual dysfunction associated with adrenergic blockers is rare (delayed ejaculation reported occasionally).

Specific changes in sexual functioning reported with various groups of cardiovascular drugs are listed in Tables 8.8–8.11. Adrenergic stimulants have been reported to cause sexual dysfunction occasionally. The types of sexual dysfunction associated with adrenergic stimulants are summarized in Table 8.8.

In theory, centrally acting adrenergic stimulants may diminish libido by depleting central neurotransmitters and decreasing norepinephrine

Table 8.6   Changes in sexual functioning associated with cardiovascular drugs

- Decreased or absent libido
- Erectile dysfunction (most frequent)
- Priapism
- Decreased vaginal lubrication
- Delayed ejaculation/orgasm
- Retrograde ejaculation
- Anorgasmia
- Premature ejaculation

Table 8.7   Reported sexual dysfunction associated with specific cardiovascular drugs

Drug	Decreased libido	Erectile dysfunction	Inhibition/ decreased lubrication	Ejaculatory/ orgasmic delay/ anorgasmia	Other
Amiodarone	−	+	−	−	−
Atenolol	−	+	−	−	−
Captopril	−	+	−	−	−
Chlorthalidone	+	+	−	−	−
Chlorothiazide	−	+	−	+	−
Clofibrate	+	+	−	−	−
Clonidine	+	+	−	+	+(1)
Diltiazem	−	+	−	+	−
Disopyramide	−	+	−	−	−
Enalapril	−	+	−	−	−
Flecainide	−	+	−	−	−
Gemfibrozil	+	+	−	−	−
Hydralazine	−	−	−	−	+(4)
Hydrochlorothiazide	+	+	+	−	−
Labetolol	−	+	−	+	+(4)
Lisinopril	−	+	−	−	−
Losartan	−	+	−	−	−
Methyldopa	+	+	−	+	+(2)
Metoprolol	−	+	−	−	+(3)
Mexiletine	−	+	−	−	−
Nadolol	−	+	−	−	−
Nifedipine	−	+	−	+	−
Phenoxybenzamine	−	−	−	+	−
Pindolol	−	+	−	−	−
Prazosin	−	+	−	−	+(4)
Propafenone	−	+	−	−	−
Propranolol	+	+	−	+	+(3)
Ramipril	−	+	−	−	−
Reserpine	+	+	−	+	−
Simvastatin	−	+	−	−	−
Solatol	−	+	−	−	−
Spironolactone	+	+	+	−	+(5)
Timolol	+	+	−	−	−
Valsartan	−	+	−	−	−
Verapamil	−	+	−	+	−

Notes:
(1) gynecomastia, retrograde ejaculation
(2) gynecomastia, lactation
(3) Peyronie's disease
(4) priapism
(5) gynecomastia, hirsutism, menstrual irregularities

activation. They also may increase serum prolactin and thus cause other problems such as gynecomastia and amenorrhea.

The incidence of sexual dysfunction associated with ACE inhibitors is lows. These drugs do not have an effect on the sympathetic nervous, and other nervous, systems. Captopril has been reported to have a lower incidence of sexual dysfunction than cardiovascular drugs such as methyldopa and propranolol.

Table 8.8 Specific types of sexual dysfunction associated with adrenergic stimulants

- Decreased libido
- Inability to maintain erection
- Ejaculatory difficulties, including retrograde ejaculation
- Difficulty achieving orgasm
- Gynecomastia
- Painful breast enlargement

Table 8.9 Specific types of sexual dysfunction associated with antilipidemics

- Decreased libido
- Erectile dysfunction
- Breast enlargement

The incidence of sexual dysfunction associated with antiarrhythmics is estimated as very low (e.g., in clinical trials with disopyramide, the incidence was less than 1%, and the causal relationship was uncertain). High plasma concentration of disopyramide was hypothesized as a cause of impotence in one case report. Amiodarone elevated serum gonadotropin levels in one study and was implicated in testicular dysfunction. Impotence and decreased libido also has been reported with amiodarone.

Sexual dysfunction occasionally occurs with antilipidemics (see Table 8.9) such as clofibrate (5–14%). Several case reports described sexual dysfunction associated with simvastatin and gemfibrozil.

Table 8.10 Specific types of sexual dysfunction associated with beta-blockers

- Erectile dysfunction
- Delayed tumescence
- Priapism
- Delayed ejaculation/orgasm

Table 8.11 Specific types of sexual dysfunction associated with diuretics

- Decreased libido
- Erectile dysfunction
- Decreased vaginal lubrication
- Failed ejaculation

Specific agents:
    chlorothiazide—erectile dysfunction, ejaculation failure
    chlorthalidone—impotence
    hydrochlorothiazide—decreased libido
    spironolactone—decreased libido, decreased vaginal lubrication,
        impotence, gynecomastia, menstrual irregularities

Sexual dysfunction associated with beta-blockers has been frequently mentioned in the literature (estimates with older drugs: 10–15%, but much lower or none with newer beta-blockers, such as bisoprolol). However, a recent reevaluation of risks of sexual dysfunction with beta-blockers and the risk of withdrawal of the drugs because of these side effects puts the risk of sexual problems associated with beta-blockers lower than previously thought (2 per 1,000 patients per year). Table 8.10 lists the sexual dysfunctions reported with beta-blockers.

Sexual dysfunction associated with some beta-blockers (e.g., propranolol) seems to be dose-related. It also appears that cardioselective beta-blockers (e.g., atenolol) are less frequently associated with sexual dysfunction. Sexual dysfunction associated with propranolol disappeared when the drug was discontinued; rechallenge led to reappearance of sexual dysfunction in a small sample. Interestingly, in one study subjects treated with labetolol (alpha/beta adrenergic blocker) reported greater reduction of vaginal lubrication than subjects taking propranolol. Another interesting finding: Sexual dysfunction (impotence, decreased libido, decreased ejaculatory volume) has been reported occasionally with the topical ophthalmic beta-blocker timolol. The etiology of sexual dysfunction associated with beta-blockers is not fully understood, but the beta-blockers may decrease beta-2 vasodilatation and unopposed alpha-2 vasoconstriction in the corpora cavernosa.

Reports of sexual dysfunction with calcium channel blockers are rare; it seems that verapamil causes erectile dysfunction less frequently than nifedipine.

Diuretics are associated with erectile dysfunction relatively frequently. Many investigators estimate the incidence of sexual dysfunction associated with thiazide diuretics to be between 10% and 20%. Specific types of sexual dysfunctions observed with diuretics are summarized in Table 8.11.

The mechanism by which erectile dysfunction occurs in association with diuretics is not fully understood, though decreased vascular resistance and depletion of zinc (important for production of testosterone) have been suggested in the etiology. The effects of diuretics on sexual dysfunction do not seem to be mediated by low serum potassium levels or low blood pressure.

Inotropic agents (e.g., digoxin) also have been associated with sexual dysfunction, specifically with decrease in sexual desire, impaired erection, and decreased frequency of sexual relations. Digoxin also seems to have an impact on plasma testosterone levels.

Sexual dysfunction associated with various cardiovascular agents is an established phenomenon; however, its frequency may be lower than

Table 8.12 Diagnostic criteria for sexual dysfunction associated with cardiovascular agents*

A. Clinically significant sexual dysfunction that results in marked distress or interpersonal difficulty predominates in the clinical picture.

B. There is evidence from the history, physical examination, or laboratory findings that the sexual dysfunction is fully explained by cardiovascular agent(s) use, as manifested by the fact that the symptoms in Criterion A developed during, or within a month of, starting cardiovascular agent administration (or substantial increase in dose).

C. The disturbance is not better accounted for by a sexual dysfunction that is not substance-induced. Evidence that the symptoms are better accounted for by a sexual dysfunction that is not substance-induced might include the following: The symptoms precede the onset of cardiovascular agent administration; the symptoms persist for a substantial period of time (e.g., about a month) after the discontinuation of the cardiovascular agent, or are substantially in excess of what would be expected given the type or amount of the cardiovascular agent used or the duration of use; or there is other evidence that suggests the existence of an independent noncardiovascular agent induced sexual dysfunction (e.g., a history of recurrent nonsubstance-related episodes).

Specify if:
  with impaired desire
  with impaired arousal
  with impaired orgasm
  with sexual pain

* Adapted from *DSM-IV*, APA, 1994.

generally believed. The overestimates may be a product of the fears and myths about coital death and an overinterpretation of mechanisms of action related to these drugs. The mechanisms of sexual dysfunction associated with various cardiovascular agents differ, as these drugs have effects on various neurotransmitters and other systems.

As is the case with other pharmacological agents, the diagnosis of sexual dysfunction associated with cardiovascular drugs requires a baseline evaluation of sexual functioning prior to starting any medication and prior to adding any medication to the standing regime (frequent in the treatment of hypertension). The diagnostic criteria in Table 8.12 may serve as a guideline for diagnosing sexual dysfunction associated with cardiovascular agents.

MANAGEMENT OF SEXUAL DYSFUNCTION ASSOCIATED WITH CARDIOVASCULAR DRUGS

The management of sexual dysfunction associated with cardiovascular drugs starts with proper diagnosis. As previously noted, proper diagnosis of sexual dysfunction attributed to any therapeutic intervention is not possible without a solid baseline pretreatment evaluation of sexual functioning. Patients also should be educated about the possibility of sexual dysfunction associated with both the cardiovascular illness and the cardiovascular drug and the possible management options available, should the dysfunction occur. A general approach to

Table 8.13 General management strategies for sexual dysfunction associated with cardiovascular drugs

- Evaluate patient's sexual functioning prior to treatment.
- Perform physical examination, giving special attention to peripheral vascular disease, testicular size, fibrotic plaques on the penis, and signs of hypogonadism.
- Order appropriate laboratory testing (e.g., thyroid hormone levels, testosterone level).
- Discuss patient's concerns regarding cardiovascular disease, cardiovascular drugs, and sexual dysfunction
- Educate patient about possible management strategies.
- Introduce lifestyle modifications:
  —cessation of smoking
  —decrease alcohol intake
  —exercise
  —diet to address possible diabetes mellitus and dyslipidemias
  —weight loss program (weight loss improved erectile dysfunction associated with thiazide diuretics)
- Warn patient about self-medication and about the dangers of over-the-counter drugs (e.g., the effects of cimetidine on sexual functioning).
- Consider initiating medication with a lower frequency of sexual dysfunction (e.g., newer beta-blockers, calcium channel blockers, ACE inhibitors).
- Select appropriate management strategy and tailor it based on the character of the dysfunction, type of cardiovascular disease, type of medication, evidence in literature, clinical situation, convenience, and patient's special needs.
- Reevaluate dysfunction and effectiveness of management strategy periodically and consider if the causative agent could be discontinued or its dose decreased.

the management of sexual dysfunction associated with cardiovascular drugs is outlined in Table 8.13. (It is important to note that there is no FDA (Food and Drug Administration) approved agent for sexual dysfunction associated with cardiovascular medications.)

The evidence for effective treatment of sexual dysfunction associated with cardiovascular drugs is scarce. The treatment options include oral, self-injection, and intraurethral suppository pharmacotherapy, vacuum constriction devices, vascular surgery, and penile prosthesis implantation.

Since surgery and penile prosthesis implantation are invasive, costly, and difficult at times, pharmacotherapy seems to be the most viable option. The possible pharmacotherapy strategies applicable to causes of sexual dysfunction associated with cardiovascular drugs are summarized in Table 8.14.

Table 8.14 Pharmacotherapy management strategies for sexual dysfunction associated with cardiovascular drugs

1. Select an agent with a low frequency of sexual dysfunction.
2. Reduce dose (could be after a certain interval, e.g., in case of some antihypertensives after a year of effective treatment).
3. Schedule sexual activity around the dose.
4. Switch to another agent with a lower frequency of sexual dysfunction.
5. Use specific agents for sexual dysfunction.

Surprisingly, the research evidence on the usefulness of the outlined approaches is quite scarce.

1. Select an agent with a low frequency of sexual dysfunction. Some authors suggest, for example, using ACE inhibitors for hypertension; or selecting the newer, selective beta-blockers over the older, nonselective ones (e.g., atenolol over propranolol); or choosing diltiazem or verapamil among the calcium channel blockers.

2. Reduce dose. Dose reduction might be an option, but, as suggested, it might occur later during the treatment of the cardiovascular disease.

3. Schedule sexual activity around the dose. This strategy might be useful in agents that are sedating or whose plasma level peaks quickly. However, there are no reports of this approach to sexual dysfunction associated with cardiovascular drugs.

4. Switch to another agent with a lower frequency of sexual dysfunction. Again, data regarding this approach are lacking. Within the group of adrenergic blockers, switching from prazosin to doxazosin or terazosin has been suggested.

5. Use specific agents for sexual dysfunction. The most frequently used agent for sexual dysfunction associated with cardiovascular and other agents has been sildenafil citrate. It is effective in erectile dysfunction of various etiologies. However, its effectiveness in sexual dysfunction in females is not clear. It is also important to note that *sildenafil is absolutely contraindicated in patients taking nitrates— fatal hypotension may occur.* The effects of sildenafil on blood pressure and heart rate in men with erectile dysfunction taking concomitant antihypertensives were small and clinically insignificant. Other possible agents applicable in this context include yohimbine and trazodone. Yohimbine has been reported to cause cardiovascular side effects, such as tachycardia, palpitations, and exacerbation of angina; however, these effects are usually mild and reversible.

Erectile dysfunction associated with cardiovascular drugs also may respond to intracavernosal injections of alprostadil, papaverine, or phentolamine, or to intraurethral alprostadil suppository. The effect of these preparations on other sexual dysfunctions, such as decreased libido or anorgasmia, is minimal or none. Cardiovascular complications of alprostadil, such as hypotension, have been rare. One case of myocardial infarction in a spinal cord injury patient treated with intracavernosal alprostadil has been reported.

Management of sexual dysfunction associated with cardiovascular agents is clearly a complicated process requiring considerable creativity by the treating physician. The seriousness of the underlying cardiovascular disease, together with patient fears and misconceptions, make it even more complicated. However, there are treatment options available, though there is scarce evidence that sexual dysfunction associated with cardiovascular drugs can be alleviated.

CONCLUSIONS

Sexual dysfunction associated with cardiovascular drugs is a serious clinical problem, even though it might occur less frequently than generally believed. Cardiovascular disease itself can cause sexual dysfunction, especially when there is associated general vascular damage. Other medications (e.g., antidepressants, hormones) could further complicate the etiology of the sexual dysfunction. The frequency of sexual dysfunction with some cardiovascular drugs (e.g., ACE inhibitors, calcium channel blockers, and even newer beta-blockers) is fairly low, but could reach 10–20% with other medications (e.g., diuretics, possibly some antilipidemics, and older, nonselective beta-blockers).

The management of sexual dysfunction associated with cardiovascular drugs should begin with a baseline evaluation of sexual functioning, patient education, and modification of patient lifestyle. The evidence of pharmacological management of sexual dysfunction associated with cardiovascular drugs is scarce. Approaches such as using an agent with low frequency of sexual dysfunction, lowering the dose, switching to another agent with a lower frequency of sexual dysfunction, using agents such as sildenafil and yohimbine, intraurethral alprostadil, or intracavernosal injections of various agents may be useful.

REFERENCES

Abramov LA. Sexual life and sexual frigidity among women developing acute myocardial infarction. *Psychosom Med.* 1976;38:418–425.

Ahmad S. Disopyramide and impotence. *South Med J.* 1980;73:958.

Ahmad S. Amiodarone and sexual dysfunction. *Am Heart J.* 1995;130:1320–1321.

Alexander JC, Christie MH, Verman KA, Fand RS, Shafer WB. Long-term experience with nadolol in treatment of hypertension and angina pectoris. *Am Heart J.* 1984;108:1136–1140.

American Psychiatric Association. *Diagnostic and Statistical Manual of Mental Disorders* (4th ed). Washington DC: American Psychiatric Association;1994.

Ananth J, Lin K-M. Propranolol in psychiatry: therapeutic uses and side effects. *Neuropsychobiol.* 1986;15:20–27.

Antonicelli R, Piani M, Paciaroni E. Evaluation of the effectiveness and tolerability of captopril in the treatment of essential arterial hypertension in nine subjects with sexual impotence secondary to the use of beta-blockers. *Curr Ther Res.* 1989;46:837–841.

Bansal S. Sexual dysfunction in hypertensive men: A critical review of the literature. *Hypertension.* 1988;12:1–10.

Barksdale JD, Gardner SE. The impact of first-line antihypertensive drugs on erectile dysfunction. *Pharmacotherapy.* 1999;19:573–581.

Bathen J. Propranolol erectile dysfunction relieved. *Ann Intern Med.* 1978;88:716–717.

Bauer GE, Hull RD, Stokes GS, Raftos J. The reversibility of side effects of guanethidine therapy. *Med J Aust.* 1973;1(19):930–933.

Bharani, A. Sexual dysfunction after gemfibrozil. *BMJ.* 1992;305:693.

Bloch A, Maeder J-P, Haissly J-C. Sexual problems after myocardial infarction. *Am Heart J.* 1975;90:536–537.

Bohlen JG, Held JP, Sanderson O, Patterson RP. Heart rate, rate-pressure product, and oxygen uptake during four sexual activities. *Arch Intern Med.* 1984;144:1745–1748.

Brass EP. Effects of antihypertensive drugs on endocrine function. *Drugs.* 1984;27:447–458.

Brock GB, Lue TF. Drug-induced male sexual dysfunction. An update. *Drug Saf.* 1993;8:414–426.

Broekman CPM, Haensel SM, Van De Ven LLM, Slob AK. Bisoprolol and hypertension: effects on sexual functioning in men. *J Sex & Marital Ther.* 1992;18:325–331.

Bruckert E, Giral P, Heshmati HM, Turpin G. Men treated with hypolipidaemic drugs complain more frequently of erectile dysfunction. *J Clin Pharm Ther.* 1996;21:89–94.

Buffum J. Pharmacosexology: The effects of drugs on sexual function. A review. *J Psychoactive Drugs.* 1982;14:5–44.

Buffum J. Pharmacosexology update: Prescription drugs and sexual function. *J Psychoactive Drugs.* 1986;18:97–106.

Bulpitt CJ, Dollery CT. Side effects of hypotensive agents evaluated by a self-administered questionnaire. *BMJ.* 1973;3:485–490.

Bulpitt CJ, Dollery CT, Carne S. Changes in symptoms of hypertensive patients after referrals to hospital clinic. *Br Heart J.* 1976;38:121–128.

Burchardt M, Burchardt T, Baer L, Kiss AJ, Pawar RV, Shabsigh A, De La Taille A, Hayek O, Shabsigh R. Hypertension is associated with severe erectile dysfunction. *J Urol.* 2000;164:1188–1191.

Burris JF. The USA experience with the clonidine transdermal therapeutic system. *Clin Auton Res.* 1996;3:391–396.

Chang SW, Fine R, Siegel D, Chesney M, Black D, Hulley SB. The impact of diuretic therapy on reported sexual function. *Ann Intern Med.* 1991;15:2402–2408.

Croog SH, Levine S, Sudilovsky A, Baume RM, Clive J. Sexual symptoms in hypertensive patients. A clinical trial of antihypertensive medication. *Arch Intern Med.* 1988;148:788–794.

Dobs AS, Sarma PS, Guarnieri T, Griffith L. Testicular dysfunction with amiodarone use. *J Am Coll Cardiol.* 1991;18:1328–1332.

Dombrowski RC, Romeo JH, Aron DC. Verapamil-induced hyperprolactinemia complicated by a pituitary incidentaloma. *Ann Pharmacother.* 1995;29:999–1001.

Drory Y, Fisman EZ, Shapira I, Pines A. Ventricular arrhythmias during sexual activity in patients with coronary artery disease. *Chest.* 1996;109:922–924.

Drory Y, Shapira I, Fisman EZ, Pines A. Myocardial ischemia during sexual activity in patients with coronary artery disease. *Am J Cardiol.* 1995;75:835–837.

Duch S, Duch C, Pasto L, Ferrer P. Changes in depressive status associated with topical Beta-blockers. *Int Ophtalmol.* 1992;16:331–335.

Duncan L, Bateman DN. Sexual function in women. Do antihypertensive drugs have an impact. *Drug Saf.* 1993;8:225–234.

Epstein RJ, Allen RC, Lunde MW. Organic impotence associated with carbonic anhydrase inhibitor therapy for glaucoma. *Ann Ophthalmol.* 1987;19:48–50.

Figueras A, Castel JM, Laporte J-R, Capella D. Gemfibrozil-induced impotence. *Ann Pharmacother.* 1993;27:982.

Foerster E-Ch, Greminger P, Siegenthaler W, Vetter H, Vetter W. Atenolol versus pindolol: side effects in hypertension. *Eur J Clin Pharmacol.* 1985;28(Suppl):89–91.

Fogari R, Zoppi A, Corradi L, Mugellini A, Poletti L, Lusardi P. Sexual dysfunction in hypertensive males treated with lisinopril or atenolol. *Am J Hypertens.* 1998;11:1244–1247.

Fogelman J. Verapamil may cause depression, confusion, and impotence. *Tex Med.* 1987;83:8.

Forsberg L, Gustavil B, Hojerback T, Olsson AM. Impotence, smoking, and beta-blocking drugs. *Fertility and Sterility.* 1979;31:589–591.

Fraunfelder FT, Meyer SM. Sexual dysfunction secondary to topical ophthalmic timolol. *JAMA.* 1985;253:3092–3093.

Frishman WH, Shapiro W, Charlap S. Labetalol compared with propranolol in patients with both angina pectoris and systemic hypertension: a double-blind study. *J Clin Pharmacol.* 1989;29:504–511.

Geissler AH, Turnlund JR, Cohen RD. Effects of chlorthalidone on zinc levels, testosterone, and sexual function in men. *Drug Nutr Interact.* 1986;4:275–283.

Greenblatt DJ, Koch-Weser J. Gynecomastia and impotence complications of spironolactone therapy. *JAMA.* 1973;223:82.

Grimm RH Jr, Grandits GA, Prineas RJ, McDonald RH, Lewis CE, Flack JM, Yunis C, Svendsen K, Liebson PR, Elmer PJ, Stamler J. Long-term effects on sexual function of five antihypertensive drugs and nutritional hygienic treatment in hypertensive men and women. Treatment of mild hypertension study (TOMHS). *Hypertension.* 1997;29:8–14.

Hellerstein HK, Friedman EH. Sexual activity and the postcoronary patient. *Arch Intern Med.* 1970;125:987–999.

Hogan MJ, Wallin JD, Baer RM. Antihypertensive therapy and male sexual dysfunction. *Psychosomatics.* 1980;21:234–237.

Jackson G. Sexual intercourse and angina pectoris. *Int Rehabil Med.* 1981;3:35–37.

Karacan I, Salis PJ, Hirshkowitz M, Borreson RE, Narter E, Williams RL. Erectile dysfunction in hypertensive men: sleep erections, penile blood flow and musculovascular events. *J Urol.* 1989;142:56–61.

Katz IM. Sexual dysfunction and ocular timolol. *JAMA.* 1986;255:37–38.

Keidan H. Impotence during antihypertensive treatment. *Can Med Assoc J.* 1976;114:874.

Kendall MJ, Beeley L. Beta-adrenoceptor blocking drugs: adverse reactions and drug interactions. *Pharmac Ther.* 1983;21:351–369.

Knarr JW. Impotence from propranolol? *Ann Intern Med.* 1976;85:259.

Ko DT, Hebert PR, Coffey CS, Sedrakyan A, Curtis JP, Krumholz HM. Beta-blocker therapy and symptoms of depression, fatigue, and sexual dysfunction. *JAMA.* 2002;288:251–357.

Kroner BA, Mulligan T, Briggs GC. Effect of frequently prescribed cardiovascular medications on sexual function: a pilot study. *Ann Pharmacother.* 1993;27:1329–1332.

Langford HG, Rockhold RW, Wassertheil-Smoller S, Oberman A, Davis BR, Blaufox MD. Effect of weight loss on thiazide produced erectile problems in men. *Trans Am Clin Climatol Assoc.* 1989;101:190–194.

Larson JL, McNaughton MW, Kennedy JW, Mansfield LW. Heart rate and blood pressure responses to sexual activity and a stair-climbing test. *Heart Lung.* 1980;9:1025–1030.

Loriaux DL, Menard R, Taylor A, Pita JC, Santen R. Spironolactone and endocrine dysfunction. *Ann Intern Med.* 1976;85:630–636.

Lynch MG, Whitson JT, Brown RH, Nguyen H, Drake MM. Topical beta-blocker therapy and central nervous system side effects. A preliminary study comparing betaxolol and timolol. *Arch Ophthalmol.* 1988;196:908–911.

Mann K, Abbott EC, Gray JD, Thiebaux HJ, Belzer EG Jr, Sexual dysfunction with beta-blocker therapy: more common than we think? *Sexuality and Disability.* 1982;5:67–77.

Mann S, Craig MWM, Gould B, Melville DI, Raftery EB. Coital blood pressure in hypertensives. Cephalgia, syncope, and the effects of beta-blockade. *Br Heart* 1982;47:84–89.

McHaffie DJ, Guz A, Johnston A. Impotence in patient on disopyramide. *Lancet.* 1977;1:859.

Miller RA. Propranolol and impotence. *Ann Intern Med.* 1976;85:682–683.

Mills LC. Drug-induced impotence. *Am Fam Physician.* 1975;12:104–106.

Morrissette DL, Skinner MH, Hoffman BB, Levine RE, Davidson JM. Effects of antihypertensive drugs atenolol and nifedipine on sexual function in older men: a placebo-controlled, crossover study. *Arch Sex Behav.* 1993;22:99–109.

Moss H.B., Procci WR. Sexual dysfunction associated with oral antihypertensive medication: a critical survey of literature. *Gen Hosp Psychiatry.* 1982;4:121–129.

Muller JE, Mittelman MA, Maclure M, Sherwood JB, Tofler GH, for the Determinants of Myocardial Infarction Onset Study investigators. Triggering myocardial infarction by sexual activity. Low absolute risk and prevention by regular physical exertion. Determinants of Myocardial Infarction Onset Study. *JAMA.* 1996;275:1405–1409.

Muller SC, El-Damanhoury H, Ruth J, Lue TF. Hypertension and impotence. *Eur Urol.* 1991;19:29–34.

Nemec ED, Mansfield L, Kennedy JW. Heart rate and blood pressure responses during sexual activity in normal males. *Am Heart J.* 1964;92:274–277.

Neri A, Aygen M, Zukerman Z, Bahary C. Subjective assessment of sexual dysfunction of patients on long-term administration of digoxin. *Arch Sex Behav.* 1980;9:343–347.

Neri A, Zukerman Z, Aygen M, Lidor Y, Kaufman H. The effect of long-term administration of digoxin on plasma androgens and sexual dysfunction. *J Sex & Marital Ther.* 1987;13:58–63.

Newman RJ, Salerno HR. Sexual dysfunction due to methyldopa. *BMJ.* 1974;4:106.

Ohman KP, Asplund J. Labetalol in primary hypertension: a long-term effect and tolerance study. *Curr Ther Res.* 1984;35:277–286.

Papadopoulos C. Cardiovascular drugs and sexuality. A cardiologist's review. *Ann Intern Med.* 1980;140:1341–1345.

Papadopoulos C, Beaumont C, Shelley SI, Larrimore P. Myocardial infarction and sexual activity of the female patient. *Arch Intern Med.* 1983;143:1528–1530.

Pedersen TR, Faergeman O. Simvastatin seems unlikely to cause impotence. *BMJ.* 1999;318:192.

Rerkpattanapipat P, Stanek MS, Kotler MN. Sex and the heart: what is the role of the cardiologist? *Eur Heart J.* 2001;22:201–208.

Riley AJ, Riley EJ. The effects of labetalol and propranolol on the pressor response to sexual arousal in women. *Br J Clin Pharmac.* 1981;12:341–344.

Rosen R. Sexual dysfunction as an obstacle to compliance with antihypertensive therapy. *Blood Press Suppl.* 1997;6(Suppl 1) 47–51.

Rosen RC, Kostis JB, Jekelis A. Beta-blocker effects on sexual function in normal males. *Arch Sex Behav.* 1988;17:241–255.

Rosen RC, Kostis JB, Jekelis A, Taska LS. Sexual sequelae of antihypertensive drugs: treatment effects on self-report and physiological measures in middle-aged male hypertensives. *Arch Sex Behav.* 1994;23:135–152.

Rosenberg KP. Sildenafil. *J Sex Marital Ther.* 1999;25:271–279.

Schart MB, Mayleben DW. Comparative effects of prazosin and hydrochlorothiazide on sexual function in men. *Am J Med.* 1989;86:110–112.

Schneider J, Kaffarnik H. Impotence in patients treated with clofibrate. *Atherosclerosis.* 1975;21:455–457.

Seidl A, Bullough B, Haughey B, Scherer Y. Understanding the effects of a myocardial infarction on sexual functioning: a basis for sexual counseling. *Rehabil Nurs.* 1991;16:253–264.

Siegel S, Streem SB, Steinmuller DR. Prazosin-induced priapism. Pathogenic and therapeutic implications. *Br J Urol.* 1988;61:165.

Smith PJ, Talbert RL. Sexual dysfunction with antihypertensive and antipsychotic agents. *Clin Pharm.* 1986;5:373–384.

Srilatha B, Adaikan PG, Arulkumaran S, Ng SG. Sexual dysfunction related to antihypertensive agents: results from the animal model. *Int J Impot Res.* 1999;11:107–113.

Stein RA. The effects of exercise training on heart rate during coitus in the post myocardial infarction patient. *Circulation.* 1977;55:738–740.

Stessman J, Ben-Ishay D. Chlorthalidone-induced impotence. *BMJ.* 1980;281:714.

Stevenson JG, Umstead GS. Sexual dysfunction due to antihypertensive agents. *Drug Intell Clin Pharm.* 1984;18:113–121.

Suzuki H, Tominaga T, Kumagai H, Saruta T. Effects of first-line antihypertensive agents on sexual function and sex hormones. *J Hypertens.* 1988;6(Suppl 4):S649–S651.

Tardif GS. Sexual activity after myocardial infarction. *Arch Phys Med Rehabil.* 1989;70:763–766.

Taylor RG, Crisp AJ, Hoffbrand BI, Maguire A, Jacobs HS. Plasma sex hormone concentration in men with hypertension treated with methyldopa and/or propranolol. *Postgrad Med.* 1981;57:425–426.

Ueno M. The so-called coition death. *Jpn J Leg Med (Nippon Hoigaku Zasshi).* 1963;17:333–340.

Veterans Administration Cooperative Study Group on Antihypertensive Agents. Comparison of prazosin with hydralazine in patients receiving hydrochlorothiazide. A randomized, double-blind clinical trial. *Circulation.* 1981;64:772–779.

Walbroehl GS. Sexual activity and the postcoronary patient. *Am Fam Physician.* 1984;29:175–177.

Warren SC, Warren SG. Propranolol and sexual impotence. *Ann Intern Med.* 1977;86:112.

Wassertheil-Smoller S, Blaufox D, Oberman A, Davis BR, Swencionis C, O'Connell Knerr M, Hawkins CM, Langford HG. Effect of antihypertensives on sexual function and quality of life: The TAIM study. *Ann Intern Med.* 1991;114:613–620.

Weiss RJ. Effects of antihypertensive agents on sexual function. *Am Fam Physician.* 1991;44:2075–2082.

Williams GH, Croog SH, Levine S, Testa MA, Sudilovsky A. Impact of antihypertensive therapy on quality of life: effects of hydrochlorothiazide. *J Hypertens.* 1987;5(Suppl):S29–S35.

Yodfat Y, Fidel J, Bloom DS. Captopril as a replacement for multiple therapy in hypertension: a controlled study. *J Hypertens.* 1985;3(Suppl 2):S155–S158.

Zusman RM, Prisant LM, Brown MJ. for the Sildenafil Study Group. Effect of sildenafil citrate on blood pressure and heart rate in men with erectile dysfunction taking antihypertensive medication. *J Hypertens.* 2000;18:1865–1869.

9. The Impact of Cancer Chemotherapy on Sexual Function

It has long been recognized that cytotoxic agents utilized in cancer treatment can have marked toxic effects on the gonads, causing amenorrhrea, ovarian and testicular failure, and early menopause. However, the major concern in cancer treatment in the past was the preservation of life, and effects on reproductive and sexual function were not systematically studied. To put the issue in perspective, successful chemotherapy of choriocarcinoma was first reported in the 1950s, and successful treatment of leukemias in the 1960s. Better life expectancy resulting from newer therapies has brought quality-of-life issues into consideration. Initial studies concerned reproductive capacity after cancer therapy. Subsequently, studies have investigated sexual functioning following cancer treatment.

Much research has focused on the psychological trauma of cancer treatment and the disturbance to body image following cancer surgery. However, both radiation and chemotherapy inflict significant internal damage, whose effects are worthy of study, such as toxicity in the gonads and neuropathies in the nerves innervating the genitals. The magnitude of sexual difficulties in patients receiving cancer treatment can be appreciated when one realizes that 80% of premenopausal women receiving MOPP (mechlorethamine, vincristine, prednisone, procarbazine) for Hodgkin's disease undergo premature menopause. Premature menopause and gonadal failure are common in women receiving alkylating agents for other types of cancer. Erectile problems and infertility are common in male cancer patients.

Table 9.1 Causes of sexual dysfunction in oncology patients

Acute stress reaction
Altered body image
Depression
Nerve damage by antineoplastic agents
Nerve damage from radiation
Surgical interruption genital innervation
Vascular damage from radiation

Long-term survival with ever-improving cancer treatment is increasingly likely, as noted. It is clearly established that many patients who survive treatment for neoplasms experience subsequent sexual difficulties. The etiology is frequently multifactorial and includes general malaise an other possible symptoms. Table 9.1 lists various possible causes of sexual dysfunction in conjunction with cancer treatment. Many antineoplastic protocols involve the combination of radiation and chemotherapy, both of which can cause sexual difficulties. In addition, many therapy regimes utilize combinations of cytotoxic agents, making determination of the responsible cytotoxic agent difficult, if not impossible.

EFFECTS OF CANCER TREATMENT

Decreased libido is often the result of cytotoxic therapy, possibly the result of hormonal alteration with gonadal failure. Amennorhea, vaginal atropy, dyspareunia, menopausal symptoms, and azoospermia are clearly associated with alkylating agents such as cystosine arabinoside, 5-fluorouracil, vinblastine, vincristine, and procarbazine. In men, antiandrogen therapy and estrogens cause gynecomastia and low libido. Men who have had previous treatment for testicular cancer or for hypothalamic–pituitary tumors usually have residual sexual problems, including impotence and decreased libido, possibly related to orchidectomy and chemotherapy. Retroperitoneal resection as well as chemotherapy can result in ejaculatory problems. Common cytotoxic agents are listed in Table 9.2.

Combination therapies such as PVB (cisplastin, vinblatine, and belomycin), MOPP, and ABVD (doxorubricin, bleomycin, vinblastine, and dacarbazine) have clearly been associated with gonadal damage. Common combination therapies are listed in Table 9.3. However, numerous individual agents have been associated with neurotoxicity as well. Neurological damage to the peripheral innervation of the genitalia

Table 9.2 Common cytotoxic antineoplastic agents

Antimetabolites	Alkylating Agents	Plant Products	Hormonal Agents	Other
azacytidine	busulfan (Myleran)	docetaxel (Taxotere)	aminoglutethide (Cytadren)	actinomycin (Cosmegen)
capecitabine (Xeloda)	carboplatin (Paraplatin)	etoposide (Vepesid)	anastrozole (Arimidex)	daunorubicin (Cerubidine)
cladribine, 2-chlorodeoxyadenosine	carmustine	irinotecan (Camptosar)	bicalutamide (Casodex)	doxorubicin (Adriamycin)
(Leustatin)	chlorambucil (Leukeran)	paclitaxel (Taxol)	dexamethason (Decadron)	epirubicin (Ellence)
cytarabine (Cytosar)	cisplatin (Platinol)	topotecan (Hycamtin)	diethylstilbestrol	idarubicin (Idamycin)
floxuridine (Fud R)	cyclophosphamide (Cytoxan)	vinblastine (Velban)	exemestane (Aromasin)	interferon-a
fludarabine phophate (Fludara)	dacarbazine (DTIC)	vincristine (Oncovin)	flutamide (Eulexin)	interleukin-2
fluouracil (5FU)	Ifofamide (Ifex)	vinorelbine (Navelbine)	goserelin (Zoladex)	mitomycin (Mutamycin)
gemcitabine (Gemzar)	lomustine		leuporide (Lupron)	mitoxanthrone (Novantrone)
hydrourea (Hydrea)	mechlorethamine (Mustargen)		prednisone	pentostatin (Nipent)
hydroxyurea (Hydrea)	melphalan (Alkeran)		tamoxifen (Nolvadex)	plicamycin (Mithracin)
metacaptopurine (Purinethol)	mesna (Uromitexan)		toremifene (Fareston)	valrubicin (Valstar)
methotrexate	phenylalanine mustard (Alkeran)			
thioguanine (Tabloid)	procarbamazine (Matulane)			
	temozolomide (Temodar)			
	thiotepa (Thioplex)			

Table 9.3 Combination chemotherapy regimes

ABVD	adriamycin, bleomycin, vinblatine, dacarbazine
AC	adriamycin, cytoxan
AP	adriamycin, cisplatin
Ara C & DNR	cytarabine, daunorubicin
ATC	adriamycin, taxol, cytoxan
C, Cb, Thio Tepa	cytoxan, carboplatin, thiotepa
CAF	cytoxan, adriamycin, fluorouracil
CCT	cytoxan, carboplatin, thiotepa
CHOP	cytoxan, doxorubicin, vincristine, prednisone
CMF	cytoxan, methotrexate, fluorouracil
CMFVP	CMF, vincristine, prednisone
COP	cytoxan, vincristine, prednisone
CP	cytoxan, cisplatin
DNR	cytarabine, daunorubicin
FU-LV	fluorouracil, leukovorin
FU-LV-P	FU-LV cisplatin
MOPP	mechlorethamine, vincristine (oncovin), prednisone, procarbazine
MVAC	methotrexate, vinblatine, adriamycin, cisplatin
TCB	taxol, carboplain
TP	taxol, cisplatin

has been hypothesized to be one of the ways cancer chemotherapy may cause sexual dysfunction. To date, no one has investigated the integrity of the genital nerves in patients postchemotherapy. Many patients experience sensory nerve damage and peripheral neuropathies. Damage to the sensory innervation of the genitalia could interrupt the erectile, lubrication, and orgasm reflexes in patients. Neoplastic agents reported to be associated with sexual dysfunction are listed in Table 9.4. Sensory neuropathy has been associated with a number of combination therapies, including fotemustine, cisplatin, etoposide; docetaxel, carboplatin, amifostine; paclitaxel and ciplatin; paclitaxel, cisplatin, and gemcitabive; paclitaxel, epirubicin, and cisplatin; oxaliplatin, fluorouracil, and folinic acid; paclitaxel, ifosfamide, and cisplatin; and paclitaxel and epirubicin. Paclitaxel, methothrexate, and thalidomide have been reported to cause peripheral neuropathies even when used in isolation. Antineoplastic drugs with neurotoxic side effects are listed in Table 9.5.

Studies of patients receiving cyclic combination therapy (MOPP) for Hodgkin's disease found that 80% reported decreased sexual function during therapy, and 89% reported a persistent decrease in libido after treatment was discontinued. Problems in libido occurred in both sexes.

Studies of CHOP therapy (cyclophosphaminde, doxorubicin, vincristine, and prednisone) for lymphomas have found that the majority of patients has persistent sexual problems with libido and arousal posttherapy.

Table 9.4 Cancer chemotherapeutic agents suspected to cause sexual dysfunction

Antimetabolites	Alkylating Agents	Other	Neuropathy
cytosine arabinoside	busulfan chlorambucil	ABVD	docetaxel–carboplatin–amifostine
5-fluorouracil	cyclophosphamide	adriamycin	fotemustine–cisplatin–etoposide
methotrexate	mechlorethamine	bleomycin	oxaliplatin–fluorouracil
	melphalan	cyclophosphamide, cisplatin (platinum, visblastine,	paclitaxel–cisplatin–gemcitabine
		bleomycin, doxorubicin, dacarbazine)	paclitaxel alone
		cyclosphosphamide	paclitaxel–epirubicin
		dacarbazine	paclitaxel–ciplatin
		isulfan	paclitaxel–epirbicin–cisplatin
		mechlorethamine	paclitaxel–ifosfamide–cisplatin
		MOPP	thalidomide
		procarbazine	
		orednisone	
		vinblatine	
		vincristine	
		vinblastine	

Table 9.5 Antineoplastic agents associated with neurotoxicity

docetaxel–carboplatin–amifostine
fotemustine–cisplatin–etoposide
oxaliplatin–fluorouracil
paclitaxel–ifosfamide–cisplatin
paclitaxel
paclitaxel–cisplatin
paclitaxel–epirubicin
paclitaxel–epirubicin–cisplatin
paclitaxel–ciplatin–gemcitabine
thalidomide

BONE MARROW TRANSPLANTATION AND HIGH-DOSE COMBINATION CHEMOTHERAPY

Several studies have shown that 20–80% of women have permanent sexual difficulties following bone marrow transplant procedures. These difficulties included decreased libido, vaginal dryness, and difficulty reaching orgasm. Prospective studies have indicated that these problems often preceded bone marrow transplantation and appeared to be related to the length and extent of exposure to high-dose chemotherapy. These studies focused predominantly on women with breast cancer, and the onset of sexual problems appeared to be related to chemotherapy. Type of surgery (mastectomy vs. breast conservation) appeared to bear little relationship to the presence of sexual dysfunction, suggesting that organic factors may be more important than psychological factors. A number of cross-sectional studies of women 3, 5, and 8 years posttreatment found that, in the absence of recurrence, most women adjusted to the diagnosis and treatment after 1 year but that sexual problems persisted. According to these studies, 90% of women will experience coitus following cancer chemotherapy, although more than 60% may experience a complete loss of libido and approximately 40% may have dyspareunia.

One study comparing women with breast cancer who had received chemotherapy with a group of women with breast cancer who had not received chemotherapy found that the postchemotherpay women had

- 5.7 times the incidence of vaginal dryness
- 3-fold increase in problems with libido
- 5.5 times the incidence of dyspareunia
- 7.1 times the incidence of difficulties reaching orgasm.

In males, bone marrow transplant has been associated with erectile disorder and low libido. Most of the males in the cancer studies had

**Table 9.6   Bone marrow transplantation
and sexual dysfunction**

Androgen therapy may reverse decreased libido
Decreased libido
Erectile dysfunction
Hypogonadism
Orgasm disorder

leukemia or lymphomas. Other studies have suggested that most of these men had high rates of sexual dysfunction preceding bone marrow transplantation, related to prior chemotherapy. In these studies, approximately 40% of men will have erectile and libido problems following high-dose chemotherpy.

A recent report suggested that high-dose chemotherapy associated with bone marrow transplant procedures may be associated with vascular damage to the corpora cavernosal walls. However, another investigator could not replicate these findings. Many clinicians routinely recommend androgen replacement to males after completing high-dose chemotherapy. Androgen therapy has been reported to increase libido, but its effects in restoring erectile function have been more limited. As might be expected, administration of human gonadotropin also increases testosterone and libido. Another study of 11 women with low sexual desire after chemotherapy for breast cancer reported a loss of libido and orgasm capacity. All had low serum testosterone levels, and their sexual functioning normalized with the addition of androgen treatment.

Table 9.6 summarizes the effects of bone marrow transplantation and high-dose combination chemotherapy on sexual function.

DIFFERING LEVELS OF TOXICITY

Combination Therapies

Some studies have suggested that the ABVD combination therapy may have less disasterous effects on gonadal function than COPP (cyclophosphamide, vincristine, procarbazine, prednisone) or MOPP therapies. A comparison of MVPP (mustine, vinblastine, procarbazine, and prednisone) with LVPP (chlorambucil, vinblastine, procarbamzine, predinose) found that both protocols had similar rates of permanent sexual dysfunction after treatment of Hodgkin's disease.

Individual Agents

In men a number of androgen-supressing drugs, including leuprorelin, avorlein, and goserelin, have been found to lead to impotence and markedly decreased libido.

Studies of tamoxifen in patients with breast cancer suggest that it may cause dyspareunia in a large number of patients. Tamoxifen, one of the most commonly prescribed cancer drugs, may increase menopausal symptoms but has estrogenic effects on bone, uterus, and cardiovacular status. The lack of vaginal lubrication on this drug has been attributed to its antiestrogenic effects on vaginal epithelium. The incidence of sexual side effects on raloxifene is probably comparable to that of tamoxifen. Both tamoxifen and raloxifene cause menopausal symptoms and are triphenylethylenes. The incidence of sexual problems on toremifine, another selective estrogen receptor modulator, is probably similar. One study found that 54% of patients on tamoxifen reported dyspareunia.

Methotrexate, used in combination therapy, was discovered to produce long-term remission of choriocarcinoma and acute leukemia. It works by competitively inhibiting the binding of folic acid to dihydrofolate reductase and is associated with neurotoxicity. Case reports have implicated this drug as associated with erectile dysfunction.

Table 9.7 lists recommendation for clinical management of drug-induced sexual side effects.

Table 9.7   Recommendations for clinical management

1. *Dyspareunia.* Advise the patient about use of vaginal lubricants. In collaboration with her oncologists and fully informing the patient, consider estrogen vaginal creams (amount of systemic absorption may vary), estradiol vaginal ring (minimal systemic absorption), or estrogen replacement.

2. *Low libido.* In males, consult with the oncologists about the risks of androgen replacement. In females, androgen therapy may be effective, but the risks of such intervention are unknown at this point.

3. *Difficulty with erections.* Consider sildenafil therapy, the vacuum erection device, or intracavernosal injection of vasoactive drugs.

4. *Difficulty with orgasm and/or ejaculation.* Consider whether the use of a vibrator in conjunction with sexual activity will augment the ability to achieve orgasm or ejaculate.

5. Consider depression or an anxiety reaction as possible etiological factors.

6. Consider alterations in body image and difficulty adjusting to diagnosis and treatment of cancer in the differential diagnosis.

7. Consider whether referral for brief counseling might be useful.

8. Consider whether education of the partner about the sexual side effects of cancer treatment might be helpful.

9. Always bear in mind that sexual dysfunction following cancer treatment can be psychogenic, organic, or of mixed etiology.

REFERENCES

Abrahamsen A, Loge J, Hannisdal E, Holte H, Kvaloy S. Socio-medical situation for long-term survivors of Hogkin's disease: a survey of 459 patients treated at one institution. *Eur J Cancer.* 1998;34:1865–1870.

Akerley, W. Paclitaxel in advanced non-small cell lung cancer: an alternative high-dose schedule. *Chest.* 2000;17(Suppl 1):152–155.

Armitage J, Fyfe M, Lewis J. Long-term remission durability and functional status of patients treated for diffuse histiocytic lymphoma with the CHOP regime. *J Clin Oncol.* 1984;2:898–901.

Baidas S, Winer E, Fleming G, et al. Phase II evaluation of thalidomide in patients with metastatic breast cancer. *J Clin Oncol.* 2000;18:2710–2717.

Barni S, Mondin R. Sexual dysfunction in treated breast cancer patients. *Ann Oncol.* 1997;8:147–153.

Boccardo F, Rubagotti A, Barichello M, et al. Bicalutamide monotherapy versus flutamide plus goserelin in prostate cancer patients: results of an Italian prostate cancer project study. *J Clin Oncol.* 1999;17:2027–2038.

Boccon-Gibod L. Are non-steroidal anti-androgens appropriate as monotherapy in advanced prostate cancer? *Eur Urol.* 1998;33:159–164.

Brogden R, Clissold S. Flutamide: a preliminary review of its pharmacodynamic and pharmacokinetic properties, and therapeutic efficacy in advanced prostatic cancer. *Drugs.* 1989;38:185–203.

Brufsky A, Fontaine-Rothe P, Berlane K, et al. Finasteride and flutamide as potency-sparing androgen-ablative therapy for advanced adenocarcinoma of the prostate. *Urol.* 1997;49:13–20.

Budman D, Weiselberg L, O'Mara, V. Severe neurotoxicity in vinorelbine-paclitaxel combinations. *J Nat Cancer Instit.* 1997;89:87–88.

Calabrese L, Fleischer A. Thalidomide: current and potential clincial applications. *Am J Med.* 2000;108:487–495.

Ceresoli G, Dell'Oro S, Passoni P, Villa E. Phase II study of paclitaxel and epirubicin as first-line treatment in patients with metastatic nonsmall cell lung cancer. *Cancer.* 2000;89:89–96.

Chapman R, Rees L, Sutcliffe S, Edwards C. Cyclical combination chemotherapy and gonadal function. *Lancet.* 1979;1(8111):285–289.

Chatterjee R, Andrews H, McGarrigle H, et al. Cavernosal arterial insufficiency is a major component of erectile dysfunction in some recipients of high-dose chemotherapy/chemoradiotherapy for hematological malignancies. *Bone Marrow Transplant.* 2000;25:1185–1189.

Chorost M, Weber T, Lee R, Rodriquez-Bigas M, Patrelli N. Sexual dysfunction, informed consent and multimodality therapy in rectal cancer. *Am J Surg.* 2000;179:271–274.

Constine L, Rubin P, Woolf P, Doane K, Lush C. Hyperprolactinemia and hypothyroidism following cytotoxic therapy for central nervous system malignancies. *J Clin Oncol.* 1987;5:1841–1851.

da Silva F. Quality of life in prostatic carcinoma. *Eur Urol.* 1993;24(Suppl 2): 113–117.

da Silva F, Reis E, Costa T, Denis L. Quality of life in patients with prostatic cancer: a fertility study. *Cancer.* 1993;71(Suppl 3):1138–1142.

Day R, Ganz P, Costantino J, Cronin W, Wickerman D, Fisher B. Health-related quality of life and tamoxifen in breast cancer prevention. *J Clin Oncol.* 1999;9:2659–2669.

Decensi A, Torrisi R, Fontana V, et al. Long-term endocrine effects of administration of either a non-steroidal antiandrogen or a luteinizing hormone-releasing hormone agonist in men with prostate cancer. *Acta Endocrinol.* 1993;129:315–321.

Dimopoulas M, Papadimitrou C, Georgoulias V, et al. Paclitaxel and cisplatin in advanced or recurrent carcinoma of the endometrium: long-term results of a phase II multicenter study. *Gynecol Oncol.* 2000;78:520–527.

Dorval M, Maunsell E, Deschenes L, Brisson J, Masse B. Long-term quality of life after breast cancer: comparison of 8-year survivors with population controls. *J Clin Oncol.* 1998;16:487–494.

Frenay M, Lebrun C, Lonjon M, Bondiau P, Chatel M. Up-front chemotherapy with fotemusine (F)/cisplatin (CDDP)/etoposide (VP16) regimen in the treatment of 33 non-removable glioblastomas. *Eur J Cancer.* 2000;36:1026–1031.

Ganz P, Cosarelli A, Fred C, Kahn B, Polinsky M, Petersen L. Breast cancer survivors: psychosocial concerns and quality of life. *Breast Cancer Res Treat.* 1996;38:183–199.

Ganz P, Rowland J, Desmond K, Meyerowitz B, Wyatt G. Life after breast cancer: understanding women's health-related quality of life and sexual functioning. *J Clin Oncol.* 1998;16:501–514.

Gatzemeier U, von Pawel J, Gottfried M, et al. Phase III comparative study of high-dose cisplatin versus a combination of paclitaxel and cisplatin in patients with advanced non-small-cell lung cancer. *J Clin Oncol.* 2000;18:3390–3399.

Gill P, McLaughlin T, Espina B, et al. Phase I study of human chorionic goandotrophin given subcutaneously to patients with acquired immunodeficincy syndrome-related mucocutaneous Kaposi's sarcoma. *J Nat Cancer Instit.* 1997;89:1797–1809.

Glisson B, Hong W. Survival after treatment of small-cell lung cancer: an endless uphill battle. *J Nat Cancer Instit.* 1997;89:1745–1747.

Goldenberg S, Gleave M, Taylor D, Bruchovsky N. Clinical experience with intermittent androgen suppression in prostate cancer. *Mol Urol.* 1999;3:287–292.

Gunel N, Akcali Z, Yamac D, et al. Cisplatin plus vinorelbine as a salvage regimen in refractory breast cancer. *Tumori.* 2000;86:283–285.

Hartmann J, Albrecht C, Schmoll H, Kuczyk M, Kollmannsberger C, Bokemeyer C. Long-term effects on sexual function and fertility after treatment of testicular cancer. *Br J Cancer.* 1999;80:801–807.

Howell S, Radford J, Smets E, Shalet S. Fatigue, sexual function and mood following treatment for haematological malignancy: the impact of mild Leydig cell dysfunction. *Br J Cancer.* 2000;82:789–793.

Janinis J, Papakostas P, Samelis G, Skarlos D, Papgianopoulos P, Fountzi G. Second-line chemotherapy with weekly oxaliplatin and high-dose fluorouracil with folinic acid in metastatic colorectal carcinoma: a Hellininc Cooperative Oncology Group (H$_e$COG) phase II feasibility study. *Ann Oncol.* 2000;11:163–167.

Juliusson G, Celsing F, Turesson I, Lenhoff S, Adriansson M, Malm C. Frequent good partial remissions from thalidomide, including best response ever in patients with advanced refractory and relapsed myeloma. *Br J Haematol.* 2000;109:89–96.

Kaisary A, Bowsher W, Gillattt D, Anderson JB, Malone P, Imbimbo B. Pharmacodynamics of a long acting depot preparation of avorelin in patients with prostate cancer. *J Urol.* 1999;162:2019–2023.

Kassabian V. erectile dysfunction in the cancer patient. *Cancer Control.* 2000;7:177–180.

Kirby R, Robertson C, Turkes A, et al. Finasteride in association with either flutamide or goserelin as combination therapy in patients with stage M1 carcinoma of the prostate gland. *Prostate.* 1999;40:105–114.

Koeman M, van Driel M, Schultz W, Mensink H. Orgasm after radical prostectomy. *Br J Urol.* 1996;77:861–864.

Komas C, Tsavaris N, Polyzos A, et al. A phase II study of paclitaxel–ifosfamide–cisplatin combination in advanced nonsmall cell lung carcinoma. *Cancer.* 2000;89:774–782.

Koukourakis M, Giatromanolaki A, Kakolyris S, et al. Phase I/II escalation study of docetaxel and carboplatin combination supported with amifostine and GM-CSF in patients with incomplete response following docetaxel chemo–radiotherapy, additional chemotherapy enhances regression of residual tumor. *Med Oncol.* 2000;17:135–143.

Kulkarni S, Sastry P, Saikia T, Parikh P, Gopal R, Advani S. Gonadal function following ABVD therapy for Hodgkin's disease. *Am J Clin Oncol.* 1997;20:354–357.

Lee M, Browneller R, Wu Z, Jung A, Ratanawong C, Sharifi R. Therapeutic effects of leuprorelin microspheres in prostate cancer. *Adv Drug Deliv Rev.* 1997;28:121–138.

Lohiya N, Sharma O, Sharma R. Testis function and sexual potentia in langur monkeys treated with combination steroidal contraceptive formulation. *Contraception.* 1986;34:417–433.

Mackie E, Hill J, Kondryn H, McNally R. Adult psychosocial outcomes in long-term survivors of acute lymphoblastic leukemia and Wilms tumor: a controlled study. *Lancet.* 2000;355:1310–1314.

Mahler C, Verhelst J, Denis, L. Clinical pharmacokinetics of the antiandrogens and their efficacy in prostate cancer. *Clin Pharmacokinet.* 1998;34:405–417.

Marks D, Crilley P, Nezu C, Nezu A. Sexual dysfunction prior to high-dose chemotherapy and bone marrow transplantation. *Bone Marrow Transplant.* 1996;17:595–599.

Marks, D, Friedman, S, Delli, C, Nezu, C, Nezu, A. A prospective study of the effects of high-dose chemotherapy and bone marrow transplantation on sexual function in the first year after transplant. *Bone Marrow Transplant.* 1997;19:819–822.

Marumo K, Baba S, Murai M. Erectile function and conturnal penile tumescence in patients with prostate cancer undergoing luteinizing hormone-releasing agonist therapy. *Int J Urol.* 1999;6:19–23.

Miyazaki M, Nagy A, Schally A, et al. Growth inhibition of human ovarian cancers by cytotoxic analogues of luteinizing hormone. *J Nat Cancer Instit.* 1997;89:1803–1809.

Moinpour C, Lovato L, Thompson I, et al. Profile of men randomized to the prostate cancer prevention trial: baseline health-related quality of life, urinary and sexual functioning and health behaviors. *J Clin Oncol.* 2000;18:1942–1953.

Mortimer J, Boucher L, Baty J, Knapp D, Ryan E, Rowland J. Effect of tamoxifen on sexual functioning in patients with breast cancer. *J Clin Oncol.* 1999;17:1488–1492.

Moyer A. Psychosocial outcomes of breast-conserving surgery versus mastectomy: a meta-analytic review. *Health Psychology.* 1997;16:284–298.

Papadimitrou C, Moulpoulos L, Vahos G. Paclitaxel, cisplatin, and epirubicin first-line chemotherapy in stage III and IV ovarian carcinoma. *Cancer.* 2000;89:1547–1554.

Pavone-Macaluso M, Cacciatore M, Daricello G, Pavonne C, Serretta V. Carcinoma of the prostate: guidelines for treatment: the role of antiandrogens. *Ann NY Acad Sci.* 1990;595:328–333.

Plosker G, Brogden R. Leuprorelin: a review of its pharmacology and therapeutic use in prostatic cancer, endometriosis, and other sex hormone-related disorders. *Drugs.* 1994;48:930–967.

Postma T, Hoekman K, van Riel J, Heimans J, Vermorken J. Peripheral neuropathy due to biweekly paclitaxel, epirubicin and cisplatin in patients with advanced ovarian cancer. *J Neurosci.* 1999;45:241–246.

Rambeaud J. Intermittent complete androgen blockade in metastatic prostate cancer. *Eur Urol.* 1998;35(Suppl S1):32–36.

Ranson M, Davidosn N, Nicolson M, et al. Randomized trial of paclitaxel plus supportive care versus supportive care for patients with advanced non-small cell lung cancer. *J Nat Cancer Instit.* 2000;92:1074–1080.

Relander T, Cavallin-Stahl E, Garwicz S, Olsson A, Willen M. Gonadal and sexual function in men treated for childhood cancer. *Med Pediatr Oncol.* 2000;35:52–63.

Rosati G, Rossi A, Nicolella G, Panza N. Second-line chemotherapy with paclitaxel, cisplatin, and gemcitabine in pre-treated sensitive cisplatin-based patients with advanced non-small cell cancer. *Anticancer.* 2000;20(3B):2229–2233.

Schroder F, Collette L, de Reijke T, Whelan P. Prostate cancer treated by anti-androgens: is sexual function preserved? *Br J Cancer.* 2000;82:283–290.

Sogani P, Whitmore W. Flutamide and other antiandrogens in the treatment of advanced prostatic carcinoma. *Cancer Treat Res.* 1988;39:131–145.

Trivedi C, Redmond B, Flaherty L, et al. Weekly 1-hour infusion of paclitaxel: clinical feasibility and efficacy in patients with hormone-refractory prostate carcinoma. *Cancer.* 2000;89:431–436.

van Basten J, Jonker-Pool G, van Driel M, et al. Sexual functioning after multimodality treatment for disseminated nonseminomatous testicular germ cell tumor. *J Urol.* 1997;158:1411–1416.

van Basten J, van Driel M, Hoefstra H, Sleifer D. Erectile dysfunction with chemotherapy. *Lancet.* 2000;356:9224–9225.

van Basten J, van Driel M, Hoekstra H, et al. Objective and subjective effects of treatment for testicular cancer and sexual function. *Br J Urol Int.* 1999;84:671–678.

vanBasten, JP, Hoekstra HJ, van Driel MF, Koops HS, et al. Sexual dysfunction in nonseminoma testicular cancer is related to chemotherapy-induced infertility. *J Clin Oncol.* 1997;15:2442–2448.

Watson M, Wheatley K, Harrison G, et al. Severe adverse impact on sexual functioning and fertility of bone marrow transplantation, either allogenic or autologous, compared with consolidation chemotherapy alone: analysis of the MRC AMI 10 trial. *Cancer.* 1999;86:1231–1239.

Wellisch D, Centeno J, Guzman J, Belin T, Schiller G. Bone marrow transplantation vs. high-dose cytorabine-based consolidation chemotherapy for acute myelogenous leukemia. *Psychosomatics.* 1996;37:144–154.

10. The Impact of Drugs Used in Obstetrics and Gynecology on Sexual Function

Although a large number of drugs routinely used in obstetrical and gynecological practice, such as oral contraceptives, hormone replacement therapy, and antiandrogen therapy, have been suspected to cause sexual side effects, there is a paucity of controlled research in this area. This lacuna is particularly puzzling in regard to oral contraceptives, which have been in use for over 40 years and even today remain the most common form of reversible contraception. Furthermore, as the lifespan increases, more and more women are concerned with the quality of life after menopause, including the quality of their sexual life. Here again there is minimal definitive evidence concerning the effects of different types of hormone replacement on sexual activity. This information is especially important as women evaluate the possible benefits of hormone replacement in the context of evidence indicating an increased risk of breast cancer and cardiovascular disease with continuous conjugated equineestrogen and medroxy progesterone. There is reason to suspect that antiandrogen therapy, oral contraception, and certain types of hormone replacement therapy might adversely affect sexual function. There is convincing data that libido in women may be related to bioavailable androgens and that many estrogens elevate serum hormone binding globulin, which decreases the amount of bioavailable androgen. Adequate estrogen levels are necessary for vaginal integrity and preventing dyspareunia. Whether estrogen directly affects clitoral sensitivity, and thus libido indirectly, is unknown. This chapter reviews the available data in a manner that is helpful to the practicing physician.

ORAL CONTRACEPTIVES

Oral contraceptives come in three major forms: combination, sequential, or progesterone-only forms. Sequential and combination oral contraceptives contain both estrogen and progestin. All birth control pills in the United States contain either ethinyl estradiol or mestranol. Estradiol is the most potent natural estrogen, and it is the major estrogen made in the ovaries. Because it is inactive if given orally, it is paired with an ethinyl group. Estrogens available in oral contraceptives are listed in Table 10.1. Synthetic progestins are used in oral contraceptives in the United States include norethindrone, ethynodiol diacetate, norgestrel, norgestimate, and levonorgestrel (Table 10.1). Norethindrone, norgestrel, and levonorgestrel are used in progesterone-only pills. Medroxyprogestereone is used in depot form, and levonorgestrel is used in an intraureterine system.

Most of the progestins are either related to norethindrone or levonorgestrel. Norethindrone is predominantly progestational, although some androgenic properties remain. Norethindrone is converted into estrogen in the body: the rate of this conversion is low and probably of minimal significance. Norethindrone and ethynodiol diacetate have weak estrogenic activity. New progestins related to levonorgestrel include desogestrel, gestodene, and norgestimate. These compounds tend to have less androgenic and more progestional effects than older progestins. Ethynodiol diacetate, norgestrel, norgestimate, and gestodene are all 19-nortestosterone progestins. Many of the progestins are converted into the parent compound in the body. For example, the activity of norethynodrel, ethynodiol diacetate, and lynestrenol is related to each's rapid conversion into norethindrone. Levonorgestrel is the

Table 10.1 Estrogens and progestins in oral contraceptives in the U.S. market

Estrogens	Progestins
ethinyl estradiol	desogestrel
mestranol	ethynodiol diacetate
	levonorgestrel
	norethindrone
	norethynodrel
	norgestimate
	norgestrel

active isomer of norgestrel, gestodene expresses its progestational effects via active metabolites, and the activity of norgestimate may be related to its metabolism into levonorgestrel. In other words, the chemical composition of estrogens and progestins in oral contraceptives is similar; hence, so are the actions. The estrogenic and androgenic activity of oral contraceptives is usually considered to be of minimal clinical significance because of the low dosages employed in oral contraceptives.

The fixed combination pills are the most widely used in this country. The estrogen–progesterone preparations available in the United States are listed in Table 10.2. The term *low-dose oral contraceptives* refers to those containing less than 50 μg of ethinyl estradiol. The term *first-generation oral contraceptives* refers to those containing more then 50 μg of ethinyl estradiol. Some of the first-generation oral contraceptives were occasionally associated with androgenic side effects. The term *new progestins* refers to desogestrel, gestodene, and norgestimate. The newer progestins have less androgenic effects. The new progestin-only, multiphasic, and low-dose estrogen products are as effective as the first-generation oral contraceptives and the higher-dose monophasic pills. The efficacy of oral contraceptives decreases slightly with the progestin-only pills.

Long-acting progestin birth control methods include norplant and depo-provera. Norplant contains levonorgestrel, which decreases serum hormone-binding globulin and thus might be expected to have a positive influence on libido—if fluctuations of free testosterone within normal limits have an effect on libido in females. Depo-provera blocks the luteinizing hormone surge and ovulation and, at high doses, interferes with testosterone metabolism; it might be expected to decrease libido—if fluctuations of testosterone above a minimal threshold amount decrease libido in females.

A number of controlled trials and extensive clinical experience have demonstrated that depo-provera is useful in the treatment of men who engage in criminal sexual behavior. Some case reports have suggested that depo-provera can be useful in controlling hypersexual behavior of female patients who have psychosis associated with bipolar disease. Trials comparing the effects of these two agents on libido are not available.

Information concerning the effect of oral contraceptives on sexual behavior is conflicting and difficult to interpret. Oral contraceptives may increase sexual activity and libido because of decreased fear of pregnancy, and social factors influencing sexual activity may partially balance or outweigh any negative biological effect on libido. The

Table 10.2   Oral contraceptives available in the United States

Brand Name	Composition	
Alesses 21 & Alesses 28	.1 mg .02 μg	levonogestrel EE*
Brevicon	.5 mg .035 μg	norethindrone EE
Cyclessa	.100 mg .125 mg .150 mg .025 μg	desogestrel desogestrel desogestrel EE
Desogen	.15 mg .03 mg	desogestrel EE
Estrostep 21	1 mg .02 μg .03 μg .035 μg	norethindrone EE EE EE
Levlen	.15 mg .03 μg	levonorgestrel EE
Levlite	.1 mg .03 μg	levonorgestrel EE
Levora	.15 mg .03 μg	levonorgestrel EE
Loestrin 21 1/20	1 mg .02 mg	norethindrone EE
Loestrin 21 1.5/30	1.5 mg .02 μg	norethindrone EE
Lo-Ovral	.3 mg .03 μg	norgestrel EE
Low-Ogestrel-28	.3 mg .03 μg	norgestrel EE
Microgestin Fe 1/20	1 mg .02 μg	norethindrone EE
Microgestin Fe 1.5/3/0	1.5 mg .03 μg	norethindrone EE
Modicon	.5 mg .035 μg	norethindrone EE
Necon 1/35–21 & Necon 1/35–28	1 mg .035 μg	norethindrone EE

Necon 10/11–21 &
  Necon 10/11–28 &
  Necon .5/35–21
  Necon .5/35–28
	.5 mg
	.035 μg
		norethindrone
		EE

Necon 1/50–21 Necon 1/50–28	1 mg .05 mg	norethindrone mestranol
Ogestrel	.5 mg .05 μg	norgestrel EE
Ortho-cept	.15 mg .03 μg	desogestrel EE
Orthicyclen	.2 mg .035 μg	norgestimate EE
Ortho-Novum 7/7/7 10/11	.5 mg .035 μg	norethindrone EE

Table 10.2   (*Cont.*)

Brand Name	Composition	
Ortho-Novum 1/35	1 mg	norethindrone
	.035 μg	EE
Ortho-Novum 1/50	1 mg	norethindrone
	.05 mg	mestranol
Ortho-tri-cyclen	.18mg	norgestimate
	.215 mg	norgestimate
	.25 mg	norgestimate
	.035 μg	EE
Ovcon 35	.4 mg	norethindrone
	.03 μg	EE
Ovcon 50	1 mg	norethindrone
	.05 μg	EE
Ovral 28	.5 mg	norgestrel
	.03 μg	EE
Progestin only		
Micronor	.35 mg	norethindrone
Nor-QD	.35 mg	norethindrone
Ovrette	.075 mg	norgestryl
Plan B	.75 mg	levonorgestrel
Tri-Levlen	.05 mg	levonorgestrel
	.075 mg	levonorgestrel
	.125 mg	levonorgestrel
	.03 μg	EE
	.04 μg	EE
	.03 μg	EE
Tri-norinyl-28	.5 mg	norethindrone
	1 mg	norethindrone
	.035 μg	EE
Tri-Norinyl-28	.5 mg	norethindrone
	1 mg	norethindrone
	.035 μg	EE
Triphasil	.05 mg	levonorgestrel
	.075 mg	levonorgestrel
	.125 mg	levonorgestrel
	.03 μg	EE
	.04 μg	EE
	.03 μg	EE
Trivora	.05 mg	levonorgestrel
	.075 mg	levonorgestrel
	.125 mg	levonorgestrel
	.03 μg	EE
	.04 μg	EE
	.03 μg	EE
Yasmin 28	3 mg	drospirenone
	.03 μg	EE
Zovia 1/50E–21 &	1 mg	ethynodiol diacetate
	.035 μg	EE
Zovia 1/50E–28	1 mg	ethynodiol diacetate
	.035 μg	EE

* EE = ethinyl estradiol

OBSTETRICS AND GYNECOLOGY

psychosocial factors certainly complicate the investigation of the effect of these agents on libido. Many clinicians are firmly convinced that oral contraceptives can decrease libido and recommend switching to a different contraceptive agent or method when women on oral contraceptives complain of new onset hypoactive sexual desire disorder.

Some estrogens increase hormone-binding globulin, which decreases the amount of bioavailable testosterone. However, progestins, in general, tend to counter the effect of estrogens on serum hormone-binding globulin. The picture is further complicated by the fact that not all estrogens and progestins are alike. Some clinicians advocate the use of sequential (multiphasic) oral contraceptive therapy for women who experience decreased libido on monophasic oral contraceptives. However, there is evidence that some multiphasic oral contraceptives may also decrease libido. Progestin-only mini-pills would be expected to have minimal influence on libido. It is important to note that the dosages of hormone contained in birth control pills are extremely small compared to the doses contained in hormone replacement medication.

There have been numerous controlled studies of the effects of oral contraceptives on sexual function. Most of these studies suggest that oral contraceptives decrease libido in some women. To date, no study has convincingly demonstrated that one agent has more deleterious effects than another. A placebo-controlled study of the effects of combined versus progesterone-only oral contraceptives was conducted in two contrasting cultures—Scotland and the Phillipines. Combined oral contraceptives had a definite adverse effect on libido in Scottish women; women from the Phillipines reported much lower levels of libido before starting the study.

A recent study by the Kinsey Institute used a different methodology to assess the effects of oral contraceptives on libido. Women were comprehensively investigated by interview and questionnaire prior to beginning the oral contraceptive trial and then reassessed at 3, 6, and 12 months after starting oral contraception. They were randomly assigned to receive Ortho-Cyclen (monophasic: .035 mg ethinyl estradiol plus .25 mg norgestimate) or Ortho Tri-Cyclen (triphasic: .035 mg ethinyl estradiol, and 18 mg, .215 mg, and .25 mg norgestimate). Discontinuation and switch rates were high on both preparations, approaching 50%, with most discontinuations occurring within 3 months of starting the drug. Women who discontinued or switched oral contraceptives reported a decrease in sexual thoughts and coital frequency. Adverse effects on mood and sexuality were predictive of discontinuation or switching agents.

MENOPAUSE AND PERIMENOPAUSE CHANGES IN HORMONES

In perimenopause, there is an elevation of follicle-stimulating hormone and a decrease in inhibin. Luteinizing hormone and estradiol may remain within normal limits. Postmenopausal women experience urogenital atrophy with decreased vaginal lubrication and loss of vaginal elasticity. The complaints of postmenopausal women (summarized in Table 10.3) are usually alleviated by restoration of estrogen.

The premenopausal ovary secretes 95% of the body's estradiol. In the premenopausal woman, the main source of estrogen are the preovulatory follicles and the corpus luteum. After menopause, the ovaries stop secreting estradiol, and estrone becomes the predominant estrogen. In premenopausal women estradiol fluctuates between 40 and 250 pg/ml in the proliferative phase and is close to 100 pg/ml in the luteal phase. By comparison, postmenopausal estradiol drops to 20 pg/ml. Estrone arises predominantly from peripheral conversion of androstenedione. The body aromatizes androgen to estrogen in fat, muscle, and lung. There is considerable individual variability in the amount and rate of aromatization. The postmenopausal woman may have a 10–20-fold increase in follicle-stimulating hormone and a 3-fold increase in luteinizing hormone.

Postmenopausal ovaries secrete androstenedione and testosterone. Androstenedione is the major androgen secreted by postmenopausal ovaries. Circulating levels of androstenedione in postmenopausal women are about 50% the level of the same hormone in premenopausal women. Testosterone usually decreases by 25% in postmenopausal women, although postmenopausal ovaries characterized by elevated gonadotrophin stimulation of the stromal tissue may produce more testosterone in some women. There is less circulating testosterone because of decreased peripheral conversion of androstenedione into testosterone. The postmenopausal woman has 1–20 pg/ml of estradiol, most of which is derived from the peripheral conversion of androstenedione. The changes in the androgen–estrogen ratio in postmenopausal woman may be accompanied by mild hirsutism. As noted,

OBSTETRICS AND GYNECOLOGY

Table 10.3   Symptoms of Hypoestrogenism

Post coital burning
Post coital spotting
Vaginal dryness
Vaginal irritation
Vaginal tightness

estrogen in the postmenopausal woman is mainly the result of extraglandular conversion of androstenedione and testosterone into estrogen. Eventually, androgen levels decrease in almost all postmenopausal women. After oophorectomy there is a precipitous drop in both estrogen and estosteone.

Low estrogen is associated with decreased vascularity to the vaginal mucosa. Atrophic vaginitis is associated with decreased lubrication, dyspareunia, and urge incontinence. Some clincians have proposed that decreased perfusion of the clitoris might contribute to difficulty with orgasm in postmenopasual women.

The brain has estrogen receptors in the pituitary, hypothalamus, and limbic forebrain, but it is unclear whether these receptors influence libido. The brain also has testosterone receptors in the preoptic area, amygdala, limbic area, hippocampus, and cortex, as well as aromatizing enzymes that convert androgen to estrogen.

HORMONE REPLACEMENT THERAPY

In 2002, the National Heart, Lung, and Blood Institute of the National Institutes of Health prematurely stopped a large multisite clinical trial of the effects of combined estrogen/progesterone replacement therapy in postmenopausal women. Women receiving .625 mg of conjugated estrogen plus 2.5 mg of medroxyprogesterone had an increased risk for breast cancer and cardiovascular disease. The full impact of these findings on recommendations for hormone replacement is still debated and it is expected that guidelines for hormone replacement will be modified in the near future. Thus the information in this section is accurate for early 2002, but is subject to revision.

Hormone replacement therapy usually involves replacing one of the estrogens. In the United States, conjugated estrogen (e.g., Premarin) is the most commonly prescribed estrogen, whereas estradiol valerate is more commonly prescribed in Europe. Commonly prescribed estrogens include conjugated estrogens, micronized estrogen, synthetic estrogen (e.g., ethinyl estradiol), estropipate, and estradiol. Both conjugated equine estrogens and esterified estrogens are derived from the urine of pregnant mares. Estropipate is estrone conjugated into piperazine. Oral estrogen is largely converted into estrone by the liver. Estrogen therapy may increase serum hormone-binding globulin, thus decreasing the amount of free testosterone. Forty-six percent of naturally menopausal women and 71% of surgically menopausal women receive hormone replacement therapy. The average duration of such therapy is about 6 years. Different types

Table 10.4   Estrogen replacement products

Brand Name	Composition
Oral	
Cenestin	synthetic conjugated estrogen tablets
	.625 mg, .9 mg, & 1.25 mg
Estinyl	ethyl estradiol tablets
	.02 mg & .05 mg
Estrace	estradiol tablets
	.5 mg, 1 mg, 2 mg
Menest	esterified estrogen
	.3 mg, .625 mg, 1.25 mg, & 2.5 mg
Ogen	estropipate tablets
	.75 mg, 1.5 mg, & 3 mg
Ortho-est	estropipate tablets
	.625 mg & 1.25 mg
Premarin	conjugated estrogen tablets
	2.5 mg, 1.25 mg, .9 mg, .625 mg, & .3 mg
Transdermal	
Alora	Estradiol transdermal system
	.05 mg, .075 mg, or .1 mg per day
Esclim	Estradiol transdermal system
	.025, .0375, .05, .075, or .1 mg per Day
Vivette	estradiol transdermal system
	.025, .0375, .05, .075, or .1 mg per day
Other	
Estrace Vaginal Cream	.01% estradiol
	.1 mg/gram
Estring	2 mg estradiol vaginal ring
Orthodienestrol Cream	2.75 oz tubes
Premarin IV	conjugated estrogen for injection
	Vial with 25 mg conjugated estrogen
Vagifem	estradiol vaginal tablets
	25 micrograms

of estrogen replacement therapy have different potencies on follicle-stimulating hormone, liver proteins, and bone density. Two types of estrogen receptors are known, and different estrogen products have different potencies at these receptor sites. Alternative methods of estrogen replacement include transdermal estradiol patches, Estring (an estradiol vaginal ring with minimal systemic absorption), and vaginal creams. Estrogen creams usually produce the systemic level if the same dose were given orally. Estrogen replacement products are listed in Table 10.4.

In women with an intact uterus, progesterone (such as medroxyprogesterone) is added to decrease uterine hyperplasia. Hormone replacement with estrogen–progesterone preparations can be given in either a combined or sequential form. Combination estrogen replacement drugs available in the United States are listed in Table 10.5. Common progesterone preparations are listed in Table 10.6. Hormone replacement can be given in either a combined or sequential form.

OBSTETRICS AND GYNECOLOGY

Table 10.5 Estrogen combinations

Brand Name	Composition*
Estratest	1.25 mg EE and 2.5 mg methyltestosterone
Estratest HS	.625 mg EE and 1.25 mg methyltestosterone
PremPhase	.625 mg EE and 5 mg medroxyprogesterone
PremPro	.625 mg EE and 2.5, or 5 mg medroxyprogesterone

* EE = ethinyl estradiol

A typical sequential regime includes estrogen daily or estrogen daily for the first 25 days, followed by progestins added on days 10–14 each month, or days 10–14 every 3 months. The estrogens used in sequential postmenopausal therapy include .625 mg conjugated estrogens, 1.25 mg estropipate, or 1 mg micronized estradiol or equivalent of other estrogens. Common progestins include .7 mg norethindrone, 200 mg micronized progesterone, or 5 mg medroxyprogesterone for 2 weeks of each month.

Continuous combination therapy usually consists of the same dose of estrogen used in the sequential medication, plus .35 mg norethindrone, or 100 mg micronized progesterone, or 2.5 mg medroxyprogesterone. The only progestins available in a transdermal preparation are norethindrone and levonorgestrel. Medroxyprogesterone, which is also used to treat male sex offenders, inhibits the secretion of gonadotrophins and has been associated with both decreased libido and anorgasmia. Progestins available worldwide are listed in Table 10.6. Estrogens may be combined in oral estrogen–androgen combination therapy.

Clearly, there are numerous mechanisms by which both oral contraceptive therapy and hormone replacement therapy might interfere with libido. The exploration of these relationships is complicated by the number of different products available, by the fact that different estrogens have different effects on serum hormone-binding globulin and androgen metabolism, and by the probability that progestins differ in their effects on libido. Theoretically, medroxyprogesterone

Table 10.6 Other progesterone products

Brand Name	Composition
Aygestin	5 mg norethindrone tablets
Crinone	4% & 8% progesterone gel
Depo-provera	150 mg/ml medroxyprosterone prefilled syringe
Mirena	levonorgestrel-relasing intrauterine system
Norplant	36 mg levonorgestael implant
Prometrium	100 & 200 mg progesterone capsules
Provera	2.5, 5, & 10 mg medroxyprogesterone tablets

may influence libido either by increasing depressed affect, decreasing testosterone, or increasing serum hormone-binding globulin, thus decreasing free testosterone. In the absence of definitive information concerning the effect on libido of changes in free testosterone levels within physiological range, it is uncertain whether differential effects of progestins on serum hormone-binding globulin account for differences in libido that have been reported on various hormone replacement regimes. Depression induced by medroxyprogesterone has been reported to be alleviated by substitution of norethindrone.

A small number of double-blind studies has examined the effects of various agents on libido in the human female. Unfortunately, many of these studies concern products not available in the United States. One study found that 1 mg ethinyl estradiol and .1 mg mestranol decreased libido. A large Swedish study found that estradiol monotherapy was more beneficial to sexual function than estradiol plus norethisterone. Other studies have reported that norethisterone decreases libido and erectile function in males. This also has been reported to decrease progestin, libido, frequency of erections, and frequency of sexual fantasies in males. Norethisterone has 50% of the affinity for the progesterone receptor as progesterone, and 45% of the affinity for the testosterone receptor as testosterone.

A large number of studies has examined the effects of various hormonal agents on serum hormone-binding globulin. In general, these studies suggest that most estrogens increase serum hormone-binding globulin by varying amounts, whereas many progestins appear to have minimal effects on, or slightly decrease, serum hormone-binding globulin. Thus the effect of any given estrogen–progesterone combination on serum hormone-binding globulin will be dependent on the specific estrogens and progestins. A study comparing levonorgesterel and desogestrel found that desogestrel decreased serum hormone-binding globulin more than levonorgestrel. Other studies have found that estradiol and levonorgestrel or estradiol and natural progesterone do not appear to influence serum hormone-binding globulin levels. A study comparing two triphasic oral contraceptives with differing doses of ethinyl estradiol and levonorgestrel found that both decreased free testosterone and increased serum hormone-binding globulin. Different estrogens have been found to have different influences on serum hormone-binding globulin: Oral equine estrogen increases it by 100%, oral estradiol increases it by 45%, and transdermal estradiol increases it by only 12%.

Estrogen–progesterone products containing medroxyprogesterone appear to increase the amount of serum hormone-binding globulin. In estrogen–progesterone replacement studies, serum hormone-binding

Table 10.7 Sexual effects of tibolone

Increase in libido
Increase in sexual activity
Increase in vaginal perfusion

globulin increased with medroxyprogesterone but not norgestrel. Hormone replacement therapy with equine estrogens and 5 mg medroxyprogesterone has been found to increase serum hormone-biding globulin.

Tibolone

Tibolone is a selective estrogen receptor modulator currently being studied for introduction into the U.S. market. It is a steroid, related to nortestosterone, used to prevent perimenopausal bone loss and hot flushes. It is metabolized into three isomers, each with varying amounts of estrogenic, progestogenic, and androgenic properties. Its effects vary with the target tissue: It has estrogenic effects on the vagina and reduces dyspareunia. Comparisons of tibolone and beta estradiol 2 plus norethisterone have found that tibolone had more postive effects on sexual activity than combined treatment. It is considered to be a selective estrogen receptor modulator.

Studies comparing tibolone against .625 mg conjugated estrogens and medroxyprogesterone found that tibilone had a more positive effect on sexual desire and frequency.

Table 10.7 summarizes the effects of tibolone and methyltestosterone on sexual function.

Methyltestosterone

Studies have shown that the addition of 5 mg of methyltestosterone may have modest effects on sexual fantasies and frequency of masturbation. Because androgens do not protect the endometrium, postmenopausal women with an intact uterus also will require progestins. Doses of androgen that have a clear effect on libido also tend to cause undesirable side effects such as acne, alopecia, and hirsutism.

GONADOTROPHIN-RELEASING HORMONE AGONISTS

Gonadotrophin-releasing hormone (GnRH) agonists are used in the treatment of precocious puberty, endometriosis, and prostate cancer. GnRH agonists, such as goserelin, leuprolide, buserelin, and nafarelin, work by depleting the pituitary of gonadotrophins. Because these

Table 10.8   Effect of GnRH agonists, antiandrogens, SERMS, and danazol on sexual function

Antiandrogens probably decease libido
Effect of danazol on libido is unclear
GnRH agonists reduce libido
SERMs may cause dyspareunia

drugs decrease sexual desire in males and interfere with nocturnal penile erections, they are employed in sex-drive reduction in paraphilics. The drugs have been reported to adversely affect libido in females. There is no definitive data comparing the incidence of sexual side effects on the various GnRH agonists. On theoretical grounds, one would expect the incidence to be comparable on all of the GnRH agonists.

Table 10.8 compares the effects of GnRH agonist, selective estrogen receptor modulators (SERMs), antiandrogens, and danazol on sexual function.

SELECTIVE ESTROGEN RECEPTOR MODULATORS

The term *selective estrogen receptor modulators* is used to describe compounds that act like estrogen in some tissues but antagonize estrogen effects in others. These drugs were formerly termed *partial estrogen agonists*. Four agents in this class are currently approved for use in the United States: clomiphene, tamoxifen, toremifene, and raloxifene. Clomiphene, a drug used to induce ovulation, apparently has minimal effects on sexual function, and it does increase serum testosterone levels. Tamoxifen and toremifene elevate serum hormone-binding globulin. Drugs like tamoxifen and raloxifene induce symptoms of menopause and have been associated with a high incidence of dyspareunia. These drugs are based on triphenylethylene or benxothiopene rings and are distinct from estrogen.

ANTIANDROGENS

Antiandrogens are used in the treatment of polycystic ovary syndrome, hirsutism, androgenic alopecia, and other androgenic disorders in females. Some of the most commonly used antiandrogen therapies are spironolactone, flutamide, cypoterone acetate, and finasteride. Spironolactone inhibits the binding of dihydrotestosterone to androgen receptors and leads to increased clearance of testosterone. In men, it causes reduced libido and erectile dysfunction, and has been linked to gynecomastia. Its effect on sexual function in women is unclear. See Table 10.8.

Table 10.9   Clinical recommendations for minimizing the negative impact of OB–GYN drugs on sexual function

1. On theoretical grounds, recommend the mini-progesterone oral contraceptives because of their low doses and lack of effect on gonadotrophins. These would be preferred to low-dose sequential oral contraceptives, which have been reported to decrease free testosterone.

2. With hormone replacement, avoid or use the lowest doses possible of medroxyprogesterone because of its adverse effect on testosterone production and its effect of increasing serum hormone-binding globulin levels. There is some reason to suspect that norgestrel and norethindrone may have minimal effects on serum hormone-binding levels.

3. Evidence suggests that testosterone replacement may be necessary to sustain libido for some women postoophorectomy. However, the exact doses needed are unclear. The dose in Estratest may or may not be sufficient.

4. Evidence suggests that oral equine estrogens and oral estradiol may have more dramatic effects on increasing serum hormone-binding globulin than transdermal estradiol.

5. Women on GnRH agonists and estrogen receptor modulators should be counseled about possible adverse consequences of this therapy on sexual activity.

6. Tibolone shows promise as a hormone replacement agent with minimal adverse effects on sexual behavior.

DANAZOL

Danazol (Danocrine) is used primarily to treat endometriosis. It is a 2,3-isoxazol derivative of 17 alpha-ethynl testosterone (ethisterone). It suppresses LH and FSH production and has only weak androgenic effect. Its effect on libido is unknown. See Table 10.8.

RECOMMENDATIONS

Definitive information regarding the impact of obstetrical–gynecological drugs on sexual function is lacking. However, certain clinical recommendations can be made by assuming that variation in free testosterone within normal levels has an effect on libido. These recommendations are listed in Table 10.9.

REFERENCES

Aden U, Jung-Hoffman C, Kuhl H. A randomized cross-over study on various hormonal parameters of two triphasic oral contraceptives. *Contraceptives*. 1998;58:75–81.

Albertazzi P, DiMicco R, Zanardi E. Tibolone: a review. *Maturitas*. 1998;30:295–305.

Alexander G, Sherwin B. Sex steroids, sexual behavior, and selective attention for erotic stimuli in women using oral contraceptives. *Psychoneuroendocrinology*. 1993;18:91–102.

Alexander G, Sherwin B, Bancroft J, Davidson J. Testosterone and sexual behavior in oral contraceptive users and nonusers: a prospective study. *Horm Behav.* 1990;24:388–402.

Aunitz AM. Injectable depot medroxyprogesterone acetate contraception: an update for U.S. clinicians. *Int J Fertil.* 1998;43:7–83.

Baker HW. Reproductive effects of nontesticular illness. *Endocrin Metab Clin.* 1998;27:1–21.

Balthazart J, Ball G. New insights into the regulation and function of brain estrogen synthase (aromatase). *Trends Neurosci.* 1998;21:243–249.

Bancroft J, Sherwin B, Alexander G, Davidson D, Walker A. Oral contraceptives, androgens, and the sexuality of young women. II: the role of androgens. *Arch Sex Behav.* 1991;20:121–135.

Basson R. Androgen replacement for women. *Can Fam Physician.* 1999;45:2100–2107.

Berman J, Berman L, Werbin T, Flaherty E, Leahy N, Goldstein I. Clinical evaluation of female sexual function: effects of age and estrogen status on subjective and physiologic sexual responses. *Int J Impot Res.* 1999;11(Suppl 1):S31–38.

Bjorn I, Bixo M, Nojd K, Nyberg S, Backstrom T. Negative mood changes during hormone replacement therapy: a comparison between two progestogens. *Am J Obstet Gynecol.* 2000;183:1–10.

Burger HG. Selective oestrogen receptor modulators. *Horm Res.* 2000;31:25–29.

Campbell B, Udry J. Implications of hormonal influences on sexual behavior for demographic models of reproduction. *Ann NY Acad Sci.* 1994;18:117–127.

Catelo-Barnaco C, Vicente J, Figueras F, et al. Comparative effects of estrogens plus androgens and tibolone on bone, lipid pattern and sexuality in postmenopausal women. *Maturitas.* 2000;34:161–168.

Celio A, Ferrari L, et al. Premenopausal breast cancer patients treated with gonadotrophin releasing hormone analog alone or in combination with an aromatic inhibitor: a comparative endocrine study. *Anticancer Res.* 1999;19:2261–2268.

Civic D, Scholes D, Ichikawa L, et al. Depressive symptoms in users and non-users of depot medroxyprogesterone. *Contraception.* 2000;61:385–390.

Couzinet B. The antigonadotrophic activity of progestins (19-nortestosterone and 19-norprogesterone derivatives) is not mediated through the androgen receptor. *J Clin Endocrin Metabol.* 1996;81:4218–4223.

Cullberg G. Pharmacodynamic studies on desogestrel administered alone and in combination with ethinylestradiol. *Acta Obstet Gynecol Scand.* 1985;133(Suppl):1–30.

Davis S, McCloud P. Testosterone enhances estradiol's effect on postmenopausal bone density and sexuality. *Maturitas.* 1995;21:227–236.

DeCherney A. Hormone receptors and sexuality in the human female. *J Women's Health Gend Based Med.* 2000;9(Suppl 1):S9–S13.

Dennerstein L, Dudley C. Sexuality, hormones, and the menopause transition. *Maturitas.* 1997;2:83–93.

Diamanti-Kandarakis E. Curent aspects of antiandrogen therapy in women. *Curr Pharm Des.* 1999;5:707–723.

Egarter C, Sator M, Berghammer P, Huber J. Efficacy, tolerability and rare side effects of tibolone treatment in postmenopausal women. *Int J Gynecol Obstet.* 1999;64:281–286.

Finkelstein J, Susman E, Chinchilli V, et al. Effects of estrogen or testosterone on self-reported sexual responses and behaviors in hypogonadal adolesents. *J Clin Endocrin Metab.* 1998;83:2281–2285.

Frey H, Aakvaag A. The treatment of essential hirsutism in women with cyproterone acetate and ethinyl estradiol. Clinical and endocrine effects in 10 cases. *Acct Obstet Gynecol Scand.* 1981;60:295–300.

Gelfand M. Role of androgens in surgical menopause. *Am J Ob Gyn.* 1999;180(3Pt 2):S325–S327.

Gelfand M. Sexuality among older women. *J Womens Health Gend Based Med.* 2000;9(Suppl 1):S15–S20.

Gelfand M, Witta M. Androgen and estrogen–androgen hormone replacement therapy: a review of the safety literature: 1941 to 1996. *Clin Therapeutics.* 1997;19:383–404.

Glick I, Bennett S. Psychiatric complications of progesterone and oral contraceptives. *J Clin Psychopharmacol.* 1981;6:350–367.

Goldstein I. Female sexual arousal disorder: new insights. *Int J Impot Res.* 2000;12(Suppl 4):152–157.

Goldstein S, Siddhanti S, Ciaccia A, Plouffe I. A pharmacological review of selective estrogen recptor modulators. *Hum Reprod Update.* 2000;6:212–224.

Graham C, Ramos R. The effects of steroidal contraceptives on the well-being and sexuality of women: a double-blind placebo-controlled two-center study of combined and progestin-only method. *Contraception.* 1995;52:363–369.

Graham C, Sherwin B. The relationship between mood and sexuality in women using an oral contraceptive as a treatment for premenstrual symptoms. *Psychoneuroendocrinol.* 1993;18:273–278.

Greendale G, Hogan P, Shumaker S. Sexual functioning in postmenopausal women: the postmenopausal estrogen/progestin interventions (PEPI) trial. *J Women's Health.* 1996;5:445–458.

Greendale G, Reboussin B, Hogan P, et al. Symptom relief and side effects of postmenopausal hormones: results from the postmenopausal estrogen/progestin interventions trial. *Obstet Gynecol.* 1998;92:982–988.

Hickok L, Toomey C. A comparison of esterified estrogens with and without methytestosterone: effects on endometrial histology and serum lipoproteins in postmenopausal women. *Obstet Gynecol.* 1993;82:919–924.

Howell R, Edmonds D, Dowsett M, Crook D, Lees B, Stevenson J. Gonadotropin-releasing hormone analogue (goserelin) plus hormone replacement therapy for the treatment of endometriosis: a randomized controlled trial. *Fertil Steril.* 1995;474–481.

Kamischke A. Potential of norethisterone enanthate for male contraception: pharmacokinetics and suppression of pituitary and gonadal function. *Clin Endocrinol.* 2000;53:351–358.

Kaplan H, Owett T. The female androgen deficiency syndrome. *J Sex Marital Ther.* 1993;19:3–24.

Kaunitz A. The role of androgens in menopausal hormonal replacement. *Endocrinol Metab Clin North AM.* 1997;26:381–387.

Kirkham C, Hahn P, van Vugt D, Carmichael J, Reid R. A randomized double-blind, placebo-controlled crossover trial to assess the side effects of medroxyprogesterone acetate in hormone replacement therapy. *Obstet Gynecol.* 1991;78:93–97.

Kochler J. Sexual dysfunction. In: Sanfilippo J., Smith R., editors. *Primary Care in Obstetrics and Gynecology.* New York: Springer;1998:487–521.

Kokcu A, Cetinkaya M, Ynik F, Alper, Malatyalioglu E. The comparison of effects of tibolone and conjugated estrogen–medroxyprogesterone acetate therapy on sexual performance in postmentopausal women. *Maturitas.* 2000;36:75–80.

Laughlin G, Barrett-Connor E, Kritz-Silverstain D, vonMuhlen D. Hysterectomy, oophorectomy, and endogenous sex hormone levels in older women: the Rancho Bernardo Study. *J Clin Endocrinol Metabol.* 2000;85:645–651.

Leedom L, Feldman M, Procci W, Zeidler A. Symptoms of sexual dysfunction and depression in diabetic women. *J Diabetic Complications.* 1991;5:38–41.

Leeton J, McMaster R, Worsley A. The effects on sexual response and mood after sterilization of women taking long-term oral contraception: results of a double-blind crossover study. *Aust NZ J Gynecol.* 1978;18:194–197.

Li C, Samsioe G, Wilaman K et al. Effect of norethisterone acetate addition to estradiol in long-term HRT. *Maturitas.* 2000;36:139–152.

Lindgren R, Berg G, Hammar M, Zuccon, E. Hormonal replacement therapy and sexuality in a population of Swedish postmenopausal women. *Acta Obstet Gynecol Scand.* 1993;72:292–297.

Meuwissen I, Over R. Sexual arousal across phases of the human menstrual cycle. *Arch Sex Behav.* 1992;21:101–118.

Moghetti P, Tosi F, Tosti A et al. Comparison of spironolactone, flutamide, and finasteride efficacy in the treatment of hirsutism: a randomized, double-blind, placebo-controlled trial. *J Clin Endocrin Metab.* 2000;85:1–12.

Murphy A, Shupnik M, Hoffman G. Androgen and estrogen (α) receptor distribution in the periaqueductal gray of the male rat. *Horm and Behavior.* 1999;36:98–108.

Myers L, Dixen J, Morrissette M, Carmichael M, Davidson J. Effects of estrogen, androgen, and progestin on sexual psychophysiology and behavior in postmenopausal women. *J Endocrinol and Metab.* 1990;70:1124–1131.

Nathorst-Boos J, Hammar M. Effects on sexual life: a comparison between tibolone and a continuous estradiol–norethisterone acetate regimen. *Maturitas.* 1997;26:15–20.

Omu A, Al-Qattan N. Effects of hormone replacement therapy on sexuality in postmenopausal women in Mideast country. *J Obstet Gynecol Res.* 1997;23:157–164.

Palacio S, Menendez C, Jurado A, Castano R, Vargas J. Changes in sexual behavior after menopause: effects of tibolone. *Maturitas.* 1995;2:155–161.

Prior J, Alojado N, McKay W, Vigna Y. No adverse effects of medroxyprogesterone treatment without estrogen in postmenopausal women: double-blind, placebo-controlled, crossover trial. *Obstet Gynecol.* 1994;83:24–28.

Rako S. Testosterone deficiency and supplementation for women: what do we need to know? *Menopause Management.* 1996;5:10–15.

Redmond G. Hormones and sexual function. *Int J Infert.* 1999;44:193–197.

Ross L, Alder E, Cawood E, Brown J, Gebbie A. Psychological effects of hormone replacement therapy: a comparison of tibolone and a sequential estrogen therapy. *J Psychosom Ostet Gynecol.* 1999;20:88–96.

Rittmaster RS. Amiandrogen treatment of Polycystic ovary disease. *Endocrinol Metab Clin North AM.* 1999;28:409–421.

Sarrel P. Psychosexual effects of menopause: role of androgens. *Am J Obstet Gynecol.* 1999;180:319–324.

Sarrel P. Effects of hormone replacement therapy on sexual psychophysiology and behavior in postmenopause. *J Womens Health Gend Based Med.* 2000;9(Suppl 1):S25–S32.

Sarrell P, Dobay B. Estrogen and estrogen–androgen replacement in postmenopausal women dissatisfied with estrogen-only therapy. *J Reproduct Med.* 1998;43:847–856.

Sherwin B. The impact of different doses of estrogen and progestin on mood and sexual behavior in postmenopausal women. *J Clin Endo Metab.* 1991;72:336–343.

Sherwin B. Sex hormones and psychological functioning in postmenopausal women. *Exp Gerontol.* 1994;29:423–430.

Sherwin B. Use of combined estrogen–androgen preparations in the postmenopause: evidence from clinical studies. *Int J Fertil Womens Med.* 1998;43:98–103.

Sherwin B, Gelfand M. The role of androgen in the maintenance of sexual functioning in oophorectomized women. *Psychosom Med.* 1987;49:397–409.

Shifren J, Braunstein G, Simon J et al. Transdermal testosterone treatment in women with impaired sexual function after oophorectomy. *New Eng J Med.* 2000;343:682–688.

Simoncini T, Genazzani A. Raloxifene acutely stimulates nitric oxide release from human endothelial cells via an activation of endothelial nitric oxide synthase. *J Clin Endo Metab.* 2000;85:2966–2969.

Slob A, Bax C, Hop W, Rowland D, van der Werff ten Bosch J. Sexual arousability and the menstrual cycle. *Psychoneuroendocrinology.* 1996;21:545–558.

Snyder K, Sparano N, Malonowski J. Raloxifene hydrochloride. *Am J Health Pharm.* 2000;57:1669–1678.

Suvanto-Luukkonen E, Sundstrom H, Pentinnen J, Kauppila A. Lipid effects on an intrauterine levonorgestrel device or oral vs. vaginal natural progesterone in post-menopausal women treated with percutaneous estradiol. *Arch Gynecol Obstet.* 1998;261:201–208.

Thorneycroft I, Stancyzk F, Bradshaw K, Ballagh SA, Nichols M, Wel M. Effect of low-dose oral contraceptives on androgenic markers and acne. *Contraception.* 1999;60:266–260.

van Goozen S, Wiegert V, Endert E, Helmond FA, van de Poll N. Psychoendocrinological assessment of the menstrual cycle: the relationship between hormones, sexuality, and mood. *Arch Sex Behavior.* 1997;26:359–382.

Warnock J, Bundren J, Morris D. Female hypoactive sexual desire disorder due to androgen deficiency: clinical and psychometric issues. *Psychopharmacol.* 1997;33:761–766.

Young R. Androgens in postmenopausal women. *Menopause Management.* 1993;2:21–24.

Zehr J, Maestripieri D, Wallen K. Estradiol increases female sexual initiation independent of male responsiveness in rhesus monkeys. *Horm Behav.* 1998;33:95–103.

Zumpe D, Claney A, Michael R. Effects of progesterone on the sexual behavior of castrated testosterone-treated male cynomolgus monkeys. *Physiol Behav.* 1997;62:61–67.

11. The Impact of Anticonvulsants on Sexual Function

ANTICONVULSANTS

INTRODUCTION

It is well known that sexual dysfunction occurs in patients treated for various forms of epilepsy (used in this chapter, *epilepsy* refers to any form of epilepsy/seizure disorder). How much of the sexual dysfunction is attributable to medications used for epilepsy is a complicated issue. Some such medications (we use the term *anticonvulsants* in this chapter) clearly have a deleterious effect on sexual and reproductive functioning. However, hyposexuality has been reported as an effect of epilepsy itself. The frequency of sexual dysfunction associated with anticonvulsants may be underestimated due to the low baseline sexual functioning in people with epilepsy. However, some reports on sexual dysfunction associated with anticonvulsants have appeared in the literature on the treatment of bipolar disorder (see also Chapter 5). These findings suggest that the incidence of sexual dysfunction attributable to anticonvulsants may be higher. The management of sexual dysfunction associated with anticonvulsants could be a complicated issue, because some management strategies (e.g., switching to another medication) may not be a viable option for a stabilized epilepsy patient. Table 11.1 lists anticonvulsants available in the United States.

This chapter discusses issues important in the assessment and management of sexual dysfunction associated with anticonvulsants. Specifically, the chapter focuses on:

- Changes of sexuality in epilepsy;
- Sexual dysfunction associated with anticonvulsants; and
- Management of sexual dysfunction associated with anticonvulsants.

Table 11.1 Anticonvulsants available in the United States

Generic Name	Brand Name	Forms and Doses (mg, unless otherwise noted)*
carbamazepine	Tegretol	tc: 100
		t: 200
		txr: 100/200/400
		o: 20/ml
	Carbatrol	cer: 200/300
clonazepam	Klonopin	t: 0.5/1/2
clorazepate dipotassium	Tranxene	t: 3.75/7.5/15
		tsd: 11.25/22.5
diazepam	Valium	t: 2/5/10
		p: 5/ml
divalproex sodium	Depakote Sprinkle	c: 125
	Depakote Tablets	t: 125/250/500
	Depakote ER	t: 500
ethosuximide	Zarontin	c: 250
		s: 50/ml
felbamate	Felbatol	t: 400/600
		o: 120/ml
fosphenytoin sodium	Cerebyx	p: 50/ml
gabapentin	Neurontin	t: 600/800
		c: 100/300/400
		o: 50/ml
lamotrigine	Lamictal	t: 25/100/150/200
		tc: 2/5/25
levetiracetam	Keppra	t: 250/500/750
lorazepam	Ativan	t: 0.5/1/2
		p: 2/ml; 4/ml
methsuximide	Celontin	c: 150/300
oxcarbazepine	Trileptal	t: 150/300/600
		o: 60/ml
pentotal sodium	Nembutal	p: 50/ml
phenobarbitone	No more available	
phenobarbital	Donnatal	t: 16.2
		c: 16.2
		e: 16.2/5ml
	Donnatal Extentabs	et: 48.6
phenobarbital elixir		e: 4/ml
phenytoin	Dilantin Infatabs	t: 50
	Dilantin Kapseal	c: 30/100
	Dilantin-125	o: 5/ml
	Dilantin SteriDose	p: 50/ml
primidone	Mysoline	t: 50/250
		o: 50/ml
tiagabine hydrochloride	Gabitril	t: 2/4/12/16/20
topiramate	Topamax	t: 25/100/200
		c: 15/25
valproate sodium	Depacon Injection	p: 100/ml
valproic acid	Depakene	c: 250
		s: 50/ml
zonisamide	Zonegran	c: 100

* c = capsules; cer = extended release capsules; e = elixir; o = oral concentrate; p = parenteral concentrate; s = syrup; t = tablet; tc = chewable tablets; tsd = single-dose tablets (slow release); txr = slow-release tablets

For sexual dysfunction associated with anticonvulsants in bipolar disorder refer to Chapter 5 on mood stabilizers.

SEXUALITY AND SEIZURE DISORDERS

Changes in sexual behavior associated with epilepsy have been studied for several decades (summarized in Table 11.2). The original observation, in 1939, of hypersexuality in monkeys after bilateral temporal lobectomy was followed by similar observations in other animals and humans. However, in 1954 hyposexuality was reported in several hundred patients with psychomotor epilepsy. The researchers described a profound disinterest in all libidinous aspects of life, including decreased or lack of sexual curiosity, erotic fantasies, and desire for sexual intercourse, as well as impotence or "frigidity." The global hyposexuality developed *after* the onset of epilepsy, usually 2 to 4 years later.

Since the 1954 report, several studies have confirmed these observations: (1) 15 cases of erectile failure in patients with temporal lobe lesions (not on excessive doses of anticonvulsants and with normal libido); (2) 11 of 21 patients with temporal lobe epilepsy and total or near total lack of sexual drive, which had developed following the onset of temporal lobe seizures; (3) 20 men with partial seizures of temporal lobe origin, 11 with diminished sexual interest or reduced potency, 9 with reproductive endocrine disorders, with features of hypogonadotropic hypogonadism in 5, hyperprolactinemia in 2, and hypergonadotropic hypogonadism in 2. Among these 9 patients were

Table 11.2   Possible changes in sexual behavior associated with epilepsy*

Both genders	
Global hyposexuality	
Men	**Women**
Lack of or lower libido (including lack of curiosity, drive)	Lack of or lower libido
Erectile failure (including abnormal nocturnal penile tumescence and rigidity)	Dyspareunia
	Lower arousal
	Vaginismus
Anorgasmia	Anorgasmia
Possible reproductive abnormalities	Lower fertility rates
	Menstrual difficulties
Lower testosterone levels?	
Lower increase of blood flow to genitalia with erotic impulse	Lower increase of blood flow to genitalia with erotic impulse

* Changes possible, but not always in all forms of epilepsy; most frequently studied regarding sexual dysfunctions has been temporal lobe epilepsy.

situations in which the reproductive abnormalities could not be attributed readily to anticonvulsant use. The researchers felt that temporal lobe epilepsy and some reproductive endocrine disorders may represent parallel effects of prenatal factors that are common to the development of both brain and the reproductive system. In another study, five of six men with temporal lobe epilepsy who complained of erectile dysfunction showed abnormal ambulatory nocturnal penile tumescence and rigidity. The researchers felt that epilepsy-related erectile dysfunction may have a substantial neurophysiological component. One group of researchers even suggested that in some men, hyposexuality and impotence may be the most immediately apparent symptoms of undiagnosed temporal lobe epilepsy.

Several studies focused on the sexual and reproductive functioning of women with epilepsy. One study reported that 28 of 50 women with partial seizures of temporal lobe origin had menstrual problems, and 19 had reproductive endocrine disorders. In their study, "polycystic ovarian syndrome and hypogonadotropic hypogonadism" occurred significantly more often in women with temporal lobe epilepsy than in the general female population. Another study assessed sexual function in 116 women. Although sexual experience was not reduced, women with epilepsy reported significantly less arousability than normal controls. Women with localization-related epilepsy reported significantly more sexual anxiety, dyspareunia, vaginismus, arousal insufficiency, and sexual dissatisfaction. Women with primary generalized epilepsy experienced anorgasmia and sexual dissatisfaction. Interestingly, sexual symptoms were not associated with seizure frequency, antiepileptic drug exposure, sexual experience, depression, or prepubertal seizure onset. The authors concluded that although their study did not show evidence of a low desire disorder, the fact that more than one-third of their female patients with epilepsy experienced disorders of sexual arousal implied a physiological deficit in sexual responsiveness. It is also estimated (Webber et al., 1996; Herzog, 1999) that the fertility rate in women with epilepsy is lower—about 70–80%—than the fertility rate in nonepileptic women.

The evidence of association between temporal lobe epilepsy and hyposexuality seems to be strong (Sorensen and Boldwig, 1987). Nevertheless, the differences between the prevalence of sexual dysfunction in various forms of epilepsy (e.g., partial vs. generalized epilepsy) are not known. As Morrell (1991) pointed out, sexual dysfunction may not be associated with all types of epilepsy. For instance, Jensen and colleagues (1990) did not find a significant difference in sexual dysfunction among epileptic patients when compared to healthy controls and patients with diabetes. Bergen and colleagues (1992) did not find a positive correlation between self-reported sexual activity or desire and the

Table 11.3 Reported types of sexual dysfunction associated with anticonvulsants

Stricter sexual morality (medication vs. illness itself?)
Impotence
Less satisfying orgasm
Loss of sensation of orgasm
Anorgasmia/ejaculatory failure
Unpleasant feelings on touching genitalia and erogenous zones

duration of epilepsy, seizure type, anticonvulsants, number or duration of anticonvulsant use, or age.

The varying estimates of sexual dysfunction prevalence in people with epilepsy could be due to numerous factors. For instance, Morrell (1991) noted that complaints of sexual dysfunction are more likely from patients who developed epilepsy later in life, after a period of normal sexual behavior. She also suggested that patients with a longer history of epilepsy may be more likely to experience sexual dysfunction. Many epileptic patients do not discuss their sexual problems with physicians and are also rarely asked about sexual functioning. In a study by Bergen and colleagues (1992), only 13% of patients reported ever being asked about their sexual functioning by a physician. Furthermore, as Pietropinto and Arora (1988) observed in their survey, only a minority of physicians is aware that patients with temporal lobe epilepsy have a lower libido than people without epilepsy—and many (35%) even believe that these patients have a higher libido. Studies of sexual dysfunction in people with epilepsy have also lacked the use of standardized questionnaires and physiological measures.

Nevertheless, sexual dysfunction, especially arousal disorder, seems to be associated with epilepsy. The strongest evidence points toward an association between temporal lobe epilepsy and hyposexuality. Sexual dysfunction associated with epilepsy can have a significant impact on the patient's quality of life, self-esteem, and intimate relationships, as well as on researchers' estimates of sexual dysfunction associated with medications used for the treatment of epilepsy (see Table 11.3).

SEXUAL DYSFUNCTION ASSOCIATED WITH ANTICONVULSANTS

Sexual Dysfunction

The reports of sexual dysfunction associated with anticonvulsants include several studies and case reports. One study compared the use of four anticonvulsants—carbamazepine, phenobarbital, phenytoin,

Table 11.4 Estimated frequency of sexual dysfunction with anticonvulsants

Carbamazepine	13%[*]
Clonazepam	
delayed ejaculation	1–2%[**]
impotence	1–3%[**]
Gabapentin (impotence)	1.5%[**]
Phenobarbital	16%[*]
Phenytoin	11%[*]
Primidone	22%[*]

[*] Mattson et al., 1985.
[**] *Physicians' Desk Reference*, 2002.

and primidone—in treating partial and secondarily generalized tonic–clonic seizures in a double-blind multicenter study. This study also focused on identifying various side effects of these drugs, including the possibility of sexual dysfunction. The frequencies of decreased libido or impotence with the four anticonvulsants, which ranged from 1% to 22%, are shown in Table 11.4. In contrast, another study did not find a positive correlation between self-reported sexual activity or desire and the number or duration of anticonvulsant use. It also compared patients on valproic acid alone with those on other anticonvulsants and did not find any significant difference in sexual function.

In an interesting study, the Sexuality Experience Scale (SES) was administered to 195 women in an epilepsy clinic (159 received anticonvulsants, 36 did not) and 48 controls. The SES has four main scales: SES 1, The Sexual Morality Scale; SES 2, The Psychosexual Stimulation Scale; SES 3, The Sexual Motivation Scale; and SES 4, The Attraction to Marriage Scale. The researchers also measured total testosterone and sex hormone-binding globulin levels and calculated free testosterone.

Women receiving anticonvulsants achieved significantly higher SES 1 and SES 2 scores than the rest, suggesting that they adhered to a stricter sexual morality and were less open to psychosexual stimulation. (Findings also suggested that women found orgasms less satisfying).

Women on anticonvulsants had significantly higher levels of total testosterone and sex hormone-binding globulin than controls and untreated women with epilepsy. However, there were no differences in free testosterone levels among the three groups. Interestingly, there was no significant correlation between free testosterone levels and the desired frequency of intercourse or enjoyment of intercourse for the three groups. The most interesting was the finding that those women on anticovulsants who had regular partners appeared to desire and enjoy intercourse as much as the control and untreated groups.

In another study, the researchers investigated the effects of anticonvulsants on sex hormone levels and sexual activity in 150 men attending an epilepsy clinic (118 on anticonvulsants, 32 not receiving anticonvulsants) and 33 controls. The SES scores showed that men receiving anticonvulsants embraced a stricter sexual morality than the controls and untreated men, and expressed greater satisfaction with their marriage/relationship than controls and untreated groups. Men with epilepsy who had a partner did not appear hyposexual. Carbamazepine-treated men had higher sex hormone-binding globulin levels than controls and lower dihydroepiandrosterone sulfate levels than controls, untreated, and valproate monotherapy groups. Phenytoin monotherapy also significantly increased sex hormone-binding globulin and total testosterone levels and lowered dihydroepiandrosterone sulphate. Valproate monotherapy had the least, if any, effect on sex hormones and sex hormone-binding globulin. The researchers emphasized that the case in favor of anticonvulsant-associated sexual dysfunction is still based on circumstantial evidence and does not take into account the fact that men are able to tolerate decreases in androgens without necessarily losing libido. These two reports illustrate the complexity of studying sexual functioning associated with medication.

Several case reports described sexual dysfunction associated with older and newer anticonvulsants. Ejaculatory failure and loss of orgasmic sensation was reported in a 61-year old male taking carbamazepine for trigeminal neuralgia; the sexual dysfunction ceased after he stopped carbamazepine. Gabapentin has been reported to cause anorgasmia in several patients treated for bipolar disorder. Recently, two cases of anorgasmia in women treated with gabapentin per epilepsy were also reported. In one case, the anorgasmia resolved after switching to valproic acid. Loss of libido and unpleasant feelings in the genitals and erogenous zones, when touched, were reported in a female patient with schizoaffective disorder treated with lamotrigine. Finally, three cases of men reporting sexual dysfunction (impotence, anorgasmia) with various anticonvulsants (combinations of phenobarbital, gabapentin, phenytoin, carbamazepine, valproate) were noted. In contrast to the preceding study, in all three cases the sexual dysfunction improved after adding or switching to lamotrigine (and, in one case, decreasing carbamazepine at the same time).

Benzodiazepines, which are also used in the treatment of epilepsy, have been occasionally reported to cause difficulties with orgasm and ejaculation or erection in special populations. However, the evidence

Table 11.5 Possible hormonal changes associated with older anticonvulsants*

	Increased	Decreased	No change
Androstendione		X	
Circulating thyroxine		X	
Dihydroepiandrosterone	X (mostly)	X	
Estrogen			X
Follicle stimulating hormone (FSH)	X		X
Free testosterone fraction	X (mostly)	X	
Free thyroxine		X	
Luteinizing hormone (LH)	X	X	
Progesterone		X	X
Prolactin	X		
Sex hormone binding globulin	X		
Testosterone	X (mostly)	X	

* Results are summarized from various studies.
1. Valproic acid may have a lower or no effects on various hormone levels.
2. The effects of newer anticonvulsants (e.g., gabapentin, lamotrigine, tiagabine) on hormone levels are unknown.

of sexual dysfunction associated with benzodiazepines is scarce, comprising only several case reports, and thus has not been established.

Sex Hormone and Other Hormone Levels

Several studies addressed the issue of antiepileptic drugs affecting the levels of various sex and other hormones and sex hormone-binding globulin. Carbamazepine was found to increase sex hormone-binding globulin and decrease testosterone, free testosterone fraction, dehydroepinadrosterone sulfate, and androstenedione within 7 days. (See Table 11.5.) In another study, carbamazepine did not significantly change the serum balance of sex hormones such as testosterone; however, it clearly affected the levels of sex hormone-binding globulin and dehydroepiandrosterone acetate. Several studies during the last two decades reported similar findings. In one study, carbamazepine monotherapy reduced the levels of testosterone and dehydroeplandrosterone and increased basal prolactin. Interestingly, valproate did not appear to affect the level of any measured hormone. However, as the authors pointed out, little is known about the relevance of these changes to sexual function, although reduced free testosterone concentrations have been associated with reduced sexual activity.

Similar findings were reported in a study that assessed circulating sex and thyroid hormones, as well as pituitary function, in 63 males with epilepsy receiving either monotherapy with carbamazepine, phenytoin, or valproate or a combination of carbamazepine plus phenytoin or carbamazepine plus valproate. All therapeutic regimens, except for valproate monotherapy, were associated with low levels of circulating thyroxine, free thyroxine, and dehydroepiandrosterone sulfate and with low values of free androgen index. The carbamazepine–valproate combination had the most pronounced effect on thyroid hormone balance and free androgen index. Again, the clinical consequences of these findings were not established.

Other researchers also found lower levels of free testosterone and higher levels of sex hormone-binding globulin, total testosterone, and bound testosterone in 51 epileptic men treated with anticonvulsant polytherapy or carbamazepine and phenytoin monotherapy, compared to normal controls. As mentioned, one study reported higher total testosterone and sex hormone-binding globulin in epileptic women treated with anticonvulsants than in controls, and significant changes in sex hormones and sex hormone-binding globulin in epileptic men treated with anticonvulsant polytherapy or carbamazepine and phenytoin monotherapy, but not with valproate. However, valproate increased serum androgen levels in a different study of epileptic men. In that study of epileptic men treated with carbamazepine dihydroepiandrosterone, sulfate levels were low and sex hormone-binding globulin levels were high while endocrine effects of oxcarbazepine seemed to be dose-dependent.

The effect of newer anticonvulsants, such as gabapentin, lamotrigine, tiagabine, and others, on sex hormones has not been properly studied and is not known.

Treatment with anticonvulsants seems to be associated with sexual dysfunction in some cases. The frequency of sexual dysfunction associated with anticonvulsants seems to be relatively low, but its estimates are conflated by sexual dysfunction associated with epilepsy itself, by a low number of studies addressing this issue, and by poor methodology in existing studies.

The etiology of sexual dysfunction associated with anticonvulsants is unclear. Changes in sex hormone levels (e.g., shortening the half-life via enzyme induction) and in sex hormone-binding globulin are most frequently implicated in sexual dysfunction associated with the older anticonvulsants, although valproic acid does not seem to affect sex hormones in the same fashion as carbamazepine, phenytoin, and phenobarbital. However, modulation of some neurotransmitters (e.g., gamma-aminobutyric acid) may play a role in sexual dysfunction associated with some newer anticonvulsants.

MANAGEMENT OF SEXUAL DYSFUNCTION ASSOCIATED WITH ANTICONVULSANTS

Whereas not very much is truly known about the frequency of sexual dysfunction associated with anticonvulsants, even less is known about the management of sexual dysfunction associated with these drugs.

Baseline sexual functioning evaluation of all patients prior to staring any therapy is extremely important, especially in view of the possible hyposexuality associated with epilepsy.

There are several management approaches to medication-associated sexual dysfunction (see also Table 11.6):

- Waiting for spontaneous remission
- Dose reduction
- Scheduling medication around sexual activity
- Switching to medication with a lower frequency of sexual dysfunction
- Taking drug holidays
- Using antidotes, vacuum erectile devices, or prosthesis
- Selecting a primary treatment agent associated with a lower frequency of sexual dysfunction.

None of these approaches has been tested in a scientific fashion and only a few has been reported successful in case reports (some of them in bipolar patients). Carbamazepine-related ejaculatory failure in a man treated for trigeminal neuralgia ceased after the discontinuation of carbamazepine. Stopping medication is probably not a viable choice in patients treated for epilepsy, however. Resolution of anorgasmia associated with gabapentin (in a bipolar patient) occurred after switching to valproic acid. The fact that, contrary to other "older" anticonvulsants, valproic acid does not change sex hormone and sex hormone-binding globulin levels also suggests the usefulness of switching to valproic acid. However, long-term treatment with valproic acid may be associated with other complications, such as polycystic ovaries. Switching to or adding lamotrigine helped with impotence and/or anorgasmia associated with various anticonvulsants (carbamazepine, gabapentin, phenobarbital, valproic acid in various combinations) in three men treated for epilepsy. Similarly, switching to clonazepam worked for sexual dysfunction associated with diazepam. Thus switching to or adding another anticonvulsant such as lamotrigine might be a viable option; however, solid evidence for this approach is lacking. Several studies also demonstrated that anticonvulsant monotherapy was associated with lesser changes in hormonal and hormone-binding protein levels. Thus limiting the number of anticonvulsants used, whenever possible, could also be helpful.

Some of the management strategies for sexual dysfunction, such as drug holidays or dose reduction, may not be an option for patients with epilepsy. Nothing substantive is known about scheduling sexual activity around the dose (i.e., sex just prior to one daily dose), using antidotes (what is their effect on seizure threshold?), and waiting for spontaneous remission. These remain possible yet untested management strategies. Selecting an anticonvulsant with a lower

Table 11.6   General strategies for management of sexual dysfunction associated with anticonvulsants

Physician	Patient
1. Establish baseline sexual functioning	1. Participate in psychoeducation
2. Eliminate other possible causes of sexual dysfunction (e.g., smoking)	2. Initiate exercise and healthy lifestyle
3. Choose monotherapy whenever possible	3. Reduce psychosocial stressors
4. Choose an anticonvulsant with low frequency of sexual dysfunction (unknown at present, maybe valproic acid) or low effect on sex hormones/sex hormone binding globulin	
5. Use alternative strategies for sexual dysfunction (e.g., psychotherapy, sex therapy)	
6. Consider switching to another anticonvulsant if possible (e.g., lamotrigine)	
7. Consider antidotes (unknown at present)	
8. Encourage patient with his/her tasks	

frequency of sexual dysfunction as the drug of first choice when starting a patient on an anticonvulsant seems to be a prudent approach. Switching to another anticonvulsant (if possible) in case of existing sexual dysfunction may be a viable option. Adding lamotrigine remains an untested possibility. As Morrell (1991) suggested, psychotherapy, behavioral therapy, and sexual therapy could be useful in epilepsy patients who also have sexual problems. Creativity and caution in selecting medications remain the basic guiding strategies in management of anticonvulsant-associated sexual dysfunction.

CONCLUSIONS

Sexual dysfunction may occur as a complication of anticonvulsant therapy and have a negative impact on self-esteem, quality of life, and intimate relationships. The exact frequency and mechanism of action of sexual dysfunction associated with anticonvulsants are not known. Hormonal changes have been implicated with older anticonvulsants, with the exception of valproic acid. The mechanism of action of sexual dysfunction associated with newer anticonvulsants may be different, however. Hyposexuality, which is frequently reported in epileptic patients, is a factor complicating both the estimates of sexual dysfunction frequency associated with anticonvulsants and its management. The management strategies for sexual dysfunction associated with anticonvulsants have not been studied. Using monotherapy, selecting anticonvulsants with a lower frequency of hormonal changes, and possibly switching to anticonvulsants with a "theoretically" lower frequency of sexual dysfunction seem to be the most prudent strategies at the present time.

REFERENCES

Balon R, Ramesh C, Pohl R. Sexual dysfunction associated with diazepam but not with clonazepam. *Can J Psychiatry*. 1989;34:947–948.

Bergen D, Daugherty S, Eckenfels E. Reduction of sexual activities in females taking antiepileptic drugs. *Psychopathology*. 1992;25:1–4.

Blumer D, Walker AE. Sexual behavior in temporal lobe epilepsy. *Arch Neurol*. 1967;16:37–43.

Brannon GE, Rolland PD. Anorgasmia in a patient with bipolar disorder type 1 treated with gabapentin. *J Clin Psychopharmacol*. 2000;20:379–381.

Brunet M, Rodamilans M, Martinez-Osaba MJ, et al. Effects of long-term antiepileptic therapy on the catabolism of testosterone. *Pharmacol Toxicol*. 1995;76:371–375.

Clark JD, Elliott J. Gabapentin-induced anorgasmia. *Neurology*. 1999;53:2209.

Connell JMC, Rapeport WG, Beastall GH, Brodie JM. Changes of circulating androgens during short-term carbamazepine therapy. *Br J Clin Pharmacol*. 1984;17:347–351.

Duncan S, Blacklaw J, Beastall GH, Brodie MJ. Sexual function in women with epilepsy. *Epilepsia*. 1997;38:1074–1081.

Duncan S, Blacklaw J, Beastall GH, Brodie MJ. Antiepileptic drug therapy and sexual function in men with epilepsy. *Epilepsia*. 1999;40:197–204.

Erfurth A, Amann B, Grunze H. Female genital disorder as adverse symptom of lamotrigine treatment. *Neuropsychobiology*. 1998;38:200–201.

Fenwick PBC, Toone BK, Wheeler MJ, Nanjee MN, Grant R, Brown D. Sexual behavior in a centre for epilepsy. *Acta Neurol Scand*. 1985;71:428–435.

Fossey MD, Hamner MB. Clonazepam-related sexual dysfunction in male veterans with PTSD. *Anxiety*. 1995;1:233–236.

Gastaut H, Collomb H. Etude du comportement sexuel chez les epileptiques psychomoteurs [Study of sexual behavior in psychomoteur epilepsy]. *Ann Med Psychol (Paris)*. 1954;112:657–696.

Grant AC, Oh H. Gabapentin-induced anorgasmia in women. *Am. J. Psychiatry*. 2002;159:1247.

Guldner GT, Morrell MJ. Nocturnal penile tumescence and rigidity evaluation in men with epilepsy. *Epilepsia*. 1996;37:1211–1214.

Herzog AG. Psychoneuroendocrine aspects of temporolimbic epilepsy. Part II: Epilepsy and reproductive steroids. *Psychosomatics*. 1999;40: 102–108.

Herzog AG, Seibel MM, Schomer DL, Vaitukaitis JL, Geschwind N. Reproductive endocrine disorders in women with partial seizures of temporal lobe origin. *Arch Neurol*. 1986a;43:341–346.

Herzog AG, Seibel MM, Schomer DL, Vaitukaitis JL, Geschwind N. Reproductive endocrine disorders in men with partial seizures of temporal lobe origin. *Arch Neurol*. 1986b;43:347–350.

Hierons R, Saunders M. Impotence in patients with temporal-lobe lesions. *Lancet*. 1966;2:761–764.

Husain AM, Carwile ST, Miller PP, Radtke RA. Improved sexual function in three men taking lamotrigine for epilepsy. *South Med J*. 2000;93:335–336.

Isojarvi JIT, Laatikainen TJ, Pakarinen AJ, Juntunen KTS, Myllala VV.

Polycystic ovaries and hyperandrogenism in women taking valproate for epilepsy. *N Engl J Med.* 1993;329:1383–1388.

Isojarvi JIT, Pakarinen AJ, Myllyla VV. Effects of carbamazepine therapy on serum sex hormone levels in male patients with epilepsy. *Epilepsia.* 1988;29:781–786.

Isojarvi JIT, Pakarinen AJ, Ylipalosaari PJ, Myllyla VV. Serum hormones in male epileptic patients receiving anticonvulsant medication. *Arch Neurol.* 1990;47:670–676.

Jensen P, Jensen SB, Sorensen PS, et al. Sexual dysfunction in male and female patients with epilepsy: a study of 86 outpatients. *Arch Sex Behav.* 1990;19:1–14.

Kluver H, Bucy PC. Preliminary analysis of functions of the temporal lobes in monkeys. *Arch Neurol Psychiatry.* 1939;42:979–1000.

Labbate LA, Rubey RN. Gabapentin-induced ejaculatory failure and anorgasmia. *Am J Psychiatry.* 1999;156:972.

Lambert MV. Seizures, hormones, and sexuality. *Seizure.* 2001;10:319–340.

Leris ACA, Stephens J, Hines JEW, McNicholas TA. Carbamazepine-related ejaculatory failure. *Br J Urol.* 1997;79:485.

Macphee GJA, Larkin JG, Butler E, Beastall GH, Brodie MJ. Circulating hormones and pituitary responsiveness in young epileptic men receiving long-term antiepileptic medication. *Epilepsia.* 1988;29:468–475.

Mattson RH, Cramer JA. Epilepsy, sex hormones, and antiepileptic drugs. *Epilepsia.* 1985;26(Suppl 1):S40–S51.

Mattson RH, Cramer JA, Collins JF, et al. Comparison of carbamazepine, phenobarbital, phenytoin, and primidone in partial and secondarily generalized tonic–clonic seizures. *N Engl J Med.* 1985;313:145–151.

Montes JM, Ferrando, L. Gabapentin-induced anorgasmia as a cause of noncompliance in a bipolar patient. *Bipolar Disord.* 2001;3:52.

Morrell, MJ. Sexual dysfunction in epilepsy. *Epilepsia.* 1991;32(Suppl 6):S38–S45.

Morrell MJ, Guldner GT. Self-reported sexual function and sexual arousability in women with epilepsy. *Epilepsia.* 1996;37:1204–1210.

Penovich PE. The effects of epilepsy and its treatment on sexual and reproductive function. *Epilepsia.* 2000;41(Suppl 2):S53–S61.

Physicians' Desk Reference. 56th ed. Montvale, NJ: Medical Economics Company; 2002.

Pietropinto A, Arora A. Epilepsy and sexual functioning:survey analysis. *Medical Aspects of Human Sexuality.* 1988;22(January):140–144.

Rattya J, Turkka J, Pakarinen AJ, et al. Reproductive effects of valproate, carbamazepine, and oxcarbazepine in men with epilepsy. *Neurology.* 2001;56:31–36.

Sorensen AS, Bolwig TG. Personality and epilepsy: new evidence for a relationship? A review. *Compr Psychiatry.* 1987;28:369–383.

Spark RF, Wills CA, Royal H. Hypogonadism, hyperprolactinaemia, and temporal lobe epilepsy in hyposexual men. *Lancet.* 1984;1:413–417.

Wang PW, Ketter TA. Pharmacokinetics of mood stabilizers and new anticonvulsants. *Psychopharmacol Bull.* 2002;36:44–66.

Webber MP, Hauser WA, Ottman R, Annegers JF. Fertility in persons with epilepsy: 1935–1974. *Epilepsia.* 1996;27:746–752.

12. The Impact of Industrial Exposure on Sexual Function

Exposure to environmental toxins can occur through acute exposure to high doses of a compound, such as occurs in an industrial accident, through chronic exposure in the manufacturing process, or through contamination in the food and water supply. Recognition of a probable causal relationship between exposure to a toxin and sexual or reproductive abnormality may be difficult to establish, especially in cases of chronic exposure and exposure involving large groups of individuals. The effects of chronic exposure may be difficult to isolate from the effects of aging and other processes. In industrial accidents, a limited number of workers exposed to high levels of a toxin may be found to have high levels of sexual abnormalities, compared to other workers of the same age group in the same setting who were not subjected to accidental exposure to the same toxin. Potential litigation for financial compensation of damages suffered from exposure in a work setting clearly distorts the usefulness of self-report. Most evidence concerning the sexual effects of exposure to toxins is derived from studies of industrial accidents and studies of chronic industrial exposure to toxins. For obvious reasons, establishment of causal relationships between environmental contamination and sexual or reproductive abnormalities is difficult.

WORK-RELATED EXPOSURE TO TOXINS

Industrial exposure to certain compounds has been reported to be related to the development of sexual disorders in humans (summarized in Table 12.1). For example, exposure to methylmercury has been

Table 12.1 Sexual problems associated with occupational exposure

Compound	Exposure Venue	Effect
Carbon disulfide	Rayon factory	Decreased libido, impotence
Chloredecone	Industry	Decreased fertility
Chlorinated hydrocarbons	Herbicides	Decreased libido, impotence
Dieldrin	Herbicides	Decreased libido, impotence
Dioxin	Industry	Decreased fertility
Disulphide	Factory	Abnormal reproductive hormones
Estrogen	Pharmaceutical factory	Impotence
Glycol esters	Factory	Abnormal reproductive hormones
Lead	Battery factories	Decreased libido, decreased fertility
Methylmercury	Dental	Decreased libido, decreased fertility
Manganese	Mining	Decreased libido, problems with ejaculation
Nitrous oxide	Dental	Impotence
Organophosphates	Herbicides	Decreased libido, impotence
Polychlorinated biphenyls	Plastics	Decreased fertility
Stilbene	Optical factory	Impotence, decreased fertility
Trinitrotoluene	Factory	Abnormal reproductive hormones
Toluene	Textile factory	Abnormal reproductive hormones
Trinitrotoluene	Munitions factory	Decreased libido, abnormal ejaculation

associated with decreased libido and abnormal sperm production. These effects can occur without other signs of mercury posioning. Certain fish, especially swordfish, have high concentrations of methylmercury. Mercury vapor is more easily absorbed than methylmercury; workers with chronic exposure to mercury vapor have been reported to have menstrual irregularities. Decreased fertility has been established in animals exposed to inorganic mercury. Because mercury is used in many dental amalgams, dental assistants experience occupational exposure to it.

Chronic lead exposure, which has been linked to hypothalamic–pituitary disturbances, typically is found in workers in battery factories and smelting industries.

Manganese has been reported to cause decreased libido and ejaculatory failure in exposed workers. Occupational exposure occurs via mining and industrial accidents. One series reported that 25% of workers in one facility had sexual problems secondary to manganese exposure, which may also be related to sexual abnormalities and difficulties in conception. One study found that approximately one-fourth of manganese mine workers in Chile had decreased libido and abnormal ejaculation. Other studies have found that workers exposed to manganese dust have lower rates of reproduction than other workers.

There is some evidence that industrial exposure to certain organic solvents may be related to sexual abnormalities. These include some glycol esters, disulphide, and trinitrotoluene. Studies in different countries have found that workers exposed to carbon disulphide, a compound used in fabric manufacture, have high rates of sexual dysfunction. A Finnish study reported that workers exposed to carbon disulphide had higher rates of decreased libido and impotence than workers not exposed to these compounds. Workers in Japanese rayon factories exposed to carbon disulphide in the manufacturing process have been reported to complain of low sexual desire. One study indicated that workers exposed to carbon disulphide, well below the Finnish threshold limit, had signs of abnormalities in the pituitary–gonadal axis. A study in Poland found that women exposed to carbon disulphide reported increased frequency of low libido and earlier menopause than women not exposed to this chemical. Levels of estradiol, progesterone, and testosterone were lower in women with chronic exposure.

Toluene is an aromatic solvent used in the manufacturing of shoes, textiles, plastics, and electronics. Hormonal abnormalities have been reported in workers exposed to this chemical. Exposure to trinitrotoluene, a worldwide environmental contaminant used in munitions manufacture, has been associated with decreased libido and erectile failure.

A variety of other compounds has been suspected of causing sexual abnormalities following occupational exposure to them; these include estrogen, nitrous oxide, and stilbene derivatives. In one series, 20% of men working in a oral contraceptive factory had hyperestrogenism, gynecomastia, decreased libido, and impotence. Interestingly, there has been one report of impotence associated with exposure to a European hair tonic containing estrogen. Prolonged exposure to nitrous oxide, reported in patients who abused the substance as well as in dentists using nitrous oxide in poorly ventilated offices, has been associated with polyneuropathy and impotence.

Stilbene derivatives are used in the manufacturing of optical brightening agents. Workers exposed to these agents show an increased incidence of impotence and low testosterone levels. There have also been reports that industrial exposure to chloredecone (kepone) resulted in abnormal spermogenesis. There is some evidence that exposure to polychlorinated biphenyls, now banned but formerly used in the manufacture of plastics and paints, may be associated with decreased fertility. Polybrominated biphenyls are used as fire retardants in plastics and are very similar structurally to the polychlorinated biphenyls. It is unclear whether these compounds have adverse effects on sexual function or reproduction.

ENVIRONMENTAL TOXINS

There have also been reports of human sexual dysfunction associated with exposure to pesticides. Several reports have suggested that certain herbicides, such as organophosphates and chlorinated hydrocarbon compounds such as dieldrin, may be associated with impotence. Exposure to 2,4,5-trichlorphenoxy acetic acid has been associated with decreased libido and impotence; this compound also has a toxic breakdown product called dioxins, which has been related to decreased fertility. Workers involved in the manufacture of dibromochloropropane and ethyline dibromide have been found to have abnormal fertility. The environmental concerns with pesticides and herbicides is that they are used in large volumes in agriculture. The water from the treated land then drains into rivers and eventually reaches reservoirs that provide drinking water and irrigation for other crops.

Substantial evidence has accumulated on the hormone-like effects of environmental chemicals, such as pesticides, on wildlife and humans. Attention has focused on the ubiquitous environmental contaminants that have weak estrogenic activity (the xenoestrogens). More recently, research has indicated that many of these compounds, labeled *endocrine disrupters*, may have effects on the androgen receptor as well. The endocrine effects of these compounds are believed to be due to their ability to mimic, antagonize, and disrupt the synthesis of endogenous hormones, and disrupt the synthesis of hormone receptors. Products such as lidane are believed to interfere with the metabolism of endogenous estrogen. In many cases, the hormone-like activity of these compounds was discovered long after they were released into the environment. Interest in the effects of environmental pollutants on human reproductive behavior began relatively recently. For example, reports of the harmful effects of the pesticide dibromomchloropropane were first reported in 1987.

Agriculture accounts for the majority of herbicide use. At least, 60% of the agricultural herbicides are theoretically capable of disrupting the endocrine or reproductive systems of animals. The possible significance of this effect becomes apparent when it is realized that U.S. agriculture used over 461 million pounds of active herbicide ingredients in 1995. A number of "inactive ingredients" have been also been identified as endocrine disrupters. For many environmental contaminants, it is assumed that a minimum concentration is necessary before the contaminant is considered harmful. Some investigators have questioned whether the theoretical assumption of threshold effect should be used in the same manner with endocrine disrupters that mimic the actions of endogenous hormones. From this perspective, environmental exposure automatically exceeds the threshold value.

Much of the research has focused on possible relationships between environmental exposure to pollutants and carcinogenesis and embryonic development. Many of these human-made chemicals bind to androgen, estrogen, and sex hormone-binding globulin. Although any given toxic substance may have a low concentration in the environment, it may have the ability to interact with several steroid-sensitive pathways. In vitro research can identify the mechanisms by which individual compounds interrupt reproductive activity. However, vertebrates are usually exposed to mixtures of endocrine disrupters. Certain environmental contaminants, such as chlorinated aromatic hydrocarbons, are ubiquitous in the environment and food chain and persist in the environment for decades. Their half-lives in humans is measured in years.

Organochlorine pesticides have received attention in the media because of their persistence in the environment. These include compounds such as DDT (dichlorodiphenyltrichloroethane) and its metabolites DDE (dichlorodiphenyldichlororethylene) and dieldrin. In addition, exposure to other compounds has been related to endocrine abnormalities in humans. Studies have demonstrated that male workers exposed to styrene in plastics manufacturing plants have elevated prolactin levels. Female dry-cleaning plant workers also have been reported to have elevated prolactin levels. Toluene exposure in printers has been associated with a decrease in gonadotropin levels.

Other human-made compounds were found to be estrogenic upon degradation. Polysterene tubes release nonylphenol, and polycarbonate flasks release bisphenol. Some detergents release estrogenic alkylphenols upon degradation during sewage treatment. Bisphenol has been found to be a contaminant in canned food in many countries; it is also used in dental sealants and composites. Other xenoestrogens have been identified in the plastizicers benzylbutylphthalate and dibutylphthalate, in the antioxidant butylhydroxyanisole, the rubber additive p-phenylphnol, and the disinfectant o-phenylphenol. Vinclozolin, an antifugal agent, has recently been shown to have antiandrogenic effects.

Exposure to endocrine disrupter pollutants has been associated with reduced fertility, disrupted mating patterns, and deformities of the reproductive tract in a variety of animal species. The evidence linking exposure to these environmental pollutants to abnormalities is clearer in wildlife than in humans. Some investigators have suggested

INDUSTRIAL EXPOSURE

that reproductive abnormalities in wildlife be regarded as important sentinels of ecosystem health of relevance to humans. The magnitude of environmental pollution with endocrine disrupters has lead some investigators to speculate that chronic exposure may result in adaptive alterations in genes that encode steroid receptors, allowing the sex hormone receptor to discriminate between natural steroids and endocrine disrupters.

Humans synthesize steroids by a pathway that involves the transformation of cholesterol to progestins, then androgens, and then estrogens. Females have elevated plasma estrogens in relation to plasma androgens, whereas males have a reverse ratio. This ratio is believed to create a sex-specific hormonal milieu such that a potent antiandrogen would have an overall estrogen-like effect. It is clear that endocrine disrupters could have varied effects, depending on their various receptor affinities. For example, a prominent metabolite of the insecticide DDT is an androgen receptor antagonist and has been shown to interfere with erectile capacity in animal models. There is reason to suspect that farm workers exposed repetitively to high doses of insecticides have a higher incidence of erectile dysfunction, decreased libido, and lowered sperm counts.

Studies suggest that many such industrial pollutants may have adverse effects on humans. However, much of this data, especially concerning carcinogenesis, is conflicting. Some of this data includes the observation of increasing incidence of hormone-dependent diseases and conditions such as hypospadias, testicular, prostate, and breast cancers, lower age of puberty, and decreasing fertility. In many cases, humans are exposed to levels of endocrine disrupters that are close to those which produce toxic effects in animals. There is minimal data on thresholds for toxic exposure in humans or for additive effects of subthreshold amounts of pollutants. A number of occupational chemical exposures, resulting in sexual dysfunction, have been reported. There is relatively little definitive information concerning the sexual effects of various industrial pollutants on humans. However, there is considerable evidence suggestive of possible adverse effects. Regulation and the threat of legal action have decreased exposure to industrial toxins in many industrialized nations. It is unclear how much effect current levels of exposure have on sexual function.

EFFECTS ON LABORATORY ANIMALS AND WILDLIFE

There is convincing evidence that many environmental pollutants cause abnormalities of sexual development and behavior in animals.

The relevance of this data to humans is unclear. Many commonly used pesticides cause sexual behavioral disturbances in animals. Pesticides such as organophosphates and compounds used as organic solvents (such as carbon disulphide) are strongly implicated. As noted, many commonly used insecticides have either estrogenic or androgenic properties, and their effects on humans are unknown. Pyrethroid insecticides such as sumithrin, fenvalerate, d-trans-allethrin, and premethrin, widely used agents for indoor pest control, are estrogenic and considered to be hormone disrupters. Fenvalerate exposure in utero disrupts male sexual behavior in offspring. Dicofol, an organochlorine pesticide, disrupts estrus cycles in laboratory animals in a dose-dependent fashion.

A number of pesticides, including the fungicides fenarimol, triadimefon, and triadimenol, are weak estrogenic receptor agonists. Fenarimol and dicofol also have effects on estrogenic receptor activation. Tris(4-chlorophenyl)methanol (TCPM) is a global contaminant that is structurally similar to DDT and binds with the androgen receptor in vitro. Antiandrogenic pesticides such as procymidone, linuron, iprodione, chlozolinate, and p,p'-DDE all cause sexual maturation problems in laboratory animals. DDT has been found to play a role in endocrine disruption. Methoxychlor, a DDT-related compound, inhibits testosterone production in rats. In vitro exposure to the pesticide methoxychlor has been found to influence sexual behavior in rat offspring. Hexachlorocyclohexane (HCH), one of the most widely used pesticides, has been reported to adversely affect reproductive activity in animals. Chlordecone, a chlorinated pesticide, activates progesterone receptors.

Reptiles exposed to industrial pollutants have been reported to show sexual reproductive abnormalities. Alligators and turtles exposed to water polluted with insecticides demonstrate abnormalities in sexual behavior. Fish near pulp mill effluents evidence alteration in reproductive patterns.

One cannot state with certainty whether human exposure to these compounds is disruptive to sexual behavior. As noted, many of the compounds known to be dangerous pollutants have become restricted, and human exposure to compounds known to cause sexual problems has been limited in developed countries.

INDUSTRIAL EXPOSURE

REFERENCES

Baccarelli A, Pesatori A, Bertazzi P. Occuptaional and environmental agents as endocrine disrupters: experimental and human evidence. *J Endocrinol Invest.* 2000;23:777–781.

Batty J, Lim R. Morphological and reproductive characteristics of male mosquito fish inhabiting sewage-contaminated water in New South Wales. *Arch Environ Contam Toxicol*. 1999;36:301–307.

Beard A, Rawlings N. Reproductive effects in mink exposed to the pesticides, lindane, carbofuran, and pentachlorophenol in a multigenerational study. *J Reproduct Fertil*. 1998;113:95–104.

Belmouden M, Asssabbane A, Ichou YA. Adsorption characteristics of a phenoxy acetic acid herbicide. *J Environ Monit*. 2000;2:257–260.

Bowerman WW, Best DA, Grubb TG, Sikarskie JG, Giesy JP. Assessment of environmental endocrine disrupters in bald eagles of the Great Lakes. *Chemosphere*. 2000;41:1569–74.

Brien S, Heaton J, Racz W, Adams M. Effects of an environmental antiandrogen on erectile function in an animal penile erection model. *J Urol*. 2000;163:1315–1321.

Brim MS, Alam SK, Jenkins LG. Organochlorine pesticides and heavy metals in muscle and ovaries of Gulf coast striped bass (Morone saxatilis) from the Apalachicola River, Florida, USA. *J Environ Sci Health B*. 2001;36:15–27.

Crews D, Willingham E, Skipper JK. Endocrine disrupters: present issues, future directions. *Q Rev Boil*. 2000;75:243–260.

Daniell W, Claypoole K, Checkoway H, Smith-Weller T, Dager S, Townes B, Rosenstock L. Neuropsychological function in retired workers with previous long term occupational exposure solvents. *Occup Environ Med*. 1999;56:93–105.

Danzo BJ. The effects of environmental hormones on reproduction. *Cell Mol Life Sci*. 1998;54:1249–1264.

Daston GP, Gooch JW, Breslin WJ, Shuey DL, Nikiforov AI, Fico TA, Gorsuch JW. Environmental estrogens and reproductive health: a discussion of the human and environmental data. *Reprod Toxicol*. 1997;11:465–481.

Degen GH, Bolt HM. Endocrine disrupters: update on xenoestrogens. *Int Arch of Occup and Environ Health*. 2000;73:433–441.

de Solla S, Bishop C, van derKraak G, Brooks R. Impact of organochlorine contamination on levels of sex hormones and external morphology on common snapping turtles. *Environ Health Perspect*. 1998;106:253–260.

Eckols K, Williams J, Uphouse L. Effects of chlordecone on progesterone receptors in immature and adult rats. *Toxicol Appl Pharmacol*. 1989;100:506–516.

Espir M, Hall J, Shirreffs J, Stevens D. Impotence in farm workers. *Br Med J*. 1979;2:423–425.

Forman R, Gilmour-White S, Forman N. Drug-induced infertility and sexual dysfunction. Cambridge, U.K.: Cambridge University Press; 1996.

Gray L, Wolf C, Lambright C, Mann P, Price M, Cooper R, Ostby J. Administration of potentially antiandrogenic pesticides (procymidone, linuron, iprodione, chlozolinate, p,p-DDE,ketoconazole) and toxic substances (dibutyl- and diethylhexyl phthalate, PCB 169 and ethane dimethane suplonate) during sex differentiation produces diverse profiles of reproductive malformations in the male rat. *Toxicol Ind Health*. 1999;15:94–118.

Guillette L, Gorss T, Masson G, Matter J, Percival H, Woodward A. Developmental abnormalities of the gonad and abnormal sex hormone concentrations in juvenile alligators from contaminated and control lakes in Florida. *Environ Health Perspect.* 1994;102:680–688.

Guillette LJ. Organochlorine pesticides as endocrine disrupters in wildlife. *Cent Eur J Public Health.* 2000;8(Suppl.):34–35.

Harrison PT, Holmes P, Humfrey CD. Reproductive health in humans and wildlife: are adverse trends associated with environmental chemical exposure? *Sci Total Environ.* 1997;205:97–106.

Healy J, Bradley SD, Northage C, Scobbie E. Inhalation exposure in secondary aluminum smelting. *Ann Occup Hyg.* 2001;45:217–225.

Hoyer AP, Jorgensen T, Broeck JW, Grandjean P. Organochlorine exposure and breast cancer survival. *J Clin Epidemiol.* 2000;53:323–30.

Jaga K. What are the implications of the interaction between DDT and estrogen receptors in the body? *Med Hypotheses.* 2000;54:18–25.

Johnson RA, Harris RE, Wilke RA. Are pesticides really endocrine disrupters? *WMJ.* 2000;99:34–38.

Kelce WR, Gray LE, Wilson EM. Antiandrogens as environmental endocrine disrupters. *Reprod Fertil Dev.* 1998;10:105–111.

Khim J, Lee K, Kannan K, Villeneuve D, Giesy J, Koh C. Trace organic contaminants in sediment and water from Ulsan Bay and its vicinity, Korea. *Arch Environ Contam Toxiocl.* 2001;40:141–150.

Khim JS, Lee KT, Villenueve DL, Kannan K, Giesy JP, Koh CH. In vitro determination of dioxin-like and estrogenic activity in sediment and water from Ulsan Bay and its vicinity, Korea. *Arch Environ Contam Toxicol.* 2001;40:151–160.

Kkebaek N, Leffers H, Meyts E. Should we watch what we eat and drink? Report on the International Workshop on hormones and endocrine disrupters in food and water: possible impact on human health. Copenhagen, Denmark, 27–30, May, 2000. Trends in Endocrinology and Metabolism, 2000, 11, 291–293.

Kloas W, Lutz I, Einspnaier, R. Amphibians as a model to study endocrine disrupters: Estrogen activity of environmental chemicals in vitro and in vivo. *Sci Total Environ.* 1999;225:59–68.

Layzer R. Myeloneuropathy after prolonged exposure to nitrous oxide. *Lancet.* 1978;1:1227–1230.

LeBlanc GA, Bain LJ, Wilson VS. Pesticides: multiple mechanisms of demasculinization. *Mol Cell Endocrinol.* 1997;126:1–5.

Luderer U, Morgan M, Brodkin C, Kalman D, Faustman E. Reproductive endocrine effects of acute exposure to toluene in men and women. *Occup Environ Med.* 1999;56:657–666.

Lutz I, KLoas W. Amphibians as a model to study endocrine disrupters: Environmental pollution and estrogen receptor binding. *Sci Total Environ.* 1999;225:49–57.

Moniz A, Cruz-Casallas P, Oliviera C, Lusisano A, Florio J, Nicolau A, et al. Perinatal fenvalerate exposure: behavioral and endocrinological changes in male rats. *Neurotoxicol Teratol.* 1999;21:611–618.

Monteiro PR, Reis-Henriques M, Coimbra J. Plasma steroid levels in female flounder (Platichthys leses) after chronic dietary exposure to single polycyclic aromatic hydrocarbons. *Mar Environ Res.* 2000;49:453–467.

Moorman WJ, Cheever KL, Skaggs S, Clark J, Turner T, Marlow K, Schrader S. Male adolescent exposure to endocrine-disrupting pesticides:vinclozlin exposure in peripubertal rabbits. *Andrologia*. 2000;32:285–293.

Munkittrick K, McMaster M, McCarthy L, Servos M, van der Kraa G. An overview of recent studies on the potential of pulp-mill effluent to alter reproductive parameters in fish. *J Toxicol Environ Health B Crit Rev*. 1998;1:347–371.

Nilsson R. Endocrine modulators in the food chain and environment. *Toxicol Pathol*. 2000;28:420–431.

Olea N, Pazos P, Exposito J. Inadvertent exposure to xenoestrogens. *Eur J Cancer Prev*. 1998;7,(Suppl 1):S17–S23.

Oyama M, Ikeda T, Lim T, Ikebukuro K, Masuda Y, Karube I. Detection of toxic chemicals with high sensitivity by measuring the quantity of induced P450 mRNAs based on surface plamon resonance. *Biotechnol Bioeng*. 2000;7:217–222.

Peck A. Impotence in farm workers. *Br Med J*. 1970;2:690.

Pieleszek A, Stanosz S. Effect of carbon disulphide on menopause in women. *Med Pr*. 1994;45:383–391.

Pieleszek, A. The effect of carbon disulphide on menopause, concentrations of monoamines, gonadotrophins, estrogens, and androgens in women. *Ann Acad Med Stetin*. 1997;43:255–267.

Quinn M, Wegman D, Greaves I, Hammond S, Ellenbecker M, Spa R, Smith ER. Investigation of reports of sexual dysfunction among male workers manufacturing stilbene derivatives. *Am J Ind Med*. 1990;18:55–68.

Safe SH. Bisphenol A and related endocrine disrupters. *Toxicol Sci*. 2000;56:251–252.

Safe SH. Endocrine disrupters and human health—is there a problem? An update. *Environ Health Perspect*. 2000;108:587–493.

Schoni P, Sumpter JP. Several environmental oestrogens are also anti-androgens. *J Endocrinol*. 1998;158:327–329.

Short P, Colborn T. Pesticide use in the US and policy implications: a focus on herbicides. *Toxicol Ind Health*. 1999;15:240–275.

Sierra-Santoyo A, Hernadez M, Albores A, Cebrian M. Sex-dependent regulation of hepatic cytochrome P-450 by DDT. *Toxicol Sci*. 2000;54:81–87.

Sinawat S. The environmental impact on male fertility. *J Med Assoc Thai*. 2000;83:880–885.

Snedeker SM. Pesticides and breast cancer risk: a review of ddt, dde, and diledrin. *Environ Health Perspect*. 2001;109:35–47.

Sonnenschein C, Soto AM. An updated review of environmental estrogen and androgen mimics and antagonists. *J Steroid Biochem Mol Biol*. 1998;65:143–150.

Soto AM, Michaelson CL, Prechtl NV, Weill BC, Sonnenschein C, Olea-Serrano F, Olea N. Assays to measure estrogen and androgen agonists and antagonists. *Adv Exp Med Biol*. 1998;444:23–28

Susskind R, Hertzberg V. Human health effects of 2,4,5-T and its toxic contaminants. *JAMA*. 1984;251:2372–2380.

Wager G, Tolonen M, Stenman U, Helpio E. Endocrinological studies in men exposed occupationally to carbon disulfide. *J Toxicology and Environmental Health*. 1981;7:363–371.

Takebayashi T, Omae K, Ishizuka C, Nomiyama T, Sakurai H. Cross sectional observation of the effects of carbon disulphide on the nervous system, endocrine system, and subjective symptoms in rayon manufacturing works. *Occup Environ Med.* 1998;55:473–479.

Vonier P, Crain D, McLachlan J, Guillette L, Arnold S. Interaction of environmental chemicals with the estrogen and progesterone receptors from the oviduct of the American alligator. *Environ Health Perspect.* 1996;104:1318–1322.

You L, Casanova M, Archibeque-Engle S, Sar M, Fan L, Heck H. Impaired male sexual development in perinatal Spraque-Dawley and Long-Evans hooded rats exposed in utero and lactactionally to p,p-DDE. *Toxicol Sci.* 1998;45:162–173.

You L, Chan S, Bruce J, Archieque-Engle S, Cassanova M, Orton J, Heck H. Modulation of testosterone-metabolizing hepatic cytochrome P-450 enzymes in developing Sprague-Dawley rats following in utero exposure to p,p-DDE. *Toxicol Appl Pharmacol.* 1999;158:197–205.

INDUSTRIAL EXPOSURE

13. The Impact of Recreational Drugs on Sexual Function

Table 13.1 summarizes the effects of nicotine, marijuana, alcohol, MDNA, cocaine, amphetamines, and heroin and methadone on sexual function.

NICOTINE

Abundant evidence indicates that smoking contributes to atherosclerosis, and population studies have demonstrated an association between smoking and the risk of erectile dysfunction or failure. The incidence of erectile dysfunction was higher in smokers in a population study of aging males in the Boston suburbs. Population studies conducted in Thailand, Australia, Italy, and Malaysia have all reported a higher incidence of erectile dysfunction in smokers. A prospective study of a sample of aging males in the Boston suburbs found that current smoking predicted subsequent development of erectile dysfunction.

Studies in laboratory animals have demonstrated a deleterious effect of nicotine on erectile function. In one study, the smoke from two or three cigarettes prevented five out of six mongrel dogs from obtaining erections after pelvic nerve stimulation. Laboratory studies in animals have shown that long-term exposure to cigarette smoke increases penile arterial blood pressure and decreases penile nitric oxide synthase. Nicotine also decreases venous constriction in laboratory animals.

Table 13.1 Recreational drugs and sexual function

Substance	Impact on Sexual Function
Nicotine	Risk factor for impotence
Marijuana	Decreased libido with chronic use
Alcohol	Small doses used acutely, may release inhibitions, whereas high doses impair performance; chronic use may be associated with impotence.
MDNA	Erectile failure, orgasmic delay, increased "libido"
Cocaine	Acute doses may increase sexual activity and preformance, whereas chronic dosing impairs performance and libido in both sexes.
Amphetamines	Increased libido
Heroin, methadone	Decreased libido in both sexes

Human laboratory studies also have demonstrated deleterious effects of nicotine on erectile function. Chronic smokers exposed to two high-nicotine cigarettes had a decreased rate of penile circumference change in response to erotic films in comparison to smokers receiving low-nicotine cigarettes. Nocturnal penile tumescence measures are different in smokers and nonsmokers, with decreased parameters of erectile function related to the number of cigarettes smoked. Smokers also have been shown to have a decreased response to intracavernosal injections of papaverine and to have decreased blood flow in the pudendal arteries. Smokers without erectile dysfunction have been demonstrated to show a dose–response relationship between smoking and changes in erectile activity during sleep; the number of cigarettes smoked correlated negatively with penile rigidity. Decreased penile tumescence time and increased rapidity of detumescence were noted in heavy smokers (more than 40 cigarettes per day).

MARIJUANA

Marijuana and its active ingredient delta-9-tetrahydrocanabinol have been shown to decrease testosterone with chronic usage. It is unclear whether chronic marijuana use has a deleterious effect on sexual function. Many chronic users of marijuana report decreased libido.

ALCOHOL

Acute use of alcohol may facilitate subjective arousal while decreasing physiological arousal. This finding has been demonstrated in well-controlled studies in both sexes. Alcohol levels of more than 120 mg have been shown to decrease various measures of nocturnal penile tumescence.

Evidence concerning the prevalence of sexual disorders in alcoholics is contradictory, perhaps as a result of methodological inconsistencies. In particular, some studies included inpatients undergoing detoxification, whereas others have engaged outpatients who were still abusing alcohol or who were had achieved sobriety for varying time periods. Furthermore, many studies have engaged subjects with varying degrees of abuse over varying time periods. These disparate variables make it difficult to isolate direct effects of alcohol from other health problems. Many studies also lacked comparison groups. Nevertheless, there is considerable evidence that long-term severe alcohol abuse is related to impotence and testicular atrophy. A number of studies have reported higher rates of impotence in men with histories of chronic alcohol abuse than in normals; the impotence may be related to peripheral neuropathy. Alcoholics with cirrhosis tend to have lower levels of testosterone and higher levels of serum hormone-binding globulin than alcoholics without cirrhosis. It is of note that animal research has documented a toxic effect of alcohol on testicular steroidogenesis. In many alcoholics, an increase in the ratio of estrogen to testosterone may occur. The hyperestrogenism appears to occur only in the presence of cirrhosis, whereas testicular atrophy may preceed the onset of cirrhosis. The highest estradiol levels are reported in patients with cirrhosis and ascites or gynecomastia.

Several facts are worth noting. Some studies have not found sexual or endocrinological abnormalities in alcoholic patients without cirrhosis. The only consistent finding is that alcoholics reported more frequent loss of erections during episodes of heavy drinking. However, these men did not report decreased sexual satisfaction during periods of heavy drinking, but their sexual partners reported decreased satisfaction. Some studies have shown that some alcohol-dependent men recover potency when discontinuing alcohol use. However, the rate of potency problems is higher in recovering alcoholics than the general population.

Entries from daily diaries kept by female volunteers suggested that acute alcohol consumption has minimal effect on sexuality. However, the same women retrospectively reported an enhanced effect of alcohol consumption on sexual activity. This contradiction has been interpreted as reflecting an expectation that alcohol will increase sexual responsiveness. Many women also report transient sexual dysfunction while intoxicated. There is clearly a relationship between alcohol use and risky sexual behavior. The rates of incest and sexual abuse reported by alcoholics tend to be higher than those in the general population. Many cases of adult sexual abuse appear to be related to alcohol use in the victum, perpetrator, or both. A number of studies has found higher rates of incest and sexual abuse in women with alcoholism. Alcohol abuse appears to have minimal effects on hormonal function in women, at least, prior to cirrhosis. Alcohol intake causes a transient increase in prolactin; with continued alcohol abuse, some elevation of estrogen may be observed, which may be related to an increased rate of testosterone aromatization or a decreased rate of estradiol-to-estrone oxidation. There may be slight increases in progesterone. Hypoactive sexual desire disorder appears to be more common in women with alcohol abuse than in the general population. With the onset of cirrhosis comes amenorrrhea and hypogonadism. It is of note that several studies have reported that sexual function improves with sobriety.

ECSTASY (MDNA)

3,4-methyfenedioxymethamphetamine (MDNA) was first synthesized in Germany as an appetite suppressant. However, it was never produced commercially, instead becoming a drug of abuse. It increases the release of serotonin, dopamine, and norephinephrine from presynaptic neurons and also inhibits the reuptake of these neurotransmitters. It also inhibits monoamine oxidase. Desirable effects of this drug include a feeling of increased empathy, interpersonal closeness, euphoria, self-esteem, and altered visual perceptions. Desire and sexual satisfaction are increased by this drug. However, the drug also causes erectile failure and orgasmic delay.

COCAINE

Acute use may be associated with increased libido and, rarely, with priapism; chronic cocaine use may be associated with impotence, anorgasmia, and hyperprolactinemia. Cocaine has been shown to decrease intracavernosal pressure in laboratory animals. This action appears to be mediated by activation of the hippocampal formation. Nitric oxide appears to mediate the effect of cocaine on penile erection. Priapism has been reported with the use of topical cocaine.

AMPHETAMINES

Laboratory studies in animals have demonstrated an excitatory effect of amphetamines on sexual function. In naïve rates amphetamine facilitates sexual behavior, as evidenced by an increase in the amount of copulation, decreased ejaculatory latency, and decreased latency to mounting behavior. The effect of amphetamines on sexual behavior in rats is related to dopamine efflux in the nucleus accumbens. Drugs that effect D1/D2 receptor blockades have been shown to decrease sexual activity in rabbits. Low doses of amphetamines may have a libido-enhancing effect in humans. Patients with a history of amphetamine abuse report intensified orgasms and prolonged coitus on amphetamines. However, chronic use may inhibit sexual activity. Some users report spontaneous orgasm on high-dose amphetamines.

HEROIN AND METHADONE

Sexual difficulties occur at high doses and with prolonged usage of all of the opiates including heroin, methadone, codeine, oxycodone, hydromorphone and propoxyphene. All opiates are associated with decreased libido, ejaculatory failure, and anorasmia. Studies of patients on heroin and methadone have consistently shown that both drugs lower libido. Female patients frequently experience amenorrhea and abnormal menstrual cycles. Upon withdrawal from heroin, male patients have reported spontaneous erections and ejaculation as well as problems with rapid ejaculation. Similar findings have been obtained in studies of the effect of intrathecal administration of morphine for chronic pain. In one series of patients receiving an average daily dose of 4.8 mg of intrathecal morphine for approximately 2 years, decreased libido and erectile problems were noted in 23 out of 24 men. Decreased libido also occurred in 22 out 32 women. Male patients were found to have low levels of testosterone and sexual function was often restored by androgen replacement therapy. Low luteinizing hormone levels were found in females receiving intrathecal opioids.

REFERENCES

Abracen J, Looman J, Anderson D. Alcohol and drug abuse in sexual and nonsexual violent offenders. *Sex Abuse*. 2000;12:263–274.

Adams ML. Interactions between alcohol- and opioid-induced suppression of rat testicular tissue steriodogenesis in vivo. *Alcoholism, Clinical and Experimental Research*. 1997;21:684–690.

Agmo A, Paredes R, Ramos J, Conteras J. Dopamine and sexual behavior in the male rabbit. *Pharmacol Biochem Behav*. 1996;55:289–295.

Beckman L, Ackerman K. Women, alcohol, and sexuality. *Recent Dev Alcohol*. 1995;12:267–285.

Chan J, Huang C, Chan S. Nitric oxide as a mediator of cocaine-induced penile erection in the rat. *Br J Pharmacol*. 1996;118:155–161.

Chang A, Chan J, Chan S. Hippocampal noradrenergic neurotransmission in concurrent EEG resynchronization and inhibition of penile erection induced by cocaine in the rat. *Br J Pharmacy*. 2000;130:1553–1560.

Chang A, Chan J, Steno L, Chan S. Differential participation of hippocampal formation in cocaine-induced cortical electroencephalographic desynchronization and penile reaction in rat. *Synapse*. 1998;30:140–149.

Chang A, Kuo T, Chan J, Chan S. Concurrent elicitation of electroencephalogram desynchronization and penile erection by cocaine in the male rat. *Synapse.* 1996;24:233–239.

Cheon J, Han H, Jung H. Mechanism of sexual dysfunction in alcohol dependence pudental SEP studies. *Biol Psychiatry.* 1996;39:626.

Cicero T, Bell R, Widest W, Allison J, Polakoski K, Robins E. Function of the male sex organs in heroin and methadone users. *New Eng J Med.* 1975;292:882–887.

Clayton D, Shen W. Psychotropic-induced sexual dysfunction disorders: diagnosis, incidence, and management. *Drug Saf.* 1998;19:299–312.

Cooper A. The effects of intoxication levels of ethanol on nocturnal penile tumescence. *J Sex Marit Ther.* 1994;20:14–23.

Crowley T, Simpson R. Methadone and human sexual behavior. *Int J Addict.* 1978;13:285–295.

Dolezal C, Carballo-Dieguez A, Nieves-Rosa L, Diaz F. Substance abuse and sexual risk behavior: understanding their actions among four ethnic groups of Latino men who have sex with men. *J Subst Abuse.* 2000;11:323–336.

Ferrari F, Giuliano D. Involvement of dopamine D2 receptors in the effect of cocaine on sexual behavior and stretching–yawning of male rats. *Neuropharamcology.* 1997;36:769–777.

Ferrari F, Ottani A, Giuliani D. Inhibitory effects of the cannabinoid agonist HU 210 on rat sexual behavior. *Physiol Behav.* 2000;69:547–554.

Fiorelli RL, Amnfrey SJ, Belkoff LH, Finkelstein LH. Priapism associated with intranasal cocaine abuse. *J Urol.* 1990;143:584–585.

Fiorino D, Phillips A. Facilitation of sexual behavior and enhanced dopamine efflux in the nucleus accumbens of male rats after d-amphetamine-induced behavioral sensitization. *J Neurosci.* 1999a;19:456–463.

Fiorino D, Phillips A. Facilitation of sexual behavior in male rats following d-amphetamine-induced behavioral sensitization. *Psychopharmacology.* 1999b;142:200–208.

Frias J, Rodriquez R, Torrs J, Ruiz E, Ortega E. Effects of acute alcohol intoxication on pituitary–gonadal axis hormones, pituitary–adrenal axis hormones, beta-endorphin and prolactin in human adolescents of both sexes. *Life Sci.* 2000;67:1081–1086.

Gambert SR. Alcohol abuse: medical effects of heavy drinking in late life. *Geriatrics.* 1997;52:30–37.

Gavaler J, Rizzo A, Rossaro L, van Thiel, D, Brezza E, Deal, S. Sexuality of alcoholic postmenopausal women. *Alcohol Clin Exp Res.* 1994;18:269–271.

Gill J. The effects of moderate alcohol consumption on female hormone levels and reproductive function. *Alcohol Alcohol.* 2000;35:417–423.

Glena S, Richest A, Lao P, Dos Reuse J. Impact of cigarette smoking on papaverine-induced erections. *J Urol.* 1998;140:523–524.

Gumus B, Yigitoglu M, Lekili M, Uyanik B, Muezzinoglu TC. Effect of long-term alcohol abuse on male sexual function and serum gonadal hormone levels. *Int Urol Nephrol.* 1998;30:755–759.

Hayahida H, Fulimoto H, Yoshida K, Tomoyoshi K, Okamura T, Toda N. Comparison of neurogenic contraction and relaxation in canine corpora cavernosum and penile artery and vein. *Jpn J Pharmacol.* 1996;72:231–240.

Heiser K, Hartmann U. Disorders of sexual desire in a sample of women alcoholics. *Drug Alcohol Depend.* 1987;19:145–157.

Hunter CL, Talcott GW, Klesges RC, Lando H, Hadock Ck. Demographic, lifestyle, and psychosocial predictors of frequent intoxication and other indicators as estimates of alcohol-related problems in Air Force basic military recruits. *Mil Med.* 2000;15:539–545.

Jaffe A, Chen Y, Kisch E, Fischel B, Alon M, Stern N. Erectile dysfunction in hypertensive subjects: assessment of potential determinants. *Hypertension.* 1996;28:859–862.

Jensen S. Sexual function and dysfunction in younger married alcoholics: a comparative study. *Acta Psychiatr Scand.* 1984;69:543–549

Jiva T, Answer S. Priapism associated with chronic cocaine abuse. *Arch Intern Med.* 1994;154:1770.

Kall K. Effects of amphetamine on sexual behavior of male IV drug users in Stockholm: a pilot study. *AIDS Educ Prev.* 1992;4:6–17.

Keene L, Davies P. Drug-related erectile dysfunction. *Adverse Drug React Toxicol Rev.* 1999;18:5–24.

Klitzman R, Pope H, Hudson J. MDNA abuse and high-risk sexual behaviors among gay and bisexual men. *Am J Psychiatry.* 2000;157:1162–1164.

Klinge E, Alaranta S, Sjostrand N. Pharmacological analysis of nicotinic relaxation of bovine retractor muscle. *J Pharmacol Exp Ther* 1988;245:280–286.

Malatesta V, Pollach R, Crotty T, Peacock L. Acute alcohol intoxication and female orgasmic response. *J Sex Res.* 1982;18:1–17.

Martinez-Riera A, Santolaria-Ferandez F, Gonzalez R, et al. Alcoholic hypogonadism: hormonal response to clomiphene. *Alcohol.* 1995;12:581–587.

Mirin S, Meyer R, Mendelson J, Ellingboe J. Opiate use and sexual function. *Am J Psychiatry.* 1980;137:909–915.

Nirenberg T, Lipeman M, Begin A, Doolittle R, Broffman, T. The sexual relationship of male alcoholics and their female partners during periods of drinking and abstinence. *J Stud Alcohol.* 1990;51:565–568.

O'Farrell T, Kleinke C, Cutter H. Sexual adjustment of male alcoholics: changes from before to after receiving alcoholism counseling with or without marital therapy. *Addictive Behaviors.* 1988;23:419–423.

Pettinati H, Rukstalis M, Luck G, Volpicelli J, O'Brein C. Gender and psychiatric comorbidity: impact on clinical presentation of alcohol dependence. *Am J Addict.* 2000;9:242–252.

Rodriquez-Blaquez H, Cardona P, Rivera-Herrara J. Priapism associated with the use of topical cocaine. *J Urol.* 1990;14:358.

Rosen R. Alcohol and drug effects on sexual response: human experimental and clinical studies. *Ann Rev Sex Res.* 1991;2:119–179.

Schiavi R, Stimmel B, Mandeli J, White D. Chronic alcoholism and male sexual function. *Am J Psychiatry.* 1995;152:1045–1051.

Seecof R, Tennant F. Subjective perceptions to the intravenous rush of heroin and cocaine opioid addicts. *Am J Drug Alcohol Abuse.* 1986;12:79–87.

Siegel RK. Cocaine and sexual dysfunction: the curse of *mana coca. J Psychoactive Drugs.* 1982;14:71–74.

Slalom E, Ohki A, Bartlett F, Ivy T, Savanna S. Priapism in sickle cell disease: possible contibution of cocaine use. *Arch Int Med.* 1993;153:2287.

Taniguchi N, Kanedko S. Alcoholic effect on male sexual function. *Nippon Rinsho*. 1997;55:3040–3044.

Teusch L, Scherman N, Bohme H, Bender S, Eschmann-Mehl G, Gaspar E. Different patterns of sexual dysfunctions associated with psychiatric and psychopharmacological treatment. *Pharmacopsychiatry*. 1995;28:84–92.

Tjandra BS, Janknegt RA. Neurogenic impotence and lower urinary tract symptoms due to vitamin B1 deficiency in chronic alcoholism. *J Urol*. 1997;157:954–955.

Valimaki M, Laitinem K, Tiitinien A, Steman U, Ylostalo P. Gonadal function and morphology in non-cirrhotic female alcoholics: a controlled study with hormone measurements and ultrasonography. *Acta Obstet Gynecol Scand*. 1995;74:462–466.

Welch S, Howden-Chapman P, Collings SC. Survey of drug and alcohol use by lesbian women in New Zealand. *Addict Behav*. 1998;23:543–548.

Xie Y, Garban H, Ng C, Rajfer J, Gonzalez-Cadavid N. Effect of long-term passive smoking on erectile function and penile nitric synthase in the rat. *J Urol*. 1997;157:1121–1126.

Yoshitsugu M, Ihori M. [Endocrine disturbances in liver cirrhosis.] *Nippon Rinsho*. 1997;55:3002–3006.

14. Miscellaneous Drugs

A large number of pharmacological agents that fall into differing therapeutic classes has been reported to be associated with sexual difficulties. In some cases, the evidence supporting a causal relationship between the drug and sexual dysfunction is strong. For other drugs, the data are limited to single case reports and have to be regarded with caution before assuming that a relationship exists between drug usage and sexual problems. Caution is especially needed when the drug is prescribed for a condition which itself is associated with a high incidence of sexual dysfunction. In the absence of adequate baseline data, it is often impossible to determine if the problem preceded the onset of a given pharmacotherapy, and patients often misattribute causality. Tables 14.1–14.3 summarize the data on drugs associated with sexual dysfunction.

ANTIFUNGAL AGENTS AND ANTIBIOTICS

Ketoconazole was introduced in the 1970s as the first orally effective azole antifungal agent. The azole compounds consist of imidazole (ketoconazole; Nizoral) and triazole groups, all of which have an azole ring with two or three nitrogens. The triazole compounds include fluconazole (Diflucan) and itraconazole (Sporanox). All of the azole drugs interfere with ergosterol synthesis in yeast cell membranes; this interference leads to the accumulation of 14-methylated ergosterol precursors and cell death. Ketoconazole is unusual in that it is a nonsteroidal compound, yet it binds to multiple steroid receptors, including androgen, and has been shown to reduce the synthesis of both free and bound testosterone. In one study, free testosterone levels fell within 4–6 hours of ketoconazole administration. The antiandrogen effect of ketoconazole has even been used to treat androgen-dependent tumors. This drug also blocks the adrenal response to corticosteroids.

Table 14.1   Drugs reported to cause erectile dysfunction

Drug	Effect
Antifungal	
griseofulvin (Grisactin)	No
itraconazole (Sporanox)	Possible
ketoconazole (Nizoral)	Yes
terbanafine (Lamisil)	No
Antiarrhythmic	
amiodarone (Cordoarone)	Numerous case reports
digoxin	Yes
disopyramide (Norpace)	Several case reports
mexiltine (Mexitil)	Case reports
propafenone (Rhymol)	Possible
sotalol (Betapace)	Possible
verapamil	Numerous case reports
Antilipid	
clofibrate (Atromid-S)	Single case report
fenofibrate (Tricor)	Case reports
genfibrosil (Lopia)	Several case reports
simvastin (Zocor)	Single case report
Ophthalmologic	
acetazolamide (Diamox)	Case reports
aminocaproic acid (Amicar)	Probable
dichlorphenamide (Bentyl)	Single case report
timolol (Timpotic)	Possible
Other	
alfa interferon 2a (Roferon)	Single case report
baclofen (Zanaflex)	Case reports
cyclobenzaprine (Flexeril)	Single case report
ethionamide (Trecator)	Single case report
etretinate (Tegison)	Single case report
hydroxyzine (Vistaril)	Single case report
indomethacin (Indocin)	Single case report
isotretionate (Accutane)	Single case report
meclizine (Antivert)	Single case report

Table 14.1   (*Cont.*)

Drug	Effect
naprosen (Anaprox)	Single case report
nizatidine (Axid)	Single case report
orphenadrine (Norflex)	Single case report
oxybutyrin (Ditropan)	Case reports
phendimetrazine (Bortril)	Case reports
primidone (Mysoline)	Single case report
propanetheline (Pro-Banthine)	Single case report
scopolamine (Transderm-Scop)	Single case report
thiabendazole (Mintezol)	Single case report

Table 14.2   Drugs reported to cause decreased libido

Drug	Effect
acetazolamide (Diamox)	Single case report
acetazolamide (Diamox)	Case reports
amiloride (Midamor)	Single case report
clofibrate (Atromid-S)	Single case report
cyclobenzaprine (Flexeril)	Single case report
democylocycline (Bentyl)	Single case report
digoxin	Probable
hydroxyzine (Vistaril)	Single case report
ketoconazole (Nizoral)	Probable
lisinopril (Zestril)	Single case report
metronidazole (Flagyl)	Single case report
mexiltine (Mextil)	Single case report
niacin (Niacor)	Single case report
phendimetrazine (Bortril)	Single case report
primidone (Mysoline)	Single case report
timolol (Timpotic)	Single case report

Table 14.3   Drugs reported to cause ejaculatory and female orgasm difficulties

Drug	Effect
aminocaproic acid (Amicar)	Numerous case reports
baclofen (Lioresal)	Single case report
isotretinon (Accutane)	Single case report
methotrexate	Numerous case reports
metyrosine (Demser)	Single case report
naproxen (Aleve)	Single case report
phendimetrazine (Bortril)	Multiple case reports

The sexual side effects are prominent only with prolonged therapy (some clinicians have recommended testosterone therapy for men on prolonged ketoconazole therapy). Ketoconazole has been consistently reported to cause diminished libido, gynecomastia, and erectile problems. The *Physicians' Desk Reference* lists the antiandrogen effect of ketoconazole but does not mention sexual side effects. Itraconazole also has been reported to be associated with impotence, though the evidence for this effect is limited to a few case reports.

In contrast to ketoconazole, terbinafine (Lamisil) shows no acute influence on the pituitary gonadal axis and does not appear to have antiandrogen effects. Terbinifine works by blocking scalene epoxidase, an enzyme necessary to make ergosterol; it has been approved for the treatment of onychomycosis. Another antifugal agent, griseofulvin (Grisactin), is an antibiotic which was first discovered as a byproduct of the penicillin mold and is now manufactured synthetically as well. It interferes with cell wall and nucleic acid synthesis in fungi and does not appear to be associated with sexual side effects.

There has been one case report of decreased libido on demecylocycline (Declomycin), a member of the tetracycline class of antibiotics used to treat Rocky Mountain Spotted Fever. A number of other antibiotics has been reported to cause abnormal spermatogenesis; these include sulfasalazin (Azulfidine), a drug used in the treatment of inflammatory bowel disease, and gentamicin and neomycin (Neosporin).

VITAMINS

Etretinate (Tegison), a vitamin-A derivative used in the treatment of psoriasis, has been reported to be associated with low libido.

Isotretinin has been associated with ejaculatory problems.

NONSTEROIDAL ANTI-INFLAMMATORY DRUGS

Naproxen (Aleve) has been reported to be associated with ejaculatory dysfunction.

Indomethacin (Indocin) has been associated with decreased libido and impotence. Researchers have hypothesized that the effect of this drug on erectile function may be related to inhibition of postaglandins. It should be noted that the incidence of sexual problems on indomethacin has never been established, and the role of prostaglandins, if it exists, in erectile function has never been elucidated.

OPHTHALMOLOGICAL AGENTS

Carbonic anhydrase inhibitors, such as acetazolamide (Diamox), have been reported to be associated with decreased libido, erectile dysfunction, and problems with ejaculation.

Timolol eye drops have been associated with erectile failure.

ANTICHOLINERGIC AGENTS

A number of drugs with anticholinergic side effects has been reported to be associated with erectile dysfunction. Given that cholinergic transmission is not believed to be essential for erectile function, these reports are difficult to interpret. Drugs reported to cause erectile problems include benztropine (Cogentin), biperiden (Akineton), hydroxyzine (Vistaril), and homatropine (Homapin).

NASAL DECONGESTANTS

Heavy use of nasal decongestants, such as phenylpropanolamine and pseudoephedrine, has been reported to be associated with erectile failure, possibly via the mechanism of vasoconstriction.

INTERFERON 2a

Interferon alfa 2a has been reported to be associated with erectile problems.

REFERENCES

Ahmad S. Disopyramide and impotence. *South Med J*. 1980;73:958.
Anath J. Impotence associated with pimozide. *Am J Psychiaty*. 1982;139:1374.
Bain SC, Lemon M, Jones AF. Gemfibrozil-induced impotence. *Lancet*. 1990;336:1389.

MISCELLANEOUS DRUGS

Berlin RG. Metoclopromide-induced reversible impotence. *West J Med.* 1986;144:359–361.

Bharani A. Sexual dysfunction after gemfibrozil. *Br Med J.* 1992;305:693.

Blackburn WD, Alarcon GS. Impotence in three rheumatoid arthritis patients treated with methotrexate. *Arthritis & Rheumatism.* 1989;32:1341–1342

Blin O. Painful clitoral tumescence during bromocriptine therapy. *Lancet.* 1991;337:1231.

Boyd IW. Comment: HMG-CoA reductase inhibitor induced impotence. *Ann Pharmacother.* 1996;30:1199.

Brock G, Lue T. Drug-induced male sexual dysfunction: an update. *Drug Saf.* 1993;8:414–426.

Bruckert E, Giral P. Men treated with hypolipidemic drugs complain frequently of erectile dysfunction. *J Clin Pharmacol and Therapeutics.* 1996;21:89–94.

Canaday BR. Amorous disinhibited behavior associated with propofol. *Clinical Pharmacy.* 1993;12:449–451.

Chapple C, Baert L, Thind P, Hofner K, Khoe K, Khoe G, Spangberg A. Tamsulosin 0.4 mg once daily: tolerability in older and younger patients with lower urinary tract symptoms suggestive of benign prostatic obstruction. *Eur Urol.* 1997;32:462–470.

Chaudhry G, Haffajee C. Antiarrhythmic agents and proarrhythmia. *Critical Care Medicine.* 2000;28:1–15.

Coleman R, MacDonald D. Effects of isotrentinon on male reproductive function. *Lancet.* 1994;344:198.

Coronary Drug Project Research Group. Clofibrate and niacin in coronary heart disease. *JAMA.* 1975;231:360–381.

Duterte JP, Soutif D, Jonville AP, Cadenn M, Valet JP, Autret E. Sexual disturbances during omeprazole therapy. *Lancet.* 1991;33:1022.

Elliott DE. Parasitic diseases of the liver and intestines. *Gastroenterology Clinics.* 1996;25:1–28.

Epstein DL, Grant WM. Carbonic anhydrase inhibitor side effects. *Arch Opthalmol.* 1977;95:1378–1382.

Evans BE, Adedort LM. Inhibition of ejaculation due to epsilon aminocaproic acid. *N Engl J Med.* 1978;298:166–167.

Fernando IN, Tobias JS. Priapism in patients on tamoxifen. *Lancet.* 1989;1:436.

Figueras A, Castel JM, LaPorte JR, Capella D. Gemfibrozil-indiced impotence. *Ann Pharmacother.* 1993;27:982.

Finger W, Lund M, Stagle M. Medications that may contribute to sexual disorders. *J Family Practice.* 1997;44:33–43.

Fogelman J. Verapamil caused depression, confusion, and impotence. *Am J Psychiatry.* 1988;145:380.

Fogelman J. Verapamil may cause depression, confusion, and impotence. *Tex Med.* 1988;83:8.

Fraunfelder FT, Meyer SM. Sexual dysfunction secondary to topical opthalmic timolol. *JAMA.* 1985;253:3092–3.

Guppy S, Salimpour P. A possible mechanism for alteration of human erectile function by digoxin: inhibition of corpus cavernossum sodium/potassium adenosine triphosphate activity. *J Urol.* 1998;159:1529–1536.

Hasegawa J, Mashiba J. Transient sexual dsyfunction in a male with Wolf-Parkinson-White patient. *Cardiovas Drugs Ther.* 1994;2:277.

Hedlet DW. Evaluation of baclofen (Lioresal) for spasticity in multiple sclerosi. *Post Grad Med.* 1975;51:615.

Heger JJ, Slow EB, Prytowsky EN, Zipes Dp. Plasma and red blood cell concentrations of amiodarone during chronic therapy. *Am J Cardiol.* 1984;53:912–927.

Heel RC. Atenolol: a review of its pharmacological properties and therapeutic efficacy in angina pectoris and hypertension. *Drugs.* 1993;17:425.

Hormonal ZT, Shilon M, Paz GF. Phenoxybenzamine-an effective male contraceptive pill. *Contraception.* 1984;29:479–491.

Housea SW, Santella ML, Brown EJ, Berger M, Katasha K, Frank MM. Long-term therapy of hereditary angioedema with danazol. *Ann Intern Med.* 1980;93:809.

Hunter DN, Thornily A, Whitburn R. Arousal from propofol. *Anesthesia.* 1988;43:170.

Ireland A, Jewel DP. Sulfasalazine-induced impotence: a beneficial resolution with olsalazine? *J Clin Gstroenterol.* 1989;11:711.

Kassianos GC. Impotence and nizatidine. *Lancet.* 1989;1(8644):963.

Katz I. Sexual dysfunction and ocular timolol. *JAMA.* 1986;255:37–38.

Kedia KR, Persky L. Efffect of phenoxybenzaome (Dibnzyline) on sexual function in man. *Urology.* 1981;18:620–622.

Keene L, Davies P. Drug related erectile impotence. *Adverse Drug React Toxicol Rev.* 1999;18:5–24.

King BD, Pitchon R, Stern EH, Schweitzer P, Schneider RR, Weiner I. Impotence during therapy with verapamil. *Arch Int Med.* 1983;143:1248–1249.

Klein N, Cunha B. New antifungal drugs for pulmonary mycoses. *Chest.* 1996;110:525–532.

Kroner BA, Mulligan T, Briggs GC. Effect of frequently prescribed cardiovascular medications on sexual function: a pilot study. *Ann Pharmacother.* 1993;27:1329–1332.

Lindquist M, Edwards IR. Endocrine adverse effects of ameprazole. *Br Med J.* 1992;305:451–2

Lombardo L. Reversible amenorrhea after ranitidine treatment. *Lancet.* 1982;1:224.

McEwen J, Meyboon RHB. Testicular pain caused by mazindol. *Br Med J.* 1983;287:1763–1764.

McHaffie DJ, Guz A, Johnson A. Impotence in a patient on disopyramide. *Lancet.* 1977;1:859.

Mann KV, Abbott EC, Gray JD, Thiebaux HJ, Belzer EG. Sexual dysfunction with beta-blocker therapy. *Sexuality & Disability.* 1982;5:67–77.

Martinez GF. Enalapril and imptence. *Aten Primaria.* 1992;9:178–179.

Miller LG. Indomethacin-associated sexual dysfunction. *J Fam Pract.* 1989;29:210–211.

Moody GA. The effects of chronic ill health and treatment with suphasalazine on fertility amongst men and women with inflammatory bowel disease in Leicestershire. *Int J Colorectal Dis.* 1997;12:220–224.

MISCELLANEOUS DRUGS

Morrissete Dl, Skinner MH, Hoffman BB, Levine RE. Effects of antihypertensive drugs atenolol and niffedipine on sexual function in older men: a placebo-controlled crossover study. *Arch Sex Behav.* 1993;22:99–109.

Neri A, Zuckerman Z. The effect of long term administration of digoxin on plasma androgens and sexual dysfunction. *J Sex Marital Ther.* 1987;13:58–63.

Oliver MF, Heady JA, Morris JN, Cooper J. A cooperative trial in the primary prevention of ischaemic heart disease using clofibrate. *Br Heart J.* 1978;40:1069–1118.

Pertusa S, Bueno JM, Quirce F. Sexual impotence caused by nifedipine. *Medicina Clinica.* 1992;98:78.

Pizarro S, Bargay J, D'Agosto P. Gemfibrozil-induced impotence. *Lancet.* 1990;336:1135.

Reynolds OD. Erctile dysfunction in etretinate treatment. *Arch Dermatil.* 1991;127:425–426.

Schaefer HG, Marsch SCU. Forewarning patients of sexual arousal following anesthesia. *Anaesthesia.* 1991;46:238–239.

Schneider J, Kaffarnik H. Impotence in patients treated with clofibrate. *Atherosclerosis.* 1975;21:455–457.

Snyder S, Karaca I, Salis PJ. Disulfiram and nocturnal penile tumescence in the chronic alcoholic. *Biol Psychaitry.* 1981;6:339.

Smith EB. The treatment of dermatophytosis: safety considerations. *J Amer Acad Pediat.* 2000;43:S113–S119.

Soto AJ, Sacristan JA, Alsar MJ. Interferon alfa-2a-induced impotence. *Drug Intell Clin Pharm.* 1991;24:1397.

Stein R, Hanaauer S. Inflammatory bowel disease. *Gastroenterolgy Clinics.* 1999;28:1–32.

Tosi S. Painful gynecomastia with ranitidine. *Lancet.* 1982;2:160.

Vukmir R. Diagnostics: cardiac arrhythmia therapy. *Am J Emergency Medicine.* 1995;13:1–24.

Wallace TR. Decreased libido-a side effect of carbonic anhydrase inhibitor. *Ann Opthalmol.* 1979;11:1563.

Wassertheil-Smoller S, Blaufox MD, Oberman A, Davis BR, Swencionis C, Knerr MO, et al. Effects of antihypertensives on sexual dysfunction and quality of life: the TAIM study. *Ann Intern Med.* 1991;114:613–620.

Wei N. Naprosen and ejaculatory dysfunction. *Ann Intern Med.* 1980;93:933.

Zanetti L. Sotalol: a new class III antiarrhythmic agent. *Clin Pharm.* 1993;12:833–891.

15. Drug Treatment of Low Libido in Women

INTRODUCTION

As mentioned in Chapter 1, female complaints of low sexual desire are common. In the National Health and Social Life Survey, a representative sample of U.S. women ages 18–59 was interviewed about their sexual activities, and 33% of the women complained of experiencing low sexual desire in the preceding year. Complaints of low libido are a frequent presenting complaint of women who seek sexual counseling. The etiology of such complaints is often elusive. In many cases, when there is not an obvious etiology, and endocrinological factors are suspected. However, the endocrinology of libido in the human female is unclear.

In lower animals, sexual desire and receptivity are related to estrogen. In rhesus monkeys who have been oophorectomized, estradiol increases sexual initiation behavior, whereas progesterone has an inhibitory effect. In the human, libido appears to be independent of estrogen, although some clinicians have suggested that estrogen sustains the clitoral perfusion necessary for sensitivity. Dyspareunia due to vaginal dryness appears to be responsive to estrogen replacement therapy, which restores vaginal cells, pH, and blood flow. For women in whom loss of libido is related to dyspareunia, estrogen replacement may be sufficient to restore libido. Progestins oppose the action of estrogen, to a certain extent, thereby contributing to vaginal dryness.

A number of studies on humans has provided suggestive evidence that libido is correlated with testosterone production. In ovulating women, testosterone tends to rise around mid-cycle and fall premenstrually. Part of the mid-cycle increase in testosterone production may be the increase in ovarian androgen production in response to luteinizing hormone. However, studies have not been consistent in finding relationships between different phases of the menstrual cycle and libido. A number of studies indicate that supraphysiological levels of androgen increase libido. It is suspected but unproven that variations in androgen levels within normal range may influence libido.

Although many clinicians are currently utilizing testosterone therapy for low sexual desire in females, it is important that clinicians be cognizant that the long-term safety of such treatment has not been established. To date, the only therapies consistently shown to be effective in increasing libido in females have employed supraphysiological doses of testosterone. In view of recent findings of an increased risk of breast cancer and cardiovascular disease in women receiving estrogen-progesterone replacement therapy for postmenopausal symptoms, caution should be employed before recommending any long term hormonal therapy.

DIFFERENTIAL DIAGNOSIS

Prior to considering the pharmacotherapy for low libido, a careful differential diagnosis is necessary. A number of psychiatric, pharmacological, and medical conditions can cause low libido. Typically, the disorder is classified as *global* or *situational* and as *acquired* or *lifelong*. *Global* means that the difficulty in present in all sexual contexts (eg., fantasy, masturbation coitus. A situational aspect to the problem is suggestive of a relationship issue. *Situational* means that the problem is not manifest in all sexual situations; an example would be a woman who does not feel sexual desire with her usual partner but who masturbates to a fantasy of a different partner.

Another factor in the differential diagnosis is whether the problem is a lifelong or acquired one. Lifelong problems are usually psychogenic in etiology, and may relate to repressing attitudes toward sexuality and/or religious prohibitions. Acquired problems can be psychogenic or organogenic. If the problem is acquired, rule out relationship discord, life stress, depression, or medication-induced etiology before considering other organic sources. Numerous population surveys have

Table 15.1 Psychiatric factors associated with low libido

Anxiety disorders
Major depressive disorder
Relationship discord
Religious prohibitions

Table 15.2 Medical factors associated with low libido

Alcohol and drug abuse	Alpha-2 agonists
Cancer chemotherapy	Anticonvulsants
Hyperprolactinemia	Beta-blockers
Hypothyroidism	Calcium channel blockers
Low testosterone?	Digitalis
Oophorectomy	Diuretics
Opiate use	Guanethidine
Oral contraceptives?	Hemodialysis
Pituitary tumors	Methyldopa
Renal dialysis	Ophthalamic solutions
	containing beta-blockers
	Oral contraceptives
	(triphasics are recommended)
	Reserpine
	Tamoxifen?

shown relationship discord to be the major predictor of decreased female sexual responsiveness. Common psychological factors associated with low libido are listed in Table 15.1. Nonpsychiatrists may find the following quick screening questions useful for identifying patients who may have major depressive disorder:

1. Have you been unable to experience pleasure for the past month?

2. Have you felt depressed or down almost ever day for the past month?

A positive answer to either question merits further investigation of probable depression.

Female sexuality also can be adversely affected by diseases, including vascular disease. Common medical causes of low libido are listed in Table 15.2. Drugs causing low libido are listed in Table 15.3.

Table 15.3 Drug therapy associated with low libido

Psychiatric Drugs	Other Drugs
Antipsychotics (prolactin-sparing antipsychotics are preferred)	Alpha-2 agonists
Benzodiazepines	Anticonvulsants
Monoamine oxidase inhibitors	Beta-blockers
Serotonin reuptake inhibitors	Calcium channel blockers
Stimulants	Digitalis
Tricyclic antidepressants	Diuretics
	Guanethidine
	Hemodialysis
	Methyldopa
	Ophthalamic solutions containing beta-blockers
	Oral contraceptives (triphasics are recommended)
	Reserpine
	Tamoxifen?

NONHORMONAL THERAPY FOR LOW SEXUAL DESIRE

The success of sildenafil (Viagara) in the treatment of erectile problems in men contributed to the search for pharmacological treatments for female sexual problems. To date, these approaches have focused primarily on the use of (1) peripheral vasodilators (e.g., sildenafil, phentolamine, etc.), (2) centrally acting dopaminergic agents, or (3) exogenous androgens. Many investigators initially assumed that peripheral vasodilators would have similar benefits in the treatment of female sexual dysfunction as it has for male sexual dysfunction. In many ways, this assumption was a logical one, given that sexual arousal in both sexes involves peripheral vasodilation.

However, research has consistently found that female arousal problems in the absence of complaints of low libido are uncommon. Similarly, a large research literature has consistently found discrepancies between self-reports of sexual pleasure and objective measures of sexual arousal in females. For example, female subjects shown erotic videotapes often demonstrate vasocongestive responses while not experiencing subjective arousal. Clinical trials have shown the ability of sildenafil and other vasoactive substances to increase genital vasocongestion. Unfortunatley, there is minimal evidence that these substances have therapeutic efficacy in women with sexual complaints. A number of studies utilizing vasoactive drugs in women with decreased libido or decreased sexual arousal has not been able to demonstrate a beneficial effect of these drugs. Indeed, increased genital perfusion was perceived as unpleasant by some postmenopausal women. A recent large multisite study of women with arousal disorder coexisting with other sexual diagnoses failed to demonstrate a beneficial effect of sildenafil.

A plethora of clinical trials is underway, investigating various treatments for female sexual disorders. Many of these involve other phosphodiesterase inhibitors. Both alpha-blockers and phosphodiesterase inhibitors increase vaginal perfusion and lubrication. However, neither agent has been shown to have clinical utility for women complaining of low sexual desire or decreased subjective sexual arousal. A recent triple crossover, double-blind, placebo-controlled study of sildenafil in young premenopausal women found that the drug improved various aspects of sexual functioning in this population. It is possible that a subpopulation of women with sexual arousal problems will be identified who are responsive to phosphodiesterase inhibitor therapy.

The findings of a recent multisite single-blind study of a select group of women with hypoactive sexual desire disorder suggest that bupropion, a drug with adrenergic and dopaminergic properties, may have libido-enhancing properties. The group studied was predominantly premenopausal, in good health, in good relationships, without psychiatric problems, and with testosterone levels within normal range. Approximately one-third of the sample subjects experienced an increase in libido, as indicated by increased thoughts of sex, more episodes of sexual arousal, and more episodes of desiring sexual activity. A double-blind investigation is currently underway.

A clitoral vacuum device was recently approved by the Food and Drug Administration. The EROS-CTD is a small battery powered device designed to increase blood flow to the clitoris. To date, there is limited data concerning its use in clinical populations.

ORAL CONTRACEPTIVE TREATMENT OF LOW LIBIDO

The relationship between oral contraceptive use and the quality of female sexual experience remains unclear, due to two key factors: (1) Interpersonal issues may be more important determinants of female sexual activity than endocrinological ones; and (2) measures of coital frequency are unreliable indices because they may reflect the partner's libido level as much as they reflect the patient's. Theoretically, hormonal contraception could influence sexual responsiveness by its effect on the amount of bioavailable testosterone. However, the effect of varying levels of bioavailable testosterone, within normal limits, on female sexual responsiveness is hypothesized but not proven. Estrogen-containing oral contraceptives increase the levels of serum hormone-binding globulin, thus decreasing the amount of free testosterone. Oral contraceptives suppress both luteinizing hormone and follicle-stimulating hormone secretion. Oral contraceptives also decrease the mid-cycle increase in testosterone. Studies have shown that women on oral contraceptives have lower levels of total, free, and bioavailable testosterone. Total testosterone levels reflect the amount of testosterone in the plasma and include the portion of testosterone bound to sex hormone-binding globulin, the portion bound to albumin, and the amount unbound. Free testosterone and testosterone bound to albumin are considered to be bioavailable and thus biologically active.

Studies of sexual activity in women on oral contraceptives compared to women not on oral contraceptives have frequently failed to show a difference between the two groups. Psychosocial factors, such as no longer fearing pregnancy, may override any biological suppression of libido, if it exists. Some studies of women on oral contraceptives have shown a correlation between free testosterone levels and sexual desire, thoughts, and anticipation of sexual activity. Different progestins in combination with low-dose estrogens produce divergent results on hormone-binding globulin. One study of patients on ethinyl estradiol

Table 15.4 Oral contraception and libido

There may be a relationship between serum free testosterone and libido
Estrogen increases serum hormone binding globulin and decreases serum
   free testosterone
Progestins have divergent effects on free testosterone

plus different progestins found that 100 μg of norethindrone acetate caused twice as much elevation of serum hormone-binding globulin than 100 μg of levonorgestrol. However, norethindrone caused more reduction of androgens, so that both caused an equal drop of bioavailable androgen. As mentioned, numerous studies of changes in sexual interest and responsivity during different phases of the menstrual cycle have shown contradictory results. Table 15.4 summarizes the use of oral contraceptives in the treatment of low libido.

USE OF EXOGENOUS ANDROGENS IN POSTMENOPAUSAL WOMEN

Studies suggesting a beneficial effect of exogenous androgen on libido in females are listed in Table 15.5.

Table 15.5 Research concerning effects of exogenous androgens

Study	Sample Size & Methodology	Finding
Greenblatt et al., 1950	Double-blind placebo-controlled postmenopausal women	Androgen/estrogen combination increased libido
Birberg & Kurzrok, 1955	N = 80 clinical series	Androgen/estrogen combination increased libido
Kupperman et al., 1955	N = 168 clinical series	Androgen/estrogen implant increased libido
Burger et al.	N = 17 clinical series	Androgen/estrogen implant increased libido
Sherwin, 1985	N = 8	Sex drive correlates with testosterone levels
Sherwin & Gerfand, 1987	N = 60 controlled study	Supraphysiological doses of androgen increase libido
Davis et al., 1995	N = 34 Single-blind study	Androgen increases libido, orgasm
Sarrel et al., 1998	N = 20 Double-blind	In women unresponsive to estrogen alone, addition of androgen increases libido
Shifren et al., 2000	N = 75 Multisite double-blind placebo-controlled study	Supraphysiological doses of androgen increase libido
Tuiten, 2000	Double-blind placebo-controlled study of normal women in laboratory	Sublingual form of testosterone increased responsivity to erotic stimuli
Meston & Heiman, 2002	N = 12 Premenopausal women, single-blind laboratory study	Acute DHEA* has no effect on response to erotic stimuli
Hackbert & Heiman, 2002	N = 12 Double-blind placebo-controlled crossover study postmenopausal women	DHEA* increases arousal to erotic stimuli

* DHEA = Dehydroepiandrosterone

These studies have shown effects, not always consistent, on different measures of sexual activity. Many studies have demonstrated a positive effect on subjective libido while not influencing actual sexual behavior. Most studies demonstrating a clear and reproducible effect have used supraphysiological doses of androgens, or androgen doses at the high end of the normal range. It is likely that these doses would have masculinizing effects with long-term usage.

The earliest study, in 1950, was a double-blind investigation that found that androgen–estrogen therapy increased libido in postmenopausal women. Similar results were reported by three other studies. It was also found that androgen increased subjective reports of libido, and that women dissatisfied with estrogen–progestin replacement therapy experienced an increase in sexual desire and satisfaction when androgen was substituted for progesterone.

Compared to women experiencing natural menopause, women who undergo oophorectomy have a 40–50% drop in free testosterone. Oophorectomy results in the abrupt cessation of gonadal hormones. Estrogen–androgen replacement therapy is recommended to reduce vasomotor flushes and to maintain libido. Androgen therapy may cause undesirable lipoprotein changes and virilizing symptoms. Estrogen causes an increase in serum hormone-binding globulin, which contributes to less bioavailable testosterone. It is of note that large-scale studies have usually found that hysterectomy has minimal impact on female sexuality.

In one series of studies, women who received androgen–estrogen therapy following total abdominal hysterectomy plus bilateral salpingo–oophorectomy had higher levels of sexual desire, sexual arousal, and fantasies than women on estrogen alone or placebo. Women scheduled for hysterectomy and bilateral oophorectomy were assessed for baseline sexual functioning. They were then randomized to one of four groups: placebo, estradiol valerate 10 mg, testosterone enanthate 200 mg, or estradiol dienenthate 7.5 mg plus estradiol benzoate 1 mg plus testosterone enanthate 175 mg. All drugs were given intramuscularly. Women who received androgen or estrogen plus androgen had higher frequencies of sexual fantasies than those on placebo or estrogen alone. In a separate but similar study, androgen plus estrogen had positive effects on coital and orgasm frequency.

More recently, research has documented the efficacy of estrogen–testosterone replacement therapy in restoring sexual libido and responsiveness. Major effects on sexual interest were seen within 2 weeks postinjection. In these studies, 7.5 mg estradiol dinanthate, 1 mg estrdiaol, and 150 mg testosterone were administered by subcutaneous injection.

Many of these studies have been criticized for using supraphysiological doses of androgens and described as studies of androgen enhancement rather than androgen replacement. Shifren and colleagues reported the results of a multicenter double-blind study of androgen–estrogen therapy in women after oophorectomy. All women received .625 mg of conjugated equine estrogen daily and either placebo, 150 μg or 300 μg testosterone transdermal patches. The 150 μg dose was not different from placebo in terms of its sexual effects. The 300 μg dose increased both subjective and objective measures of sexual libido. This dose level produced above-normal total testosterone levels and free testosterone levels near the upper limit of normal. It is likely that continued treatment at these dose levels would have resulted in masculinization. It is possible that the brain does not respond to changes in testosterone that are within the normal range. Most studies have demonstrated an increase in libido with supraphysiological levels of testosterone.

A recent study has demonstrated a relationship between acute androgen administration and short-term changes in arousal. In a double-blind randomized crossover study, eight women were shown sexually explicit film strips before and after being given .5 mg testosterone undeconoate or placebo. Plasma testosterone peaked in about 90 minutes. Genital responsivity peaked about 3–4 hours later. On the day of treatment, subjects also reported increased sexual sensations and increased libido.

Studies using small samples or women with low libido have found evidence of efficacy of dehydroepiandrosterone (DHEA) in enhancing libido in postmenopausal women.

ANDROGEN LEVELS DURING MENOPAUSE

Clinicians are urged to use caution before instituting any long-term hormonal therapy of low sexual desire. There is no long-term safety data concerning the use of androgen in women. The importance of caution is highlighted by the recent finding that estrogen/progesterone replacement increases the risk of breast cancer and cardiovascular disease.

Premenopausal women with menstrual cycles produce ovarian testosterone, which is an essential precursor of estradiol. In premenopausal women, there is a mid-cycle peak in testosterone. In ovulatory cycles, 60% of testosterone is derived from the adrenal cortex and adrenal precursors (DHEA-dehydro-3-epiandrosterone and androstenedione) and 40% from the ovary and ovarian precursors during the follicular phase. During the luteal phase, the majority is ovarian in origin.

Table 15.6 Androgens and menopause

Postmenopausal ovary still produces testosterone
There is a drop in testosterone at menopause
Postmenopausal testosterone may gradually return to premenopausal levels
Exogenous testosterone in supraphysiological levels increases libido in women
    with surgical menopause

Studies show that postmenopausal ovaries remain a source of testosterone. In a large community-based study (the Rancho Bernardo Study), most women were found to experience a drop in testosterone at menopause. However, testosterone levels increased to premenopausal levels by 10 years. Other studies suggest that a substantial increase in testosterone occurs within 2 years of menopause. There appears to a decline around menopause, followed by increased ovarian production of testosterone. Androgen therapy in premenopausal women may be associated with virilizing effects and alteration of plasma lipids. There may be an increase in facial oiliness, acne, and alopecia. Androgen replacement in naturally postmenopausal women may have little or no effect on sexual motivation.

Table 15.6 summarizes the changes in androgen levels during menopause and their effects on sexual function.

ANDROGEN DEFICIENCY SYNDROME

The concept of an androgen deficiency syndrome was introduced by Helen Singer Kaplan, who reported that some women who either had received chemotherapy for cancer or had had oophorectomy experienced a deficiency of sexual desire, which was improved by androgen therapy. The diagnosis of androgen deficiency syndrome is a hypothetical and unproven clinical diagnosis. This syndrome is expected to occur mainly in women who are surgically oophorectomized. It also may occur in some postmenopausal women whose ovaries are producing minimal amounts of androgen.

LIFELONG HYPOACTIVE SEXUAL DESIRE DISORDER AND ANDROGEN LEVELS

Evidence concerning levels of free testosterone in women with hypoactive sexual desire is inconsistent. A recent study reported that mid-cycle free testosterone was significantly lower in women with lifelong hypoactive sexual desire disorder than in women without problems with sexual desire. Hypoactive sexual desire disorder was operationally defined as the lack of need for sexual activity of any sort, the absence of sexual daydreams, and an inability to generate sexual fantasies. In this study, coital frequency also correlated with mid-cycle free testosterone levels. A previous study using a different definition of sexual desire disorder did not find a difference between free testosterone levels in women with hypoactive sexual desire disorder and women without the disorder.

HORMONAL EFFECTS ON CENTRAL NERVOUS SYSTEM

The rat midbrain periaqueductal area contains neurons that are immunoreactive for both the androgen and estrogen receptors (alpha type). These receptors are concentrated in the caudal two-thirds of the periaqueductal gray, which may be the major site of the central nervous system responsible for steroid-mediated changes in reproductive behavior. Interaction of central monoaminergic systems and steroid hormones plays a major role in the control of sexual behavior in lower animals. A number of studies has reported high prolactin levels to be associated with low sexual desire.

PHARMACOTHERAPY

There are no androgens approved for the treatment of hypoactive sexual desire disorder in females, and there are no well-established guidelines for the dosages that should be employed. However, many clinicians are using androgens to treat women with complaints of low sexual desire, and compounding pharmacies can provide androgen in various doses and delivery forms. Table 15.7 lists androgen–estrogen preparations available in the United States. Some clinicians utilize testosterone gels and creams. Varying doses have been recommended by different clinicians. Many recommend doses between .25 and 2 mg testosterone per day: The use of 2% testosterone cream can be applied three times a week; testosterone gel containing 2.5 mg methyltestosterone can be reformulated by a 10-fold dilution, because female androgens are usually about one-tenth of male levels. Oral methyltestosterone tablets also can be reformalated into smaller doses. Because the degree of systemic absorption is uncertain, hormone assays of free testsoterone after 30 days treatment are recommended.

Table 15.7 Estrogen–androgen combination formulations

Estratest
    1.25 mg esterified estrogens
    2.5 mg methyltestosterone
Estratest HS
    .625 mg esterified estrogens
    1.25 mg methyltestosterone

Other approaches of unproven efficacy include taking l-argentine and yohimbine and the use of EROS-CTD, a clitoral therapy device (made by Urometrics) that consists of a small pump. Fifty mg of dehydroepiandrosterone (DHEA) has been recommended by some clinicians as helpful in increasing libido; however, this relationship has not been documented convincingly using large numbers of women.

Table 15.8   Information concerning hormonal treatment of low libido in women

1. Androgen treatment for hypoactive sexual desire disorder is not approved by the FDA.
2. The risks and benefits of long-term treatment have not been established.
3. The criteria for use of androgen therapy, doses, routes, and indications have not been established.
4. To date, the rationale for the use of androgen therapy in premenopausal women is extremely controversial.
5. Patients must be advised that the treatment is experimental.
6. If androgen therapy is being considered, first determine if estrogen therapy relieves postmenopausal symptoms, negating need to consider androgen therapy.
7. In women who have significant risk associated with systemic estrogen therapy, consider an estradiol ring or estrogen cream.
8. Prior to androgen therapy, determine serum free testosterone or bioavailable testosterone levels.
9. Calculate free testosterone level or use direct testosterone assay.
10. Do not consider exogenous androgen unless the free testosterone is below, or in the lower levels of, normal for women in reproductive years.
11. Consider obtaining a second measure if your laboratory does not routinely measure free testosterone levels in females.
12. Inform patient of possible alopecia, acne, hirsutism, and other side effects.
13. Oral methyltestosterone, IM testosterone, and testosterone gel are available.
14. The long-acting testosterone esters have minimal hepatotoxicity because they bypass the liver.
15. Typical doses of IM testosterone are 50–100 mg q 4 weeks.
16. Oral testosterone, such as 2.5 mg methyltestosterone, may have adverse effects on lipoproteins as well as hepatotoxicity.
17. Methyltestosterone undergoes minimal peripheral conversion to estrogen in breast tissue; it is unclear whether this is true of other forms of androgen.
18. Testosterone patches for women are in clinical trials.
19. Affecting libido probably requires a dose close to the upper limit of normal.
20. It may be necessary to titrate efficacy against the risk of masculinizing effects.
21. Fluid retention and virilization are possible on excessive doses.
22. Adverse lipoprotein effects are possible with oral androgen.
23. It is unknown if androgen has an effect on the risk of breast cancer.
24. Androgen receptors are commonly found in breast tumors.
25. Androgel (a 1–2% topical testosterone cream) can be reformulated for females.
26. Androgel avoids the transient supraphysiological levels associated with intramuscular testosterone; it is unclear whether testosterone in this form undergoes peripheral conversion to estrogen.

Caution should be employed in androgen therapy in terms of monitoring breast cancer risk, deep vein phlebitis, liver disease, and changes in serum lipids. Table 15.8 summarizes hormonal treatment of women with low libido.

REFERENCES

Aaresranta TKI, Polo-Kantola P, Helenius H, Polo O. Prolonged endocrine responses to medroxyprogesterone in postmenopausal women with respiratory insufficiency. *Obstet Gynecol.* 2000; 96:243–249.

Althof SE, Turner LA, Levine SB, Bodner D, Kursh ED, Resnick MI. Through the eyes of women: the sexual and psychological responses of women to their partner's treatment with self-injection or external vacuum therapy. *J Urol.* 1992;147(4):1024–1027.

Althof SE, Turner LA, Levine SB, et al. Sexual, psychological, and marital impact of self-injection of papaverine and phentolamine: a long-term prospective study. *J Sex Marital Ther.* 1991;17(2):101–112.

Andersson KEA, Stief C. Neurotransmission and the contraction and relaxation of penile erectile tissue. *World J Urol.* 1997;10:14–20.

Aydin S, Odabas O, Ercan M, Kara H, Agargun MY. Efficacy of testosterone, trazodone, and hypnotic suggestion in the treatment of non-organic male sexual dysfunction. *Br J Urol.* 1996;77:256–260.

Banos R, Bosch F, Farre M. Drud-induced priapism: its etiology, incidence, and treatment. *Med Toxicol.* 1989;10:45–58.

Brain E, Kreiger J. Pharmacological priapism: comparison of trazodone and papaverine associated cases. *Int Urol Nephrol.* 1990;5:147–152.

Basson R. Clarifying the complaint of low sexual desire in men and women. *Med Asp Hum Sex.* 2001;1:39–42.

Basson R, McInnes R, Smith M, Hidgson G, Spain T, Koppiker, N. Efficacy and safety of sildenafil in estrogenized women with sexual dysfunction associated with female arousal disorder. *Obstet Gynecol.* 2000;95(4 Suppl 1): 554.

Berman J, Berman L. *For Women Only.* New York:Henry Holt; 2001.

Berman J. Goldstein I. Female sexual pysfunction. *Urol Clin North Am.* 2001;28:405–416.

Birnberg CH, Kurzrok R. Low density androgen estrogen therapy in the older age group. *J Am Geriatr Soc.* 1955;3:656–660.

Boolell M, Gepl-Attee S, Gingell JC, Allen MJ. Sildenafil, a novel effective oral therapy for male erectile disorder. *Br J Urol.* 1996;78:257–261.

Brindley G. Cavernosal alpha-blockade: a new technique for investigating and treating erectile impotence. *Br J Psychiat.* 1983;143:332–337.

Burger HG, Hailes J, Menelaus M, Nelson J, Hudson B, Balasz N. The management of persistent menopausal symptoms with oestradiol testosterone implants: Clinical, lipid, and hormonal results. *Matutritas.* 1984;6:351–358.

Cheitlin M, Hutter A. Use of sildenafil in patients with cardiovascular disease. *Circulation.* 1999;99:168–171.

Chiang PH, Wu SN, Tsai EM, Wu CC, Shen MR, Huang CH, Chiang CP. Adenosine modulation of neurotransmission in penile erection. *Br J Clin Pharmacol.* 1994;38:357–362.

Clayton AH, Owens JE, McGarvey EL. Assessment of paroxetine-induced sexual dysfunction using the changes in sexual functioning questionnaire. *Psychopharmacol Bull.* 1995;31:397–413.

Culberg G. Pharmacodynamic studies on desogestrel administered alone and in combination with ethinylestrdiol. *Acta Obstet Gynecol Scand.* 1985;133:1–30.

Danjou P, Alexandre L, Warot D, Lacomblez L, Peuch AJ. Assessment of erectogenic properties of apomorphine and yohimbine in man. *Brit J Clin Pharmacol.* 1988;26:733–739.

Davis SR, McCloud P, Strauss B, Burger H. Testosterone enhances estradiol's effect on postmenopausal bone density and sexuality. *Matuitas.* 1995;21:227–232.

DeCherney A. Hormone receptors and sexuality in the human female. *J Women's Health Gend Based Med.* 2000;9(Suppl 1):9–13.

Gall H, Sparwasser C, Bahren W, Scherb W, Irion R. Long-term results of corpus cavernosum autoinjection therapy for chronic erectile dysfunction. *Andrologia.* 1992;24(5):285–292.

Garcia-Campayo J, Sant-Carrilloc. Lobo A. Orgasmic sexual experiences as a side effect of fluoxetine: a case report. *Acta Psychiatr Scand.* 1995;9:69–70.

Georgitis WJ, Merenich JA. Trial of pentoxifylline for diabetic impotence. *Diabetes Care.* 1995;18(3):345–352.

Gold DP, Justino FD. Bicycle kickstand phenomena: prolonged erections associated with antipsychotic agents. *Southern Medical Journal.* 1988;81:792–794.

Goldstein I, Lue T. Oral sildenafil in the treatment of erectile dysfunction. *New Engl J med.* 1998;338:379–404.

Greenblatt RB, Barfield WE, Garner JF, Calf GL, Harrod JP. Evaluation of an estrogen, androgen, estrogen-androgen combination and a placebo in the treatment of menopause. *J Clin Endocrinol.* 1950;10:1547–1558.

Guay AT. Advances in the management of androgen deficiency in women. *Med Asp Hum Sex.* 2001;1:32–38.

Hackbert L, Heiman J. Acute dehydroepiandrosterone (DHEA) effects on sexual arousal in postmenopausal women. *J Womens Health Gend Based Med.* 2001;11:155–162.

Kaplan S, Reis R, Kohn I, Ikeguchi E, Laor E, Te A, Martins A. Safety and efficacy of sildenafil in postmenopausal women with sexual dysfunction. *Urology.* 1999;53(3):483–486.

Katz RC, Jardine D. The relationship between normal sexual aversion and low sexual desire. *J Sex Marital Ther.* 1999;25:293–296.

Kim SC, Azadzoi K. A nitirc acid-like factor mediating noradreneic, noncholinergic neurogenic relaxation of penile corpus cavernosum smooth muscle. *J Clin Investigation.* 1991;88:112–118.

Kim SC, Seo KK. Efficacy and safety of fluoxetine, sertraline, and clomipramine in patients with premature ejaculation: A double-blind, placebo controlled study. *J Urol.* 1998;159(2):425–427.

Knoll J. The facilitation of dopaminergic activity in the aged brain by (-)deprenyl: A proposal for a strategy to improve the quality of life in senescence. *Mech. Ageing Dev.* 1985;30/2:109–122.

Kokeu A, Cetinkaya M, Yanik F, Alper T, Malatyalioglu E. The comparison of effects of tibolone and conjugated estrogen–medroxyprogesterone acetate therapy on sexual performance in postmenopausal women. *Maturitas.* 2000;36:75–80.

Kupperman HS, Wetchler BB, Blatt M. Contemporary therapy of the post-menopausal syndrome. *JAMA.* 1959;171:1627–1629.

Lal S. Apomorphine in the evaluation of dopaminergic function in man. *Prog Neuro-psychopharmacol & Biol Psychiatry.* 1988;12:117–164.

Lal S, Rios O, Thavundayil JX. Treatment of impotence with trazodone: a case report. *J Urol.* 1990;143:819–820.

McLean JD, Forsythe RG, Kaplin LA. Unusual side effects of clomipramine associated with yawning. *Can J Psychiatry.* 1983;28:569–570.

Meinhardt W, Schmidt PI, Kropman RF, et al. Trazodone, a double-blind trial for treatment of erectile dysfunction. *Int J Imp Res.* 1997;9(3),163–165.

Meston CM, Gorzalka BB. Psychoactive drugs and human sexual behavior: the role of serotonergic activity. *J Psychoactive Drugs.* 1992;24(1):1–40.

Meston C, Heiman J. Acute dehydroepiandrosterone effects on sexual arousal in premenopausal women. *J. Sex Marit Ther.* 2002;28:53–60.

Michael A, Owen A. Venlafaxine-induced increased libido and spontaneous erections. *Brit J Psychiatry.* 1997;170:193.

Michelson D, Bancroft B, Targum S, Kim Y, Tepner R. Female sexual dysfunction associated with antidepressant administration: a randomized, placebo-controlled study of pharmacologic intervention. *Am J Psychiatry.* 2000;157:239–241.

Modell JG. Repeated observations of yawning, clitoral engorgement, and orgasm associated with fluoxetine administration. *J Clin Psychopharmacol.* 1989;9(1):63–65.

Morales A, Condra M, Owen JA, Surridge DH, Fenemore J, Harris C. Is yohimbine effective in the treatment of organic impotence?: results of a controlled trial. *J Urology.* 1987;137:1168–1172.

Morales A, Surridge DH, Marshall PG. Yohimbine for treatment of impotence in diabetes. *N Engl J Med.* 1981;305:1221.

Myers L, Dixen J, Morrissette M, Carmichael M, Davidson J. Effects of estrogen, androgen, and progestin on sexual psychophysiology and behavior in postmenopausal women. *J Clin Endocrinol Metabol.* 1990;70:1124–1131.

Nachtigall L, Raju U, Banerjee S, Wan K, Levitz M. Serum estradiol-binding profiles in postmenopausal women undergoing three common estrogen replacement therapies. *Menopause.* 2000;7:243–250.

Nemeth A, Arato M, Treuer T, Vandlik E. Treatment of fluvoxamine-induced anorgasmia with a partial drug holiday. *Am J Psychiatry.* 1996;153:1365.

Pehek EA, Thompson JT, Hull E M. The effects of intrathecal administration of the dopamine agonist apomorphine on penile reflexes and copulation in the rat. *Psychopharmacol.* 1989;99:304–308.

Pescatori ES, Engelman JC, Davis G, Goldstein I. Priapism of the clitoris: a case report following trazodone use. *J Urol.* 1993;149:1557–1559.

Purcell P. Trazodone and spontaneous orgasms in an elderly postmenopausal woman: a case report. *J Clin Psychopharmacol.* 1995;15:293–294.

Reid K, Surridge DH, Morales A, Condra M, Harris C, Owen J, Fenemore J. Double-blind trial of yohimbine in treatment of psychogenic impotence. *Lancet.* 1987;2:421–423.

Rhodes JC, Kjerulff KH, Langerberg PW, Guzinski GM. Hysterectomy and sexual functioning. *JAMA*. 1999;282:1934–1941.

Riley AJ, Kellet JM, Orr R. Double-blind trial of yohimbine hydrochloride in the treatment of erection inadequacy. *Sexual and Marital Therapy*. 1989;4:17–26.

Riley AJ, Riley EJ. The effect of single dose diazepam on female sexual response induced by masturbation. *Sexual and Marital Therapy* (UK). 1986;1:49–53.

Rodriquez-Aleman F, Torres J, Cuadros J, Ruiz E, Ortiz E. Effect of estrogen–progesterone replacement therapy on plasma lipids and lipoprotein postmenopausal women. *Endocr Res*. 2000;26:263–273.

Rosen RC, Ashton AK. Prosexual drugs: empirical status of the new aphrodisiacs. *Arch Sex Behav*. 1993;22:521–543.

Rosen RC, Phillips NA, Gendarme NC, Ferguson DM. Oral phentolamine and female sexual arousal: a pilot study. *J Sex Marital Ther*. 1999;25:137–144.

Schreiner-Engel P, Schiavi RC. Lifetime Psychopathology in individuals with low sexual desire. *J Nern Ment Dis*. 1986;174:646–651.

Schreiner-Engel P, Schiavi RC, White D, Ghizzani A. Low sexual desire in women; The role of reproductive hormones. *Horm Behave*. 1989;23:221–234.

Schlatter EKE, Lal S. Treatment of alcoholism with Dent's oral apomorphine method. *Quart J Studies Alcohol*. 1972;33:430–436.

Schlegel W, Petersdorf L, Junker R, Schulte H, Ebert C, von Eckardstein I. The effects of six months of treatment with a low dose of conjugated estrogens in menopausal women. *Clin Endocrinol*. 1999;51:63–51.

Segraves RT. Pharmacological enhancement of human sexual behavior. *J Sex Education and Therapy*. 1991;17:283–289.

Segraves RT, Segraves K. Pharmacotherapy for sexual disorders: advantages and pitfalls. *Sex Marital Ther (UK)*. 1998;13(3):295–309.

Segraves RT, Segraves K, Spirnak P. Effect of apomorphine on penile tumescence in men with psychogenic impotence. *J Urol*. 1991;145:1174–1175.

Sherwin B. The impact of different doses of estrogen and progestin on mood and sexual behavior in postmenopausal women. *J Clin Endo Metab*. 1991;72:336–343.

Sherwin BB, Geldfand MM, Brendler W. Androgen enhances sexual motivation in females: A prospective crossover study of sex steroid administration in the surgical menopause. *Psychosom Med*. 1985;47:339–351.

Smith DM, Levitte SS. Association of fluoxetine and return of sexual potency in three elderly men. *J Clin Psychiatry*. 1993;54:317–319.

Sondra LP, Mazor R, Chancellor MD. The role of yohimbine in the treatment of erectile impotence. *J Sex and Marital Therapy*. 1990;16:15–21.

Stevenson RW, Solyom L. The aphrodisiac effect of fenfluramine: two case reports of a possible side effect to the use of fenfluramine in the treatment of bulimia. *J Clin Psychopharmacol*. 1990;10(1):69–71.

Susset JG, Tessier CD. Effect of yohimbine hydrochloride on erectile impotence: a double-blind study. *J of Urology*. 1989;141:1360–1363.

Swenson JR. Fluoxetine and sexual dysfunction. *Canad J Psychiatry*. 1993;38:297.

Tuiten A. Time course of effects of testosterone administration on sexual arousal in women. *Arch Gen Psychiatry.* 2000;57:149.

Turner LA, Althof SE. The clinical effectiveness of self-injection and external vacuum devices in the treatment of erectile dysfunction: a six-month comparison. *Psychiatr Med.* 1992;10(2):283–293.

Turner LA, Althof SE, Levine SB, Bodner DR, Kursh ED, Resnick MI. Twelve-month comparison of two treatments for erectile dysfunction: self-injection versus external vacuum devices. *Urol.* 1992;39(2):139–144.

van Ahlen H, Piehota HJ, Kias HJ, Brennerman W, Klingmiller D. Opiate antagonists in erectile dysfunction: a possible new treatment option? *Eur Urol.* 1995;28:246–250.

Waldinger M, Hengeveld MW, Zwinderman AH. Ejaculation retarding properties of paroxetine in patients with premature ejaculation. *Brit J Urol.* 1997;79:592–595.

Zimmerman T, Detrich H, Wisser K, Hoffman H. The efficacy and tolerability of Valette. *Eur J Contracept Reprod Health Care.* 1999;4:155–164.

16. Drug Treatment of Low Libido in Men

INTRODUCTION

Potency enhancing properties have been attributed to a variety of food substances such as mandrake root, ginseng, olives, oysters, truffles, and orchid root. Medical text books in the late 1800s had lists of recommended aphrodisiacs. Susuta of India advocated ingestion of animal testicular tissue to increase potency. In 1889, the famous French neurologist, Charles-Edward Brown-Sequard, at the age of 72, self-administered an aqueous extract of dog testicular tissue and reported an increase in vigor and potency. Subsequently, other physicians advocated the transplantation of testicular grafts from apes into human testicular tissue or into the subtunical space. It is doubtful that any of these procedures had physiological effects on libido, although the psychological benefits of such procedures may have been strong.

The relationship of endogenous androgen levels to sexual performance has remained an area of considerable interest to physicians since testosterone was identified.

A number of investigators has found that testosterone replacement in hypogonadal men leads to a dramatic increase in sexual desire, nocturnal erections, and fantasy-associated erections. Findings from studies of testosterone supplementation in eugonadal men have suggested that a relatively low level of androgen is sufficient to maintain normal sexual activity, and that there is no demonstrable relationship between sexual function and variations of testosterone above this threshold value. The absolute value of this threshold amount is unknown for any given patient. However, it is generally assumed that changes in testosterone, within normal limits, have minimal effect on sexual function. The minimal levels of androgens necessary

215

Table 16.1   Testosterone and male sexuality

Androgen replacement restores erectile function in hypogonadal men
Exogenous testosterone has minimal effect in eugonadal men
Threshold level testosterone is sufficient to maintain sexual function
Major effect of testosterone is on libido and ejaculation
In hypogonadal men, androgen replacement leads to marked increases in sexual
   desire, nocturnal erections, and fantasy-associated erections
Supraphysiological levels of androgens have minimal effects on sexual function

for normal sexual function are probably between 200–350 ng/dl. With testosterone augmentation, one can observe changes in sexual behavior untill serum levels approach 450 ng/dl above that level, it is difficult to demonstrate a relationship between testosterone and sexual activity.

Suppression of testosterone in eugonadal men results in reduced libido and a decrease in nocturnal erections. Gonadotropin-releasing hormones and other drugs that suppress endogenous production of testosterone have been utilized successfully to treat men with criminal sexual behavior. The suppression of sexual behavior appears to occur as serum testosterone levels fall below normal limits. Conversely, some investigators have found that supraphysiological doses of testosterone administered to eugonadal men lead to a modest increase in libido and enhancement of nocturnal erection turgidity but has no demonstrable effect on daytime sexual function.

Interestingly, there is some evidence that sexual activity, per se, may increase testosterone. A recent study found that successful treatment of erectile dysfunction, leading to an increase in sexual activity, activated a dramatic increase in both total and free serum testosterone. This increase occurred regardless of etiology and treatment approach.

In summary, the available evidence indicates that testosterone is the hormone responsible for normal male sexual libido and that testosterone replacement in hypogonadal men leads to restoration of libido. The major effect of androgens on sexual function are felt to be mediated through libido.

Table 16.1 summarizes the role of testosterone in male sexuality.

PHYSIOLOGY OF TESTOSTERONE SECRETION

Testosterone is felt to exert effects at the level of the medial pre-optic nucleus and the motor neurons of the spinal cord. It may also have a direct effect on the penis. Both the testes and adrenal glands secrete androgens, with testosterone being the most potent;

dehydroepiandrosterone is the most common androgen produced by the adrenal gland. Testosterone receptors are present throughout the body and central nervous system. Secretion of testosterone occurs in pulsatile bursts, with a morning peak and late-afternoon trough. Secretion is regulated by negative feedback from the hypothalamus and pituitary. The half-life of testosterone in the blood is approximately 20 minutes. Most testosterone is protein-bound; one-half may be loosely bound to albumin, and the rest is bound to serum hormone-binding globulin. Testosterone diffuses into target cells, where it is converted into one of two active metabolites: dihydrotestosterone or estradiol. The enzymes responsible for these conversions are 5 alpha-reductase and aromatase. Dihydrotestosterone exerts its effect on the external genitalia; conversion to estradiol may be required for some of testosterone's effects to the central nervous system.

Testicular functioning involves a complex, interrelated interaction between the central nervous system, the anterior pituitary, and the testes. Neural activity in the medial basal hypothalamus stimulates the release of gonadotrophin-releasing hormone (GnRH). GnRH, in turn, promotes release of luteinizing hormone (LH) and follicle-stimulating hormone (FSH) from the anterior pituitary. FSH primarily stimulates the Sertoli cells, which produce spermatozoa. LH stimulates the interstitial cells to produce and secrete sex steroids, testosterone, dihydrotestosterone, and estradiol. Testosterone feedback to the hypothalamus and pituitary regulates GnRH secretion. The negative feedback on GnRH secretion is assumed to come from estradiol, which is formed by the aromatization of testosterone in the central nervous system. In the circulation, testosterone is bound to serum hormone-binding globulin, beta globulin, and albumin. Only nonprotein-bound testosterone is biologically active; nonprotein-bound testosterone represents about 3% of total serum testosterone.

TESTOSTERONE AND AGING

Adult testosterone levels usually peak at age 20 and decline by 1% a year after age 40. This age-related decline occurs through a reduction in Leydig cell function and a reduction in hypothalamic–pituitary system function. Bioavailable testosterone decreases with age and serum hormone binding globulin (SHBG) increases with age. There also appears to be a decline in end organ response; in particular, testicular response to LH decreases. The early A.M. peak is reduced and LH usually increases. In 80-year-old men, for example, free testosterone is 50% of what it was at age 20. There has been speculation that the decline in libido that accompanies aging may also reflect a decreased receptor sensitivity to androgen, particularly in the central nervous system.

Table 16.2   Testosterone changes that accompany aging

Decreased testosterone production
Decreased number of Leydig cells
Decreased bound and free testosterone
Decreased testicular response to luteinizing hormone
Increased serum hormone-binding globulin
Increased estradiol
Increased follicle-stimulating hormone
Increased luteinizing hormone

Hypogonadism is a common clinical syndrome that is characterized by decreased libido, decreased ejaculatory demand, decreased sexual activity, lack of vigor, reduced musculoskeletal mass, impaired fertility, dysphoria, fatigue, irritability, and appetite loss. These effects of hypogonadism are reversed by exogenous testosterone administration. Testosterone changes that accompany aging are listed in Table 16.2.

TESTOSTERONE REPLACEMENT

There is disagreement concerning the indications for hormone replacement in the male. There is not a common agreement about how low androgen levels should be for various age groups before androgen replacement should be considered. Most clinicians are reluctant to begin androgen replacement before androgen levels fall below normal limits. Some clinicians have questionned this approach, pointing out that statistically based normal limits are not clinically derived and that the meaning of a given laboratory value is usually observed without knowledge of the baseline for each particular individual. If a decrease in receptor sensitivity occurs with aging, a logical argument can be made for ignoring normal limits. With decreased receptor sensitivity, testosterone levels at the lower end of the normal range may be insufficient to maintain normal libido.

When considering testosterone replacement therapy, a number of clinical concerns are relevant. For example, testosterone stimulates erythropoieses and reduces high-density cholesterol. It also is thought to stimulate the growth of prostatic adenocarcinoma. It is worth noting that the danger of inducing polycythemia has never been proven, nor has it been proven that testosterone promotes prostatic cancer or worsens prostatic hypertrophy. It also has never been demonstrated that high testosterone levels worsen cardiovascular disease. Many clinicians refuse to administer testosterone to men with PSA (prostate-specific antigen) levels greater than 3 ng/ml, or to men whose rectal exam is abnormal. Other clinicians will administer testosterone but monitor PSA levels at regular intervals. Table 16.3 lists the available

Table 16.3   Testosterone products

Androderm Transdermal System	2.5 or 5 mg testosterone daily
Androgel 1%	Daily application of 50, 75 or 100 mg
Delatestryl	Testosterone enanthate injection in 1 1 ml single dose syringes & 5 ml vials
Testoderm	Testosterone transdermal system 4, 5, or 6 mg daily
Testopel Pellets	Each pellet has 75 mg testosterone
Testred	10 mg methyltestosterone capsules

forms of androgen therapy. Table 16.4 lists further factors to be considered in choice of type of replacement therapy.

TESTOSTERONE AND PROLACTIN SCREENING

A recent study involving serum testosterone and prolactin screening in 1,022 men with erectile dysfunction found abnormally low testosterone (less than 4 ng/ml) in 4% of men less than age 50 and 9% more than age 50. Determining testosterone levels only in cases of low sexual desire or abnormal physical exam would have missed 37% of those with low testosterone. Prolactin was abnormal upon repeat measurement in only two men, one of whom had a prolactinoma. It was concluded that because of the low frequency of abnormal testosterone levels in men with erectile dysfunction, testosterone should only be drawn in men under age 50 who have low libido or an abnormal physical examination. It should be obtained routinely in men after age 50. It was recommended that prolactin levels be determined in men with low sexual desire and or gynecomastia. Only the free portion of testosterone is biologically active, so men can have total testosterone within normal limits while having abnormally low levels of free testosterne. It is prudent to obtain a free testosterone level in men with ideopathic loss of sexual desire. As mentioned, testosterone that is bound to serum hormone-binding globulin is inactive. Thus conditons that increases the amount of serum hormone-binding globulin available (e.g., thyrotoxicosis, estrogens, cirrhosis, alcoholism, and the use of certain anticonvulsants) or decrease it (e.g., exogenous, androgens, acromegaly, and hypothyroidism) can alter the action of testosterone without influencing the level of total testosterone. The relationship of

Table 16.4   Choice of testosterone product

1. Oral androgens are associated with heptatotoxicity

2. Intramuscular forms produce supraphysiological levels followed by subnormal levels

3. Transdermal delivery systems are preferred

Table 16.5 Routine screening of testosterone and prolactin in patients with erectile dysfunction

Testosterone should be checked in men over 50
Prolactin should be checked if testosterone is less than 200 ng/dl
The patient can be hypogonadal with a normal low total testostereone if serum hormone binding globulin is markedly elevated
Testosterone bound to serum hormone binding globulin is inactive

serum testosterone and serum hormone binding globulin is summarized in Table 16.5.

Table 16.6 summarizes routine screening recommendations.

CLINICAL PRESENTATION OF HYPOGONADISM

A decrease in ejaculatory volume may be the first objective indication of decreased libido from hypogonadism. Stimulation of prostate and seminal vesicle secretion requires high levels of testosterone. The presence of normal ejaculatory volumes suggests that hypogonadism is not responsible for the complaint of low libido. In some patients, a complaint of decreased libido may be a first sign of hypogonadism preceding gynecomastia or changes in shaving. Male castrates experience decreased libido and decreased sexual activity, both of which are restored by external androgens. Antiandrogen drugs such as cyproterone acetate, spironolactone, and flutamide suppress sexuality in men. Studies of male castrates, in countries that employ surgical castration of violent sexual offenders, indicate that some remain capable of sexual activity. It is possible that small amounts of androgens from the adrenals play a role in this continued activity.

The amount of plasma testosterone required for normal libido appears to be low. Significant relationships between libido and testosterone have only been demonstrated up to certain limit, somewhere in the 200–450 ng/ml range. Above these levels, the relationship between testosterone and libido is much weaker and more difficult to demonstrate.

Table 16.7 summarizes the clinical presentation of hypogonadism.

Table 16.6 Routine screening of testosterone and prolactin in patients with low libido

Obtain free testosterone regardless of age
Obtain serum prolactin regardless of age

Table 16.7   Presentation of hypogonadism

Decreased libido
Decreased ejaculatory volume
Change in libido may precede change in shaving by years
Threshold amount of testosterone to sustain sexual activity
between 200 and 400 nanograms per dl

Adrenal Androgen

Dehydroepiandrosterone (known in the lay press as DHEA) is the major androgen produced by the adrenal glands. In 1994 the Massachusetts Male Aging Study, a large population-based study in the Boston area, found an inverse correlation between dehydroepiandrosterone levels and the incidence of erectile dysfunction. Subsequent study by different investigators found that this relationship existed only for men under 60 years of age. Since that time, several controlled studies have produced suggestive evidence that exogenous dehydroepiandrosterone may have mild effects on sexual function. To date, no carefully controlled study of dehydroepiandrosterone's effect on libido has been conducted.

Prolactin

The clinical presentation of hyperprolactinemia in men is usually decreased libido and erectile dysfunction. The mechanism by which hyperprolactinemia disrupts sexual behavior is incompletely understood and probably involves both central and peripheral effects. Because prolactin levels can vary, it is recommended that three separate levels be obtained before diagnosing hyperprolactinemia. On laboratory exam, plasma testosterone is also usually below normal limits or at low normal levels in men with hyperprolactinemia. However, administration of exogenous testosterone does not restore sexual function, whereas bromocriptine therapy is effective even before gonadal steroid levels are restored to normal levels, suggesting that the sexual effects of hyperprolactinemia involve more than a direct effect on the gonads. This hypothesis is supported by a recent study of experimental hyperprolactinemia in rats, which found that hyperprolactinemia inhibited male rat erectile responses without affecting testosterone levels. Hyperprolactinemia may inhibit sexual behavior in men by a central mechanisms of action. Prolactin secretion is primarily regulated by the secretion of inhibitory hypothalamic dopamine originating in the tubero-infundibular neurons of the arcuate nucleus. A number of different states can induce hyperprolactinemia—indeed, anything that prevents the hypothalamic dopamine from reaching the pituitary lactotroph membrane. Hypothalamic lesions, pituitary stalk lesions, compression of portal vessels, and drug therapy with dopamine blockers

Table 16.8   Hyperprolactinemia

1. Can present as decreased libido and erectile problems
2. May also have headache and decreased ejaculatory volume as associated symptoms
3. Usually serum testosterone is also low
4. May be drug-induced or due to prolactinoma
5. First rule out drug-induced etiology
6. If hyperprolactemia persists, obtain endocrinolgy consult

all can cause hyperprolactinemia, as can prolactinomas. Drugs commonly associated with elevated prolactin levels include risperidone, metoclopromide, and the phenothiazines.

Symptomatic treatment of hyperprolactinemia can be accomplished with bromocriptine or cagergoline, both of which are dopamine D2 agonists. It is important to diagnose prolactinomas early, as approximately 40% of these patients presenting also will show visual field defects. Typical evaluation of hyperprolactinemia involves a skull x-ray, computerized tomography, or an MRI. Formal visual field testing is usually performed as well as basic pituitary function tests.

Table 16.8 summarizes the clinical presentation of hyperprolactinemia.

Hypergonadism

High gonodotropin levels associated with elevated testosterone suggest a possible diagnosis of androgen insensitivity syndrome or gonadotropin-secreting pituitary tumor.

Evaluation of Hypogonadism

If hypogonadism is detected, it is critical to determine if it is of testicular (secondary to primary gonadal failure) or hypothalamico–pituitary origin, because the treatments for these conditions are quite different. Initial laboratory evaluation would involve morning levels of serum hormone-binding globulin, testosterone, luteinizing, hormone, follicle-stimulating hormone, estradiol, and prolactin. Also rule out

Table 16.9   Basic facts of androgen function

1. All androgens have similar biological effects.
2. All androgens work on the same receptor.
3. Androgens may have different effects in different tissues because of differing metabolism.
4. Five alpha-reductase metabolizes testosterone to 5 alpha-dihydrotestosterone.
5. Aromatase metabolizes testosterone to estradiol, which acts on the estrogen receptor.

Table 16.10   Evaluation of hypogonadism

1. Primary goal is to distinguish between testicular or hypothalamic disease
2. Obtain total testosterone plus serum hormone binding globulin, LH, FSH, estradiol, prolactin at 9 AM
3. Also obtain ferritin, iron binding capacity to rule out hemochormatosis

hemochormatosis as a possible etiological factor. The combination of low serum testosterone, high gonadotrophin levels, and a high estrogen level suggests primary gonadal failure, for which the treatment is hormone replacement.

This diagnosis can be confirmed by provocative testing with human chorionic gonadotrophin 4000 units IM for 4 days. Provocative testing in primary gonadal failure will not result in the expected doubling of serum testosterone. However, this test is rarely needed to make the diagnosis of primary hypogonadism.

The combination of low testosterone, low gonadotrophin, and high estradiol levels suggests the possibility of an estrogen-secreting tumor or an adrenal tumor. The presence of low testosterone in the presence of low gonadotrophins should alert the clinician to search for possible hypothalamic–pituitary disease. In this case, a skull radiogram to detect an abnormal pituitary fossa or suprastellar calcification should be performed, as well as an MRI of the hypothalamic–pituitary region. Other evaluations would include a GnRH test to measure pituitary gonadotrophin reserve, and a clomiphene test of the integrity of the hypothalamic–pituitary axis. Normally, one would observe a doubling of luteinizing hormone with clomiphene. A positive response to GnRH coupled with nonresponse of luteinizing hormone to clomiphene suggest GnRH deficiency. Table 16.9 summarizes androgen function. Tables 16.10 and 16.11 summarize the primary differential diagnosis of hypogonadism. Table 16.12 summarizes considerations in androgen replacement therapy.

Table 16.11   Differential diagnosis of hypogonadism

Laboratory finding	Probable diagnosis
Low testosterone High LH, FSH, estradiol	Primary gonadal failure
Low testosterone Low FSH, LH	Hypothalamico–pituitary disease
Low testosterone Low FSH, LH High estradiol	Rule out estrogen-secreting adrenal or testicular tumor

Table 16.12   Considerations in androgen replacement therapy

1. First establish that the problem is androgen deficiency of gonadal origin
2. Transdermal routes of testosterone replacement are preferred
3. Physical examination should document body hair distribution, musculature, testicular volume, gynecomastia
4. Goal is to restore physiological levels of androgen
5. Return of LH to normal levels indicates adequate testosterone replacement
6. Routine monitoring of serum lipids, hematocrit, prostate specific antigen recommended
7. Adverse effects can include acne, weight gain, gynecomastia, hair loss, plycythemia, and urinary problems

REFERENCES

Beuna F, Swerdloff R, Steiner B, et al. Sexual function does not change when serum testosterone levels are pharmacologically varied within the normal range. *Fertil Steril.* 1993;59:1118–1123.

Burge M, Lanzai R, Skarda S, Eaton R. Idiopathic hypogonadotropic hypogonadism in a male runner is reversed by clomiphene citrate. *Fertil Steril.* 1997;67:783–785.

Boolell M, Gepi-Attee S, Gingell JC, Allen MJ. Sildenafil, a novel effective oral therapy for male erectile disorder. *Br J Urol.* 1996;78:257–261.

Brindley G. Cavernosal alpha-blockade: a new technique for investigating and treating erectile impotence. *Br J Psychiat.* 1983;143:332–337.

Brown GA. Endocrine responses to chronic androstenedione intake in 30 to 56 year old men. *J Clin Endocrinol Metab.* 2000;85:4074–4080.

Cohan P. Erectile dysfunction. *J Clin Endocrinol Metab.* 2001;86:2391–2394.

Eri L, Tveter K. Safety, side effects and patient acceptance of the luteining hormone releasing hormone agonis leuprolide in treatment of benign prostatic hyperplagia. *J Urol.* 1994;152(2 Pt 1):448–452.

Feldman HA, Goldstein I, Hatzichriston DG. Impotence and its medical and psychological correlates: Results of the Massachusetts male aging study. *J Urol.* 1994;151:54–56.

Feldman HA, Johannes CB, Aranjo AB. Low dehydroepiandrosterone and iscemic heart disease in middle-aged men. *Am J Epidermiol.* 2001;153:78–89.

Feldman HA, Longcape C, Derby CA, et al. Age trends in the level of serum testosterone and other hormones in middle-aged men: Longitudinal results from the massachusetts male aging study. *J Clin Endocrinol Metab.* 2002;87:589–598.

Freda PU. Long term treatment of prolactin secreting macroadenomas with pergolide. *J Clin Endocrinol Metab.* 2000;85:8–13.

Gall H, Sparwasser C, Baehren W, Scherb W, Irion R. Long-term results of corpus cavernosum autoinjection therapy for chronic erectile dysfunction. *Andrologia.* 1992;24(5):285–292.

Guay A, Bansal S, Heatley G. Effect of raising endogenous testosterone levels in impotent men with secondary hypogonadism: double blind placebo-controlled trial with clomiphene citrate. *J Clin Endocrinol Metab.* 1995;80:3546–3552.

Jannini EA. Lack of sexual activity from erectile dysfunction is associated with a reversible reduction in serum testosterone. *Int J Androl.* 1999;22:385–392.

Johri A, Heaton JP, Morales A. Severe erectile dysfunction is a marker for hyperprolactinemia. *Int J Impot Res.* 2001;13:176–182.

Kaiser FE. Erectile dysfunction in the aging man. *Med Clin North Am.* 1999;83:1213–1229.

Kamischke A, Diebacker J, Nieschlag E. Potential of norethisterone enanthate for male contraception: pharmacokinetics and suppression of pituitary function. *Clin Endocrin.* 2000;53:351–358.

Lewis R. Epidemiolgy of erectiel dysfunction. *Urol Clin North Am.* 2001;28:363–375.

Lim V, Fang V. Restoration of plasma testosterone levels in uremic men with clopihene citrate. *J Clin Endocrinol Metab.* 1976;43:1370–1377.

Loosen P, Purdon S, Pavlou S. Effects on behavior of modulation of gonadal function in men with gonadotropin releasing hormone antagonists. *Am J Psychiatry.* 1994;151:271–273.

Losa M. Surgical treatment of prolactin secreting pituitary adenomas. *J Clin Endocrinol Metab.* 2002;87:3180–3186.

Master VA. Ejaculatory physiology and f dysfunction. *Urol Clin North Am.* 2001;28:363–375.

Morley JE. Testosterone replacement in older men and women. *J Gend Specif Med.* 2001;4:59–53.

Murialdo G, Galimberti C, Fonzi S, et al. Sex hormones and pititary function in male epilpetic patients with altered or normal sexuality. *Epilpesia.* 1995;36:360–365.

Randeva HS, Davison R, Bouloux M. Endocrinolgy. In C Carson, R Kirby, I Goldstein, eds. *Textbook of Erectile Dysfunction.* Oxford, U.K.: Isis; 89–104.

Reiter WJ. Dehydroepiandrosterone in the treatment of erectile dysfunction: a prospective, double-blind, randomized, placebo-controlled study. *Urology.* 1999;53:590–594.

Reiter WJ. Serum dehyroepiandrosterone sulfate in men with erectile dysfunction. *Urology.* 2000;55:755–758.

Reiter WJ. A placebo controlled dehydroepiandrosterone substation in elderly men. *Gynakol Geburtshilfliche Rundsch.* 1999;39:208–209.

Schill WB. Fertility and sexual life of men after their forties and in older age. *Asian J Androl.* 2001;3:1–7

Seidman S, Spitz E, Rizzo C, Roose SP. Testosterone replacement therapy for hypogonadal men with major depressive disorder. *J Clin Psychiatry.* 2001;62:406–412.

Thibaut F, Cordier B, Kuhn J. Drug modulation of libido and sexual activity. *Ann Endocrinol.* 1994;55:229–233.

Vermuelen A. Androgen replacement therapy in the aging amle. *J Clin Endocrinol Metab.* 2001;86:2380–2390.

Vickery B, McRae G, Briones W, Worden A, Seidenberg R, Schanbachen B, Falvo R. Effects of an LHRH agonist analogue upon sexual function in male dogs. *J Androl.* 1984;5:28–41.

Wang C. Pharmacodynamics of transdermal testsoterone gel in hypogonadal men. *J Clin Endocrinol Metab.* 2000;18:47–61.

17. Drug Treatment of Erectile Dysfunction

The pharmacological treatment of male erectile disorder has evolved rapidly over the past decades. In the 1970s effective pharmacotherapies for organic erectile problems were unavailable, and the major intervention was penile prosthesis surgery. In the 1980s intracavernosal injection of vasoactive substances was discovered and became the major intervention. The substances originally employed were phentolamine and papaverine. In 1997, alprostadil was introduced and used either as monotherapy or part of combination therapy. In the same year, the treatment of erectile dysfunction was revolutionized by the introduction of sildenafil, an effective oral agent for erectile dysfunction. Prior to that time, the only oral agent available in the U.S. market was yohimbine, a drug of questionable efficacy in organogenic impotence. At the time of publication of this text, numerous agents are being investigated as oral erectogenic agents. Many such as vardenafil and talalafil are similar to sildenafil in their mechanisms of action, except apomorphine. Whereas sildenafil has a peripheral mechanism of action, prolonging the vasodilation induced by nitrous oxide in the corposa cavernosa, apomorphine has a central mechanism of action, working as a dopaminergic agonist stimulating oxytocinergic pathways originating in the paraventricular nucleus of the hypothalamus.

EVALUATING COMPLAINTS OF ERECTILE DYSFUNCTION

Many men use imprecise terms in the description of their sexual problems, and they also have unrealistic expectations of their sexual performance. Therefore, the clinician needs to conduct a careful clinical assessment to ascertain the exact complaint, then establish the medical and psychosocial contexts in which the problem occurs. During the first visit, a physical examination and routine laboratory tests are recommended. With the sexual history and physical exam, the clinician observes secondary sex characteristics, peripheral pulses, penile sensation, bulbocavernosus reflex, testicular size, and firmness. The clinician also wants to obtain information about other sexual functioning, libido, and the partner's role and impact. For example, if the patient reports frequent turgid early morning and masturbatory erections but erectile failure with the spouse, an interpersonal etiology to the problem is likely. The history and physical exam also would identify possible conditions that might interfere with erectile function (e.g., diabetes mellitus, multiple sclerosis, antihypertensive medication, hypercholesterolemia, smoking, pelvic trauma, previous laminectomy, radical prostatectomy, hypogonadism, and psychiatric conditions).

Recommended routine laboratory examinations vary according to different protocols. Most protocols suggest a serum testosterone, glucose, and lipids. Routine screening of testosterone in men less than 50 years old will have minimal yield. A prostate specific antigen also is usually recommended by most urologists. Specialized testing, such as penile ultrasound and angiography, are usually reserved for patients in whom history suggests the possibility of a correctable vascular lesion.

Findings are usually reviewed with the patient on the second visit and referral considered in certain situations. Referral would obviously be considered in men with serious psychiatric problems, in those with suspected correctable vascular lesions, and in those whose laboratory results are inconsistent with known syndromes.

Table 17.1 describes the steps in a clinical evaluation of erectile dysfunction.

Table 17.1 Clinical evaluation of erectile dysfunction

Careful history of the complaint
    Assessment of libido
    Assessment of ejaculatory function
    Assessment of relationship with partner
    History of erections upon awakening or with masturbation
Physical examination
    Secondary sex characteristics
    Peripheral pulses
    Penile sensation
    Bulbocavernosus reflex
    Testicular firmness
Routine laboratory examination
    Serum testosterone if 50 years old or older
    Serum glucose
    Serum lipids

INTERVENTIONS FOR ERECTILE DYSFUNCTION

Counseling is recommended as the first line of treatment for problems in which the major etiology is interpersonal in nature. In all patients, the physician will want to identify modifiable factors, such as smoking, excessive alcohol intake, and any ongoing pharmacological regimes that interfere with sexual function. In the majority of cases, a clearly correctable pathology will not be identified, and treatment is empiric. In these cases, first-line treatment recommendations include sildenafil or a vacuum erection device. If sildenafil and the vacuum erection device are ineffective, contraindicated, or unacceptable to the patient and partner, second-line treatments include the intraurethral and intracorporeal injectable erectogenic agents. Penile prosthesis implantation is clearly the treatment of last resort.

Table 17.2 summarizes interventions for erectile dysfunction.

Sildenafil (Viagra)

Sildenafil, an oral vasoactive drug, is usually the preferred first-line intervention. In response to sexual stimulation, nitric oxide is released from epithelia and nerve cells and activates guanylate cyclase, which converts 5-guanosine triphosphate into 3,5 cyclic guanosine monophosphate (GMP). This chemical acts as a cellular second messenger and elicits smooth muscle relaxation, producing vascular engorgement and erection. The action of cyclic GMP is terminated by phosphodiesterase (PDE) type 5. Sildenafil works by inhibiting phosphodiesterase type 5. Thus sildenafil works peripherally either to prolong or magnify the effect of erectogenic stimuli. Sildenafil is a pyrazolopyrimidine with predominant affinity for phosphodiesterase 5. It is relatively selective for PDE type 5 but also has some affinity for PDE type 6, which is in the retina. This mechanism probably explains

Table 17.2   Interventions for erectile dysfunction

Identify modifiable factors
   Smoking
   Excess alcohol use
   Drug-induced sexual dysfunction
First-line approaches
   Counseling for psychogenic problems
   Androgen replacement if hypogonadal
   Oral erectogenic agents (e.g., sildenafil citrate)
   Vacuum erection devices
Second-line approaches
   Intraurethral erectogenic agents
   Intracorporeal erectogenic agents
Third-line interventions
   Penile prosthesis surgery

Table 17.3 a   Significant pharmacological properties of sildenafil

1. Sildenafil is rapidly absorbed and achieves peak plasma levels within one hour of ingestion.
2. Sildenafil has a mean plasma value of 411/h and reaches a steady state volume distribution of 105 liters.
3. The absolute bioavailabilty of a 50 mg capsule is 41%.
4. The terminal half-life is 3–4 hours.
5. A high-fat meal may slow the absorption of sildenafil; it is unclear whether this factor has clinical significance.
6. Sildenafil is metabolized by cytochrome P450 3A4. Drugs inhibiting the metabolism of sildenafil include cimetidine, ketoconazole, and erythromycin. It is unclear whether this effect is clinically significant.
7. The response to sildenafil appears to be dose-related, between 25 and 100 mg. There appears to be no advantage in giving a dose higher than 100 mg.

the side effect of sildenafil on color vision. Table 17.3a summarizes the pharmacological properties of sildenafil. Table 17.3b summarizes sildenafil's mechanism of action.

The efficacy of sildenafil is well established and impressive. In a group of men with idiopathic erectile disorder, 69% of coital attempts were successful on 100 mg sildenafil, as opposed to 22% on placebo. Sildenafil was effective in a variety of patient populations, including those with hypertension, depression, diabetes mellitus, and hyperlipidemia. Lower efficacy rates were obtained in patients with diabetes mellitus and men who had undergone nerve-sparing radical prostatectomy. Older men appeared to have similar success rates as younger men.

Common side effects with sildenafil include headache, flushing, rhinitis, dyspepsia, and transient visual abnormalities. Priapism is rare side effect of sildenafil. More alarming, a large number of deaths has occurred on sildenafil. Many clinicians feel that the deaths are the result of cardiac exertion during sex in men who have predominantly sedentary lifestyles. Other clinicians point out the relative absence of deaths reported regarding other sexually active drugs. These clinicians feel that sildenafil may have an increased risk for cardiovascular death because it augments the hypotensive effect of nitrates. This effect is secondary to nitrates stimulating the release of nitric oxide, thus augmenting the formation of cGMP (cyclic guanosine monophosphate). Any clinician prescribing sildenafil must consider the personal meaning of sexuality to the patient and the interpersonal context in which

Table 17.3 b   Mechanism of action of sildenafil

With sexual stimulation, nitric oxide is released
Nitric oxide stimulates formation of cyclic guanosine monophosphate (cGMP)
C GMP elicits smooth muscle relaxation, vasocongestion, and erection
The action of cGMP is terminated by phosphodiesterase type 5
Sildenafil inhibits phosphodiesterase type 5, effectively magnifying or prolonging effect of sexual stimuli on erectile response

Table 17.4   Clinical recommendations regarding prescription of sildenafil

1. Sildenafil is absolutely contraindicated in patients taking any nitrate drug.

2. All patients prescribed sildenafil should be informed of the risk of combining this drug with nitrates or of taking this drug within 24 hours of nitrate use.

3. Patients with coronary disease should be cautioned about the possible risk of cardiac exertion associated with sexual activity.

4. Caution should be used in prescribing sildenafil to patients on multiple antihypertensive agents.

5. Extreme caution should be used in prescribing sildenafil to someone with unstable angina.

6. Sildenafil should be used with caution in men with retinitis pigmentosa because the drug also inhibits PDE6, which regulates signal transduction in the retinal photoreceptors.

7. The symbolic meaning of sexual activity to the patient and partner should be explored prior to drug prescription.

this drug will be used. There have been case reports of severe discord and divorce precipitated by the successful restoration of erectile function. Other trials have found that as many as 14% of men in long-term relationships who experience sildenafil-mediated restoration of erectile function do not return to partner-related sexual activity. For many individuals and couples, sexuality and sexual intimacy may be an activity about which they have ambivalent feelings. Table 17.4 summarizes the clinical recommendations for prescribing sildenafil. Organic nitrates which are contraindicated with sildenafil are listed in Table 17.5. Drugs that theoretically interfere with the metabolism of sildenafil are listed in Table 17.6.

Apomorphine SL (Uprima)

The erectogenic effect of apomorphine was discovered by Sam Lal, a Canadian psychiatrist, who utilized the emetic effect of the apomorphine drug in conditioning therapy treatment of alcoholics. An incidental finding of his research was that the drug induced penile erections as a side effect. The erectogenic effect of apomorphine was confirmed in controlled studies in Paris, France, and Cleveland, Ohio. The drug is a central D1/D2 agonist. Lal subsequently performed a number of studies to identify the mechanism of apomorphine's action. He concluded that the erectogenic effect of apomorphine is the result of the drug's effect on central nervous system dopamine. His research includes studies demonstrating the following:

1. The erectogenic effect of apomorphine is blocked by central dopamine blockers.

2. This effect is not blocked by peripheral dopamine blockers, opioid antagonists, anticholinergic drugs, or antiserotonergic drugs.

Table 17.5 Organic nitrates contraindicated with sildenafil

Isosorbide Nitrate	Nitroglycerin	Isosorbide Mononitrate	Pentaerythritol Tetranitrate	Erythrityl Tetranitrate	Illicit Substances
Dilacrate-SR	Deponit	Imdur	Peritrate	Cardilate	Poppers
Iso-Bid	Minitran	Ismo	Peritrate SA	Isosorbide Dinitratel-Phenobarbital	
Isordil	Nitrok	Isosorbide mononitrate		Isordil w/PB	
Isordil tembids	Nitro-Bid	Monoket			
Isosorbide dinitrate	Nitrocine				
Isosorbide dinitrate LA	Nitrodenn				
Sorbitrate	Nitro Disc				
Sorbitrate SA	Nitro-Dur				
	Nitroeard				
	Nitroglycerin				
	Nitroglycerin T/R				
	Nitro-Ivn				
	Nitrolingual spray				
	Nitrol ointment				
	Nitrong				
	Nitro-Par				
	Nitropress				
	Nitro SA				
	Nitrospan				
	Nitrostat				
	Nitro-Time				
	Nitro transdermal				
	Nitro-trans system				
	Transiderm-Nitro				
	Tridil				

3. Animal studies suggest that apomorphine probably impacts the paraventricular nucleus.

Apomorphine was originally used in medicine as an emetic. A sublinqual slow-release form was developed that substantially reduced the nausea associated with this drug. Other advantages of this drug: it does not interact with nitrates, and there are no known drug–drug interactions. Properties of apomorphine are summarized in Table 17.7.

Efficacy data from large-scale clinical trials are impressive: 60% of patients taking 4 mg of apomorphine achieved erections on at least 50% of attempts; on this same dose, 49% of attempts at intercourse was successful. Time from administration to time of erection is 15–25 minutes, and the window of sexual opportunity is approximately 2 hours after dosing. Table 17.7 summarizes the pharmacokinetics of apomorphine.

Table 17.6   Drugs that are metabolized by, or that inhibit, cytochrome P450 3A4

Antibiotic/Antifungal	HMG	Psychotropics	Other
biaxin (clarithromycin)	Baycol (cerivastatin)	Dilantin (phenytoin)	acetaminophen
clotrimazole	Lipitor (atorvastatin)	Halcion (triazolam)	cyclosporine
ditlucan	Mevacor (lovastatin)	Luvox (fluvoxamine)	dexamethasone
erythromycin	Zocor (simvastatin)	phenobarbital	ethinyl estradiol
ketoconazole		Prozac (fluoxetine)	hismana (astemizole)
miconazole		Serzone (nefazodone)	naringenin (grapefruit
noroxin		Tegretol	juice)
sporanox		(carbamazepine)	Prilosec (omeprazole)
troleandomycin		Tofranil (imipramine)	Propulsid (cisapride)
		Zanax (alprazolam)	Protease inhibitors
		Zoloft (sertraline)	(Crixivan [indinavir],
			Norvir [ritonavir],
			Viracept [nelfinaavir],
			Invirase [saquinavir])
			Rezulin (troglitazone)
			rifampin
			Seldane (terfenadine)
			Tacrolimus
			Tagamet (cimetidine)
			theophylline
			Viagra (sildenafil)

Adverse events include nausea, dizziness, sweating, somnolence, yawning, and vomiting. Only 1% of patients with nausea has severe nausea. Syncope occurs in .6% of patients; prodromal symptoms include feeling lightheaded. Syncope appears to be vagal–vagal, without cardiac implications. On rechallenge syncope does not recur. Table 17.8 summarizes the properties and side effects of apomorphine.

Apomorphine has efficacy in a variety of diseases. Because sildenafil and apomorphine studies utilized different outcome measures, it is impossible, at this point, to state the relative efficacy of the two drugs. At the time of publication, apomorphine had not been approved by the FDA for use in the United States.

Phentolamine (Vasomax)

Alpha-adrenergic stimulation promotes vasoconstriction in the corpora cavernosa and thus detumescence. Drugs that oppose the effect of alpha-adrenergic activity tend to elicit vasodilation and thus erection. Phentolamine is a nonspecific alpha-blocker, used to treat

Table 17.7   Pharmacokinetics: 4 mg apomorphine

Tmax (hr)	.8
C max (ng/ml)	1.26
T1/2 (hr)	1.04

Table 17.8 Properties and side effects of apomorphine

Properties

Oral erectogenic agent under investigation in United States
Central nervous system dopamine agonist
Effect within 15–25 minutes
No interaction with nitrates
Side effects of nausea, dizziness, syncope

Symptom	Percentage
Nausea	16.9
Dizziness	8.3
Yawning	7.9
Sweating	5.0
Somnolence	5.8
Vomiting	3.7

arterial hypertension, which causes arterial smooth muscle relaxation. Alpha-adrenergic blockers probably increase erectile rigidity by opposing the endogenous vasoconstrictor influence of adrenergic activity. Double-blind studies of alpha-adrenergic blockers show mild improvement in men with minimal erectile dysfunction. Adverse effects include nasal congestion, dizziness, flushing, and headaches. Development of this drug is on hold, because early toxicology studies suggested possible high rates of fatty tumors. At this point, it is doubtful that phentolamine will be brought to the U.S. market.

Table 17.9 summarizes the properties and possible side effects of phentolamine.

Yohimbine (Yocon)

Yohimbine is an alpha-2 adrenoceptor antagonist that has clear positive effects on sexual behavior in lower animals, but the evidence for efficacy in humans is less clear. A number of studies of varying methodological sophistication has found suggestive evidence of modest efficacy with this drug. Meta-analyses of multiple studies suggest that yohimbine may have a modest effect in men with pychogenic impotence. The American Urological Association guidelines state that there is no evidence for the efficacy of yohimbine in the treatment of

Table 17.9 Properties and possible side effects of phentolamine

Oral erectogenic agent being investigated
Nonspecific alpha-adrenergic antagonist
Opposes endogenous vasoconstrictor activity
Approved in some foreign markets
Efficacy less than sildenafil or apomorphine
Toxicology studies in animals indicates high rate of fatty tumors

Table 17.10   Properties and side effects of yohimbine

Properties

Oral erectogenic agent
Alpha-2 adrenoceptor antagonist
Probable mild efficacy in humans

Side Effects

Anxiety
Insomnia
Elevated blood pressure
Use not recommended by American Urological Association

erectile disorder. Yohimbine in clinical series appears to be useful in reversing anorgasmia induced by serotonergic antidepressants. Side effects of yohimbine include anxiety, insomnia, and elevated blood pressure.

Table 17.10 summarizes the properties and side effects of yohimbine.

Other Agents

A number of agents is in various stages of development, including other phosphodiesterase inhibitors, prostaglandin E-1 topical gel, and other dopaminergic agonists. In laboratory animals, central 5HT2c agonists have been shown to induce penile erections. Inhibitors of rho kinase also have been shown to induce erections in laboratory animals. The rho kinase system regulates phosphorylation of myosin phosphate and thus regulates smooth muscle contraction by way of a calcium-independent erectile pathway. Other agents being investigated are listed in Table 17.11.

Topical Therapy

An Egyptian research group reported that a topical cream of three vasodilators—aminophylline, isosorbide dinitrate, and co-dergocrine mesylate—improved erectile function. This finding was confirmed in a double-blind study. However, a research group from South Africa

Table 17.11   Other agents under study

Other phosphodiesterase inhibitors
Prostaglandin E-1 topical gel
Other topical vasodilator creams
Other dopaminergic drugs
5HT2c agonists
Rho kinase inhibitors

Table 17.12   Intraurethral therapy

Properties

Intraurethral administration of alprostadil causes vasodilation
    of penile arteries
Semisolid pellet inserted into distal urethra
High drop-out rate
Difficulties with inconsistent rigidity

Side Effects

Urethral pain
Occasional problems with syncope, hypotension, and
    vaginities in partner

was unable to replicate these results, reporting no difference between active cream and placebo.

Intraurethral Therapy (MUSE)

Prostaglandin E-1 (alprostadil) causes arterial dilation when administered intraurethrally. Prostaglandins work via the adenyl cyclase second messenger system, rapidly absorbed. A semisolid pellet is placed into the distal 3 cm of the urethra by an applicator. This treatment has a high drop-out rate secondary to penile, urethral, testicular, and perineal pain, and some partners have symptoms of vaginitis after coitus. Hypotension and syncope may occur in 1–4% of patients. A major problem with this approach is frequent inadequate and inconsistent rigidity. Some clinicians have experimented with combinations of prostaglandin E-1 and prazosin; these combinations have higher efficacy but also a higher incidence of hypotension.

Table 17.12 summarizes the properties and side effects of intraurethral therapy.

Intracorporeal Injection Therapy

The most commonly used intracorporeal injections in the United States are papaverine, papaverine plus phentolamine, prostaglandin E-1, and triple mix. Their success rates are listed in Table 17.13.

The first injection is usually performed by the clinician to demonstrate the technique. The injection location is the dorsolateral area

Table 17.13   Average success rates of various intracorporeal injection therapies

Papaverine	54%
Papaverine/phentolamine	71%
Prostaglandin E-1	73%
Triple mix (all of above)	75%

Table 17.14   Intracorporeal injection

Properties
Initial injection in clinic to establish dose
Injection into dorsolateral, proximal penis
Rotation of injection sites
High drop-out rate
Education about risk of priapism

Side Effects
Priapism
Bleeding
Hematoma
Fibrosis
Infection

Dosage
Alprostadil: Start at 5 to 10 micrograms; maximum dose usually 40 micrograms
Papaverine/phentolamine: Doses range from .25 to 7.5 mg papaverine and .8 to 30 mg phentolamine.

of the proximal part of the penis. The conditions should be aseptic, and the injection site should be changed each time. It is recommended that only one injection be given daily. Side effects include priapism, bleeding, hematoma, fibrosis, and infection.

The recommended starting dose with papaverine/phentolamine injection therapy ranges from .25 to 7.5 mg ml papaverine, and from .8 to 30 mg phentolamine. The recommended starting dose of prostaglandin E-1 is 5–10 μg. In severe vascular disease, the clinician may want to start with 10–20 μg; the maximum dose is usually 40 μg. Table 17.14 summarizes the side effects and dosing protocol for intracorporeal injection therapy.

There is usually a high drop-out rate associated with injection therapy. Patients undergoing intraurethral injection of vasoactive substances should be educated about the possibility of priapism and told to contact a physician if they have an erection lasting 3–8 hours. Recommended treatment is corporeal aspiration with a large bore butterfly needle. After 20–50 ml of venous blood has been withdrawn, there usually is a noticeable reduction in pain. If the erection recurs, irrigation of the corpus cavernous with one of the following is recommended:

Adrenaline   10 to 20 microgram
Phenylephrine   100–200 microgram

Chapter 18 elaborates on the treatment of priapism.

Endocrine Therapy

A minimum level of testosterone is necessary for libido and ejaculatory function. Some hypogonadal men experience erectile problems. It is believed that the association of erectile dysfunction with low testosterone levels is mediated largely by the effect of androgens on libido. The amount of testosterone necessary to maintain erectile function must be extremely low, as some castrates remain sexually active. Because hypogonadal men have been observed to obtain erections in response to erotic stimuli but not to internal fantasies, it has been hypothesized that hypogonadal men lack the ability to generate internal sexual stimuli to augment sexual arousal. There is no evidence that the addition of exogenous testosterone, in the presence of normal levels of bioavailable testosterone, facilitates erectile function, although it may have a small effect on libido.

It is not cost-effective to monitor testosterone and prolactin in all men with complaints of erectile dysfunction. There is a low incidence of endocrinological causes of erectile problems in men under the age of 50 years old. Hence, routine assessment of testosterone and prolactin in men of this age group is not recommended. However, if the patient also has low libido, testosterone and prolactin levels should be obtained. After age 50, testosterone should be monitored in all men with erectile problems. Typically, prolactin levels only need to be obtained if the man also has low libido, gynecomastia, or testosterone levels below normal or at the lower end of the normal range.

Various assays of testosterone are available. Total testosterone measures both free testosterone and testosterone bound to serum hormone-binding globulin and the portion bound to albumin. Testosterone bound to serum hormone-binding globulin is thought to be inactive. An elevation in serum hormone-binding globulin can reduce the level of bioavailable testosterone, although the level of total testosterone will remain within normal limits. Thus, total testosterone is an imprecise measure of the activity of androgen. More precise assays include serum free testosterone and serum bioavailable testosterone. However, the more precise measures are also more expensive. A recent recommendation of the First International Consultation on Erectile Dysfunction was that all men with erectile dysfunction of unknown etiology have a single morning total testosterone assay. If that value is low or borderline low, it is recommended that a second testosterone level be obtained as well as luteinizing hormone and serum hormone-binding globulin levels. This will allow for the determination of bioavailable testosterone.

Androgen replacement therapy is usually lifelong and should only be started after documenting the presence of hypogonadism. A variety of androgen replacement products is available in the U.S. market, including oral, intramuscular, and transdermal preparations. Oral androgens are associated with heptatic toxicity, and intramuscular delivery systems lead to initial supraphysiological levels. Transdermal

Table 17.15   Endocrine therapy: General considerations

Absolute contraindications: breast and prostate cancer
Relative contraindications: androgen-sensitive epilepsy, migraine, sleep apnea,
  polycytemia
Minimal level androgen necessary for sexual function
Androgen insufficiency unlikely if plasma testosterone above 20 nmol/l
Check serum testosterone and prolactin in men with low libido
If testosterone is low, do free testosterone and check LH
Oral androgens associated with hepatotoxicity
Intramuscular androgens associated with supraphysiological peaks
Transdermal methods preferred

preparations are preferred. Contraindications include prostate and breast cancer. Androgen-sensitive epilepsy, migraine, sleep apnea, and polycytemia are additional factors which need to be considered prior to androgen therapy. Information concerning androgen therapy is summarized in Table 17.15.

REFERENCES

Alexander G, Sherwin B. The association between testosterone, sexual arousal, and selective attention for erotic stimuli. *Horm Behav.* 1991;25:367–381.

Althof SE, Turner LA, Levine SB, Risen CB, Bodner D, Kursh ED, et al. Sexual, psychological, and marital impact of self-injection of papaverine and phentolamine: a long-term prospective study. *J Sex Marital Ther.* 1991;17(2):101–112.

Althof SE, Turner LA, Levine SB, Bodner D, Kursh ED, Resnick MI. Through the eyes of women: the sexual and psychological responses of women to their partner's treatment with self-injection or external vacuum therapy. *J Urol.* 1992;147(4):1024–1027.

Amadeo M. Antiandrogen treatment of aggressivity in men suffering from dementia. *J Geriatr Psychiatry Neurol.* 1996;9:142–145.

Andersson K, Stief C. Neurotransmission of the contraction and relaxation of penile erectile tissue. *World J Urol.* 1997;15:14–20.

Aydin S, Odabas O, Ercan M, et al. Kara H, My, A. Efficacy of testosterone, trazodone, and hypnotic suggestion in the treatment of non-organic male sexual dysfunction. *Br J Urol.* 1996;77:256–260.

Ansong K, Punmancy R. An assessment of the clinical relevance of serum testosterone level determination in the evaluation of men with low sexual drive. *J Urol.* 1999;162(3 Pt 1):719–721.

Beutal M. Psychosomatic aspects in the diagnosis and treatment of erectile dysfunction. *Andrologia.* 1999;31(Suppl 1):37–44.

Burns-Cox N, Gingell JC. Erectile dysfunction: endocrinological therapies, risks and benefits of treatment. In: Carson C, Kirby R, Goldstein I; editors. *Textbook of erectile dysfunction.* Oxford, U.K.: Isis;1999:327–344.

Buvat J & Lemaire A. Endocrine screening in 1,022 men with erectile dysfunction: clinical significance and cost effective strategy. *J Urol.* 1997;158:1764–1767.

Banos R, Bosch F, Farre M. Drug-induced priapism: its etiology, incidence, and treatment. *Med Toxicol Advers Drug Exp.* 1989;4:46–58.

Bardin E, Kreiger J. Pharmacological priapism: comparison of trazodone and papaverine associated cases. *Int Urol Nephrol.* 1990;5:147–152.

Berkovitch M, Keresteci A. Efficacy of prilocaine–lidocaine cream in the treatment of premature ejaculation. *J Urol.* 1996;156:1783–1784.

Boolell M, Gepi-Attee S, Gingell J, Allen M. Sildenafil, a novel effective oral therapy for male erectile disorder. *Br J Urol.* 1996;78:257–261.

Briken P, Berner W, Noldus J, Nika E, Michl U. Treatment of paraphilias and sexually aggressive impulsive behavior with the LHRH-agonist leuprolide acetate. *Nervenarzi.* 2000;71:380–385.

Brindley G. Cavernosal alpha-blockade: a new technique for investigating and treating erectile impotence. *Br J Psychiat.* 1983;143:332–337.

Brooks J, Wailar M. Inappropriate masturbation and schizophrenia. *J Clin Psychiatry.* 2000;61:451.

Brufsky A, Fontaine-Rothe P, Berlane K, Riefer P, Jiroutek M, Kaplan I, et al. Finasteride and flutamide as potency-sparing androgen-ablative therapy for advanced adenocarcinoma of the prostate. *Urol.* 1997;49:913–920.

Carraro J, Raynaud J, Koch G, Chisholm G, DiSilverio F, Teillac P. Comparison of physiotherapy with finasteride in the treatment of benign prostate hyperplagia. *Prostate.* 1996;29:231–240.

Carani C, Granata A, Fustini M, Marrama P. Prolactin and testosterone: their role in male sexual function. *Int J Androl.* 1996;19:48–54.

Conway A, Handelsman D, Lording D, Stuckey B, Zajac J. Use, misuse and abuse of androgens. *Medical J Australia.* 2000;172:220–224.

Cooper AJ. Progesterone in the treatment of male sexual offenders: a review. *Can J Psychiatry.* 1986;31:73–79.

Cheitlin M, Hutter A. Use of sildenafil in patients with cardiovascular disease. *Circulation.* 1999;99:168–171.

Chiang P, Wu SN, Tsai EM, et al. Adenosine modulation of neurotransmission in penile erection. *Br J Clin Pharmacol.* 1994;38:357–362.

Clayton A, Owens J, McGarvey E. Assessment of paroxetine-induced sexual dysfunction using the Changes in Sexual Functioning questionnaire. *Psychopharmacol Bull.* 1995;31:397–413.

Constant M, Abrams C, Chasalow F. Gonadotrophin associated psychosis in perimenstrual behavior disorder. *Horm Res.* 1993;40:141–144.

Cooper A. Progestins in the treatment of male sex offenders: a review. *Can J Psychiatry.* 1986;31:73–79.

Cooper A, Sandhu S, Losztyn S, Cernovsky Z. A double-blind placebo controlled trial of medroxyprogesterone acetate and cyproterone acetate with seven pedophiles. *Can J Psychiatry.* 1992;37:687–693.

Cordova O, Chapel J. Medroxyprogesterone acetate antiandrogen treatment of hypersexuality in a pedophiliac sex offender. *Am J Psychiatry.* 1983;140:1036–1039.

Danjou P, Alexandre L, Warot D, Lacomblez L, Peuch AJ. Assessment of erectogenic properties of apomorphine and yohimbine in men. *Brit J Clin Pharmacol.* 1988;26:733–739.

Dickey R. The management of a case of treatment-resistant paraphilia with a long-acting LHRH agonist. *Can J Psychiatry*. 1992;37:567–569.

Doody K, Bain J. The effect of oral medroxyprogesterone acetate and methyltestosterone on sexual functioning in a male contraceptive trial. *Contraception*. 1985;31:65–70.

Fahmy A, Mitra S, Blacklock A, Desai K. Is the measurement of serum testosterone routinely indicated in men with erectile dysfunction? *BJU Int*. 1999;84:482–484.

Govier F, McClure R, Kramer-Levien D. Endocrine screening for sexual dysfunction using free testosterone determinations. *J Urol*. 1996;156:405–408.

Guay A, Bansal S, Heatley G. Effect of raising endogenous testosterone levels in impotent men with secondary hypogonadism: double blind placebo-controlled trial with clomiphene citrate. *J Clin Endocrinol Metabol*. 1995;80:2546–2552.

Gall H, Sparuasser C, Bahren W, et al. Long-term results of corpus cavernosum autoinjection therapy for chronic erectile dysfunction. *Andrologia*. 1992;24(5):285–292.

Georgitis W. J, Merenich J A. Trial of pentoxifylline for diabetic impotence. *Diabetes Care*. 1995;18(3):345–352.

Giraud B. Interim report of a large French multicentre study of efficacy and safety of 3.75 mg leuprorelin depot in metastatic prostatic cancer. *J Int Med Res*. 1990;18(Suppl 1):84–89.

Girman C, Kolman C, Liss C, Bolognese J, Binkowitz B, Stoner E. Effects of finasteride on health-related quality of life in men with symptomatic benign prostatic hypertrophy. *Prostate*. 1996;29:83–90.

Gold D P, Justino F D. Bicycle kickstand phenomena: prolonged erections associated with antipsychotic agents. *South Med J*. 1988;81:792–794.

Goldstein I, Lue T. Oral sildenafil in the treatment of erectile dysfunction. *New Engl J Med*. 1998;338:379–404.

Gomaa A, Shalaby M, Osman M, et al. Topical treatment of erectile dsyfunction: randomized double-blind placebo controlled trial of cream containing aminophylline, isosorbide dinitrate, and co-dergocrine mesylate. *Br Med J*. 1996;312:1512–1515.

Heaton J. Apomorphine: an update on clinical trial results. *Int J Imp Res*. 2000;12(Suppl 4):67–73.

Hajjar R, Kaiser F, Morley J. Outcomes of long-term testosterone replacement in older hypogonadal males: a retrospective analysis. *J Clin Endocrinol Metab*. 1997;82:3793–3796.

Kim SC, Azadzoi K. A nitric acid-like factor mediating noradrenergic, noncholinergic neurogenic relaxation of penile corpus cavernosum smooth muscle. *J Clin Investigation*. 1991;88:112–118.

Kim SC, Seo KK. Efficacy and safety of fluoxetine, sertraline, and clomipramine in patients with premature ejaculation: double-blind, placebo controlled study. *J Urol*. 1998;159(2):425–427.

Kloner R. Cardiovascular risk and sildenafil. *Am J Cardiol*. 2000;86 (2 Suppl 1):57–61.

Kirby R, Carson C, Goldstein I. *Erectile Dysfunction*. Oxford: Isis; 1999.

Knoll J. The facilitation of dopaminergic activity in the aged brain by (-)deprenyl. A proposal for a strategy to improve the quality of life in senescence. *Mech Ageing Dev*. 1985;30(2):109–122.

Lal S, Rios O, Thavundayil JX. Treatment of impotence with trazodone: a case report. *J Urol.* 1990;143:819–820.

Lal S. Apomorphine in the evaluation of dopaminergic function in men. *Prog Neuro-psychopharmacol & Biol Psychiatry.* 1988;12:117–164.

Le Roux P, Naude J. Topical vasoactive cream in the treatment of erectile failure. *Br J Urol.* 1999;83:810–811.

Lewis R. Review of intraurethral suppositories and ionophoresis therapy for erectile dysfunction. *Int J Imp Res.* 2000;12(Suppl 4):86–90.

Marum K, Baba S, Murai M. Erectile function and nocturnal penile tumescence in patients with prostate cancer undergoing luteinizing hormone-releasing hormone agonist therapy. *Int J Urol.* 1999;6:19–23.

Michael R, Zumpe D. Medroxyprogesterone acetate decreases the sexual activity of male cynomolgus monkeys(Macaca fascicularis): an action on the brain. *Physiol Behav.* 1993;53:783–788.

Mulhall J, Goldstein I. Oral agents in the management of erectile dysfunction. In Carson C, Kirby R, Goldstein I, editors. *Textbook of Erectile Dysfunction.* Oxford: Isis;1999:309–316.

McLean JD, Fgrsytue RG, Kapkin IA. Unusual side effects of clomipramine associated with yawning. *Can J Psychiatry.* 1983;28:569–570.

Meinhardt W, Schmidt PI, Kropman RF, et al. Trazodone, a double-blind trial for treatment of erectile dysfunction. *Int J Imp Res.* 1997;9(3):163–165.

Meston CM, Gorzalka BB. Psychoactive drugs and human sexual behavior: the role of serotonergic activity. *J Psychoactive Drugs.* 1992;24(1):1–40.

Michael R, Zumpe D. Medroxyprogesterone acetate decreases the sexual activity of male cynomolgus monkeys: an action on the brain. *Physiol Behav.* 1993;53:783–788.

Michael A, Owen A. Venlafaxine-induced increased libido and spontaneous erections. *Brit J Psychiatry.* 1997;170:193.

Michelson D, Bancroft J, Targum S, Kim Y, Tepner R. Female sexual dysfunction associated with antidepressant administration: a randomized, placebo-controlled study of pharmacological intervention. *Am J Psychiatry.* 2000;157:239–243.

Modell JG. Repeated observations of yawning, clitoral engorgement, and orgasm associated with fluoxetine administration. *J Clin Psychopharmacol.* 1989;9(1):63–65.

Morales A, Surridge D, Marshall PG. Yohimbine for treatment of impotence in diabetes. *New England J of Medicine.* 1981;305:1221.

Morales A, Condra M, Owen JA, et al. Is yohimbine effective in the treatment of organic impotence?: results of a controlled trial. *J Urol.* 1987;137:1168–1172.

Morales A. Yohimbine in erectile dysfunction: the facts. *Int J Impot Res.* 2000;12(Suppl 1):S70–74.

Mydlo J, Volpe M, Macchia R. Initial results using combination therapy for patients with a suboptimal response to either alprostadil or sildenafil therapy. *Eur Urol.* 2000;38:30–34.

Nemeth A, Arato M, Treuer T, et al. Treatment of fluvoxamine-induced anorgasmia with a partial drug holiday. *Am J Psychiatry.* 1996;153:1365.

Onu P. Depot medroxyprogesterone in the management of benign prostatic hyperplagia. *Eur Urol.* 1995;28:229–235.

Ott B. Leuporide treatment of sexual aggression in a patient with dementia and the Kluver-Bucy syndrome. *Clin Neuropharmacol.* 1995;18:443–447.

Oakley N, Allen P, Moore, K. Vacuum devices for erectile dysfunction. In Carson C, Kirby R, Goldstein I, editors. *Textbook of Erectile Dysfunction.* Oxford, U.K.: Isis;1999:371–382.

Osteroh I, Eardley I, Carson C, Padma-Nathan H. Sildenafil: a selective phophodiesterase 5 inhibitor for the treatment of erectile dysfunction. In Carson C, Kirby R, Goldstein I, editors. *Textbook of Erectile Dysfunction.* Oxford U.K.: Isis;1999:285–308.

Padma-Nathan H. Intra-urethral and topical agents in the management of erectile dysfunction. In Carson C, Kirby R, Goldstein I, editors. *Textbook of Erectile Dysfunction.* Oxford U.K.: Isis;1999:323–326.

Pehek EA, Thompson JT, Hull EM. The effects of intrathecal administration of the dopamine agonist apomorphine on penile reflexes and copulation in the rat. *Psychopharmacol.* 1989;99:304–308.

Pescatori E, Engelman J, Davis G, Goldstein I. Priapism of the clitoris: a case report following trazodone use. *J Urol.* 1993;149:1557–1559.

Porst H. Current perspectives on intracavernosal pharmacotherapy for erectile dysfunction. *Int J Imp Res.* 2000;12(Suppl 4):91–100.

Purcell P. Trazodone and spontaneous orgasms in an elderly postmenopausal woman: a case report. *J Clin Psychopharmacol.* 1995;15:293–294.

Reid K, Surridge D, Morales A, et al. Double-blind trial of yohimbine in treatment of psychogenic impotence. *Lancet.* 1987;2:421–423.

Rich S, Ovsiew F. Leuprolide acetate for exhibitionism in Huntington's disease. *Mov Disord.* 1994;9:353–357.

Rosen RC, Phillips NA, Gendrano NC. Oral phentolamine and female sexual arousal: a pilot study. *J Sex Marital Ther.* 1999;25:137–144.

Rosen RC, Ashton AK. Prosexual drugs: empirical status of the new aphrodisiacs. *Archives of Sexual Behavior.* 1993;22:521–543.

Rosler A, Witztum E. Treatment of men with paraphilias with a long-acting analogue of gonadotropin-releasing hormone. *N Engl J Med.* 1998;338:416–422.

Rousseau L, Couture M, Dupont A, Labrie F, Couture N. Effect of combined androgen blockade with an LHRH agonist and flutamide in one severe case of male exhibitionism. *Can J Psychiatry.* 1990;35:338–341.

Randeva H, Davisin R, Bouloux P. Endocrinology. In Carson C, Kirby R, Goldstein I, editors. *Textbook of Erectile Dysfunction.* Oxford,U.K.: Isis;1999:89–104.

Reiter W, Pycha A, Schatzl G, et al. Serum dehydroepiandrosterone sulfate concentrations in men with erectile dysfunction. *Urol.* 2000;55:755–758.

Spahn M, Manning M. Juenemann K. Intracavernosal therapy. In Carson C, Kirby R, Goldstein I, editors. *Textbook of Erectile Dysfunction.* Oxford U.K.: Isis;1999:345–354.

Schlatter EK, Lal S. Treatment of alcoholism with Dent's oral apomorphine method. *Quart J Studies Alcohol.* 1972;33:430–436.

Segraves RT. Pharmacological enhancement of human sexual behavior. *J Sex Education and Therapy.* 1991;17:283–289.

Segraves R, Bari M, Segraves KB, Maguire E. Effect of apomorphine on penile tumescence in men with psychogenic impotence. *J Urology.* 1991;145:1174–1175.

Segraves R, Segraves K. Pharmacotherapy for sexual disorders: advantages and pitfalls. *Sex Marital Ther* (UK). 1998;13(3):295–309.

Smith DM, Levitte SS. Association of fluoxetine and return of sexual potency in three elderly men. *J Clin Psychiatry*. 1993;54:317–319.

Sondra L, Mazo R, Chancellon MD. The role of yohimbine in the treatment of erectile impotence. *J Sex Marital Ther*. 1990;16:15–21.

Stevenson RW, Soliom L. The aphrodisiac effect of fenfluramine: two case reports of a possible side effect to the use of fenfluramine in the treatment of bulimia. *J Clin Psychopharmacol*. 1990;10(1):69–71.

Susset JG, Tessier CD, Wincze J, et al. Effect of yohimbine hydrochloride on erectile impotence: a double-blind study. *J Urol*. 1989;141:1360–1363.

Swanson JR. Fluoxetine and sexual dysfunction. *Canad J Psychiatry*. 1993;38:297.

Thibaut F, Cordier B, Kuhn J. Effect of a long lasting gonadotrophin hormone releasing hormone agonist in six cases of severe male paraphilia. *Acta Psychiatrica Scand*. 1993;87:445–450.

Tenover J. Testosterone replacement therapy in older adult men. *Int J Androl*. 1999;22:300–306.

Thibaut F, Kuhn J, Cordier B, Petit M. Hormone treatment of sex offenses. *Encephale*. 1998;24:132–137.

Turner LA, Althof SE. The clinical effectiveness of self-injection and external vacuum devices in the treatment of erectile dysfunction: a six-month comparison. *Psychiatr Med*. 1992;10(2):283–293.

Turner LA, Althof SE, Lenine SB, et al. Twelve-month comparison of two treatments for erectile dysfunction: self-injection versus external vacuum devices. *Urology*. 1992;39(2):139–144.

van Ahlen H, Piehota HJ, Kias HJ, Brennerman W, Klingmiller D. Opiate antagonists in erectile dysfunction: a possible new treatment option? *Eur Urol*. 1995;28:246–250.

Waldinger M, Hengeveld MW, Zwinderman AH. Ejaculation retarding properties of paroxetine in patients with premature ejaculation. *Brit J Urol*. 1997;79:592–595.

Webb D, Muirhead G, Wulff M, Sutton J, Levi R, Dinsmore W. Sildenafil citrate potentiates the hypotensive effects of nitric oxide donor drugs in male patients with stable angina. *J Am Coll Cardiol*. 2000;36:25–31.

Wessells H, Levine N, Hadley M, Dorr R, Hruby V. Melanocortin receptor agonists, penile erection, and sexual motivation: human studies with melanotin II. *Int J Imp Res*. 2000;12(Suppl 4): 74–79.

Wincze J, Bansal S, Malamud M. Effects of medroxyprogesterone acetate on subjective arousal, arousal to erotic stimulation and nocturnal penile tumescence in male sex offenders. *Arch Sex Behavior*. 1986;15:293–305.

Willke R, Glick H, McCarron T, Erder M, Althof S, Linet O. Quality of life effects of alprostadil therapy for erectile dysfunction. *J Urol*. 1997;157:2125–2128.

Winters S. Current status of testosterone replacement in men. *Arch Fam Med*. 1999;8:257–263.

Wortsman J, Rosner W, Duau M. Abnormal testicular function in men with primary hypothyroidism. *Am J Med*. 1987;82:207–212.

Wyllie M, Andersson KE. Orally active agents: the potential of alpha-adreneceptor antagonists. In Carson C, Kirby R, Goldstein I, editors. *Textbook of Erectile Dysfunction*. Oxford,U. K.: Isis;1999:317–322.

18. Priapism and Its Treatment

OVERVIEW OF THE CONDITION

Priapism is a prolonged, usually painful, persistent erection that does not subside with orgasm. Twenty-eight per cent of reported priapism cases have been associated with psychiatric drugs, especially antipsychotics and trazodone. Priapism is a medical emergency warranting urological consultation if the erection persists more than 4–6 hours. Priapism can result in endothelial and trabecular necrosis, as well as widespread smooth muscle destruction. Most episodes of priapism occur early in the morning. Approximately 50% result in permanent erectile failure.

The arterial blood supply to the penis comes from the pudendal artery, which is trifurcated. One branch, the cavernous artery, divides into helicine branches that supply trabecular tissue. With erection, the lacunae and trabecular walls expand against the tunica albuginea, trapping the blood within the corpora. Venous drainage occurs by venules between the tunica and peripheral sinusoids. Blood then exits by emissary vein and the deep dorsal vein. Erection occurs by dilation of the arterial smooth muscle and trapping of the incoming blood by a venoocclusive mechanism. This mechanism is hypothesized to occur by expansion of the lucunar spaces against the tunica albuginea, stretching the subtunical venules and thereby greatly increasing their resistance to outflow. In the flaccid state, the helicine arteries are contracted and only a small amount enters the sinusoidal spaces.

Failure of detumescence mechanisms produces priapism. Because alpha-adrenergic stimulation controls detumescence, many drugs that block alpha-adrenergic processes are associated with priapism.

Table 18.1 Drugs associated with priapism

Antidepressants	Antipsychotics	Antihypertensives	Other
Trazodone	Chlorpromazine Clozapine Olanzapine Risperidone Thioridazine	Hydralazine Prazosin Quanethidine	Cocaine Papaverine Phentolamine

Other hypotheses concerning the mechanism of priapism involve adrenergic–cholinergic balance, the histaminic system, and the beta-adrenergic system.

There are two types of priapism: high-flow and low-flow. High-flow priapism is usually the result of trauma. Low-flow priapism is more common and is usually associated with pain, secondary to tissue ischemia. Penile priapism can result in permanent impotence, whereas clitoral priapism is painful but does not appear to interfere with subsequent sexual function. Low-flow priapism can be a side effect of pharmacotherapy. Medications causing priapism are listed in Table 18.1. Nonpharmacological causes of low-flow priapism include sickle cell anemia and metastatic lesions.

Differential diagnosis of high- from low-flow priapism is critical, because low-flow priapism causes trabecular destruction in 24 hours and widespread smooth muscle necrosis by 48 hours.

Low-flow priapism, associated with full rigidity of the corpus cavernosum, is a painful condition in which the glans penis remains soft. In high-flow priapism, the penis is only semirigid and pain is unusual. In uncertain cases or for malpractice coverage, penile blood gases can be drawn to establish the differential diagnosis.

TREATMENT

Low-flow priapism can be treated by corporeal aspiration of blood with a large bore butterfly needle and irrigation with nonheparinized saline. After 20–50 ml of venous blood are withdrawn, the patient will usually experience a reduction in pain. If the first intervention is ineffective or if the erection recurs after aspiration, the treatment of choice is irrigation of the corpus cavernosum with phenylephrine 100–200 μg, which can be repeated every 5 minutes. Other agents that can be used include epinephrine (10–20 μg), metaraminol (2–4 mg), phenylephrine (100–200 μg), or norephinephrine (10–20 μg). Surgical shunt procedures are necessary for patients who do not respond to pharmacological procedures. Table 18.2 summarizes the treatment for priapism.

Table 18.2   Treatment of low-flow priapism

Treat as medical emergency
Corporeal aspiration 20–50 ml venous blood
Pain should subside
If priapism recurs, injection with 100–200 μg of phenylephrine
Repeat q 5 minutes
If unresponsive to above, consider surgical shunt

Recent research has investigated the differential effectiveness of oral medications for the treatment of priapism. In one study, patients were given intracorporeal prostaglandin E-1 to induce erections, and various agents were utilized to produce detumescence. Oral terbutaline was more effective than pseudoephedrine. As deaths have occurred with metaraminol, most clinicians avoid this agent.

REFERENCES

Broderick GA, Gordon D, Hypolite J, Levin RM. Anoxia and corporeal smooth muscle dysfunction: a model for ischemic priapism. *J Urol.* 1994;151:259–262.

Evans C. Complications of intracavernosal therapy for impotence. In Carson CC, Kirby RS, Goldstein I (editors). *Textbook of erectile dysfunction.* Oxford, U.K.: ISIS; 1999:365–370.

Levine JF, Saenz de Tejada I, Payton TR, Goldstein I. Recurrent prolonged erections and priapism as a sequela of priapism; pathophysiology and management. *J Urol.* 1991;145:746–747.

Lowe FC, Jarow JP. Placebo-controlled study of oral terbutaline and pseudoephedrine in management of prostaglandin E1—induced prolonged erection. *Urology.* 1993;42:51–54.

Pryor JP. Management of priapism, Current opinion in urology.1994;4:343–345.

Serel S, Melman A. Priapism. In Carson CC, Kirby RS, Goldstein I (editors). *Textbook of erectile dysfunction.* Oxford, U.K.: ISIS; 1999:529–539.

Shifren JL, Braunstein GD, Simon JA, Casson R, Buster J, Redmond J, Burki R, Ginsberg ES, Rosen R, Leiblum S, Caranelli K, Mayer N. Transdermal testosterone treatment in women with impaired sexual function after oophorectomy. *N Engl J Med.* 2000;343:682–686.

Stackl W, Bondril P, Cartmill R, Knoll D, Pescatori ES. Priapism. In Jardin A, Wagner G, Khoury S, Giuliano F, Padma-Nathan H, Rosen R (editors). *Erectile dysfunction.* Plymouth, U.K.: Health Publications; 2000:557–572.

Thavundayil JX, Hambalek R, Kin NM. Prolonged penile erections induced by hydroxyzine: possible mechanism of action. *Neuropsychobiology.* 1994;30:4–6.

P
R
I
A
P
I
S
M

19. Treatment of Female Sexual Arousal Disorder

INTRODUCTION

Human sexual response is a complex, multidimensional process. The response cycle has been described and divided, perhaps a bit artificially, into four phases: desire/libido, arousal/excitement, orgasm/release, and resolution/plateau. Impairment of sexual functioning can occur during any phase of the response cycle. Even though this chapter focuses on the impairment or disorder of the arousal/excitement phase, it is important to realize that impairment does not usually occur only during one phase of the sexual response cycle. Female sexual arousal disorder (FSAD) may coexist with female sexual desire disorders (decreased or absent libido) and/or female orgasmic disorder.

The chapter focuses specifically on:

- Description, epidemiology, diagnosis, and physiology of female sexual arousal disorder
- Treatment with hormone replacement
- Treatment with sildenafil
- Treatment with other agents (alprostadil, apomorphine, L-arginine, phentolamine, yohimbine)
- Use of various lubricants
- Treatment with other modalities
- The importance of combining psychopharmacological and psychotherapy treatment modalities in the management of this disorder
- Management of the disorder when it is medication-induced.

Table 19.1 Pharmacological agents discussed in this chapter

Generic Name	Brand Name	Doses (mg) and Forms
Hormonal Preparations: systemic		
conjugated estrogen	Premarin	t: 0.3; 0.625; 0.9; 1.25; 2.5
estrogen + methyltestosterone	Estratest	t: 0.625/1.25; 1.25/2.5
Hormonal Preparations: topical/vaginal		
conjugated estrogen	Premarin vaginal cream	cr: 0.625 per gram
estradiol	Estrace	cr: 0.01%
	Estring	r: 2
	Vagifem	vt: 25 μg
Oral Vasoactive and Other Agents		
alprostadil	Caverject	pw: 5/10/20/40 μg/vial
	MUSE	supp: 125/250/500
		1000 μg/supp
apomorphine		
phentolamine		
yohimbine hydrochloride	Aphrodyne	cp: 5.4
sildenafil	Viagra	t: 25/50/100
Nutritional Supplement		
L-arginine	ArginMax	

cp = caplet; cr = cream; pw: = powder; r = vaginal ring; supp = suppository; t = tablets; vt = vaginal tablets.

Table 19.1 lists the pharmacological agents discussed in this chapter.

It is important to note that none of the agents/devices in Table 19.1 has been approved by the FDA for the treatment of female sexual arousal disorder (probably due to the lack of solid evidence from rigorous studies and the cost associated with the FDA approval process).

DESCRIPTION, EPIDEMIOLOGY, DIAGNOSIS, AND PHYSIOLOGY

According to the *DSM-IV* (American Psychiatric Association, 1994), the "essential feature of female sexual arousal disorder is a persistent or recurrent inability to attain, or to maintain until completion of the sexual activity, an adequate lubrication–swelling response of sexual excitement. The arousal response consists of vasocongestion in the pelvis, vaginal lubrication and expansion, and swelling of the external genitalia. The disturbance must cause marked distress or interpersonal difficulty. The dysfunction is not better accounted for by another Axis I disorder (except for another sexual dysfunction) and is not due exclusively to the physiological effect of a substance (including medications) or general medical condition."

The definition of sexual arousal disorder by an international panel of experts (Basson et al., 2001) is basically the same: "persistent or recurrent inability to attain or maintain sufficient sexual excitement, causing personal distress, which may be expressed as a lack of subjective excitement, or genital (lubrication/swelling) or other somatic responses." In addition to the lack or diminished lubrication, FSAD may include decreased clitoral or labial sensation, decreased clitoral and labial engorgement, or lack of vaginal smooth muscle relaxation.

According to the National Health and Social Life Survey, the prevalence of female arousal problems is 14% (+7% of sexual pain disorder). Estimates of sexual arousal disorder in women in other studies vary from 11% to 48%. In the national survey, the incidence of "trouble lubricating" and "sex not pleasurable" for women between 18 and 59 years old was estimated at 18.8% and 21.2%, respectively. In one study, lack of lubrication was reported in 13.6% of 329 women treated in an outpatient gynecological clinic. Earlier reports suggested that FSAD is a very frequent, if not the most frequent (around 50%), complaint among women seeking sex therapy.

The diagnosis of female sexual arousal disorder is made along three dimensions:

- Lubrication–swelling response
- Presence of marked distress or interpersonal difficulty
- Lack of direct effect of another Axis I disorder (except another sexual dysfunction), or direct effect of a substance (e.g., of abuse), or a general medical condition.

Table 19.2   Prevalence of female sexual arousal difficulties

General population	
Community studies (Spector & Carey, 1990)	11–48%
National Health and Social Life Survey (Laumann et al., 1999)	14% (+7% sexual pain disorder)
OB/GYN clinics	
Lack of lubrication (Rosen et al., 1990)	13.6%
Painful intercourse (Rosen et al., 1990)	11.3%
Sex therapy clinics	
(Spector & Carey, 1990)	over 50%
Women seeking marital therapy	
(Frank et al., 1976)	up to 80%

FEMALE SEXUAL AROUSAL DISORDER

Table 19.3 Issues in the diagnosis of FSAD

1. Individual
   a. Anxiety?
   b. Depression?
   c. Fatigue?
   d. History of sexual abuse?
   e. Life stressors?
   f. Menopause?
   g. Religious taboos?

2. Couple (if possible to obtain)
   a. Different expectations, desires?
   b. Lack of/short foreplay?
   c. Poor communication?
   d. Psychosocial issues?
   e. Relationship issues?

3. Sexual history
   a. Anorgasmia?
   b. Delayed orgasm?
   c. Lack of desire?

4. Review of medical systems
   a. Endocrine
   b. Genitourinary (surgery, trauma)
   c. Neurological diseases
   d. Vascular diseases

5. Medications
   a. Anticholinergisc?
   b. Antidepressants?
   c. Antihistamines?
   d. Antihypertensives?
   e. Antipsychotics?
   f. Chemotherapeutic agents?
   g. Hormonal supplements?

6. Lifestyle issues
   a. Alcohol abuse?
   b. Lack of exercise?
   c. Smoking?
   d. Substance abuse?

7. Physical examination, including gynecological examination

8. Laboratory tests
   a. Complete blood count
   b. Estrogen, testosterone, prolactin, sex hormone binding globulin, FSH and LH levels, thyroid hormones (TSH, T3, T4)
   c. Glucose level
   d. Liver function tests
   e. Urinalysis
   f. Vaginal cultures

9. Special tests in specialist office
   a. Genital blood flow (Doppler ultrasonography, vaginal photoplethysmography)
   b. Genital sensation
   c. Vaginal lubrication measurements

Further subclassification is based on course (lifelong vs. acquired type), situation (generalized vs. situational type), and possible etiology (due to psychological factors vs. combined factors).

The diagnosis of female sexual arousal disorder (see Table 19.3) is based on a clinical interview of the individual, the couple (if possible), sexual history review of medical systems, review of medications and lifestyle, and (in most cases) general physical examination. Various routine and specialized laboratory tests should be performed, whenever indicated. There are several instruments available to assist in the evaluation of subjective sexual functioning (e.g., Brief Index of Sexual Function Inventory, Female Sexual Function Index); however, most of them are not used in routine clinical practice and are not necessary to confirm the diagnosis of sexual arousal disorder. There also are various vascular tests for measuring sexual arousal (e.g., vaginal photoplethysmography, duplex Doppler ultrasonography) available. However, these tests are research tools and their clinical applicability and normative data are yet to be determined.

The physiology of female sexual arousal is quite complex and not fully understood. Numerous anatomical structures, genital and nongenital, and neural connections are involved in female sexual arousal. (see Table 19.4.) The regulation of female sexual arousal includes

Table 19.4 Systems/mechanisms involved in physiology/regulation of FSAD

Central and peripheral nervous systems
  Bulbocavernous reflex
  Spinal cord—brainstem—hypothalamus—amygdala—cortex
  Spinal cord reflex mechanisms
  Sympathetic and parasympathetic stimulation
  Vaginal and clitoral autonomic nerve stimulation

Muscular system
  Smooth muscle relaxation
  Vaginal prolongation

Vascular system
  Vaginal and clitoral engorgement and vasocongestion

Glandular system involved in lubrication
  Bartholini, vaginal, and cervical glands
  Plasma transudation through vaginal epithelium

Hormones
  Gonadal, possibly thyroid, and others

Neurotransmitters
  Acetylcholine
  Adenosin triphosphate
  Nitric oxide
  Norepinephrine
  Serotonin (centrally)
  Substance P
  Vasoactive intestinal polypeptide

the central and peripheral nervous systems (spinal cord, brainstem, hypothalamus, amygdala, input from the cortex), and several spinal cord reflex mechanisms (e.g., bulbocavernosus reflex, vaginal and clitoral autonomic nerve stimulation) are involved. Sexual stimulation generally results in smooth muscle relaxation, increased blood flow (vaginal and clitoral engorgement and vasocongestion), and increased vaginal lubrication (from increased transudation of plasma through the vaginal epithelium and secretion from several glands, such as the Bartholini glands and vaginal and cervical glands), and vaginal prolongation. Various neurotransmitters, such as acetylcholine, adenosin triphosphate, nitric oxide, substance P, vasoactive intestinal peptide, norepinephrine, serotonin (centrally), and others are involved in the regulation of sexual arousal. In addition, gonadal and other hormones modulate sexual arousal response.

Until fairly recently, various forms of psychotherapy and treatment of underlying medical diseases have been the mainstay in the treatment of FSAD because psychological factors and medical diseases have been viewed as the main etiological factors. Pharmacology of FSAD has developed only during the last several years (except for various lubricants and use of hormones).

Nonpharmacological treatment approaches to FSAD include the Masters and Johnson program involving sensate focus strategy, various imagery techniques, and individual and couple psychotherapy. The outcome of these techniques in the treatment of FSAD has not been clear. Outcome studies have been criticized for their selection bias, lack of solid outcome measures, and other methodological problems.

TREATMENT

Lifestyle changes (cessation of smoking, discontinuation of substance abuse, initiation of exercise), treatment of possible underlying medical and/or mental diseases, and patient–partner education about sexual functioning should be initiated prior to starting pharmacotherapy for female sexual arousal disorder (see Table 19.5).

Table 19.6 summarizes the treatments currently in use in the treatment of sexual arousal disorder.

Hormone Replacement

Hormonal replacement for female sexual arousal disorder has been used mainly in postmenopausal or otherwise estrogen-deficient women. The vaginal mucosa in these women becomes dry and thin.

Table 19.5   What could be done therapeutically prior staring pharmacotherapy of FSAD

1. Patient education about sexual functioning and sexual response

2. Lifestyle changes
   a. Discontinuation of substance abuse
   b. Initiation of exercise
   c. Smoking cessation

3. Treatment of possible underlying medical and/or mental disease
   a. Anxiety
   b. Depression
   c. Diabetes mellitus
   d. Hypertension

4. Evaluate existing medication use
   a. Consider discontinuation (if possible)
   b. Recommend change when appropriate

Lubricants have been used to address the dryness, but they do not help to increase the thickness or elasticity of the mucosa. Estrogens have been used either systemically or locally. In menopausal women, the systemic administration of estrogens may have multiple beneficial effects, such as relieving hot flashes, increasing libido, and prevention of osteoporosis systemically, and decreased dryness, decreased pain and burning, and improved clitoral sensitivity locally. Testosterone

Table 19.6   Summary of possible treatments currently in use for FSAD

1. Hormones
   a. Systemic (mostly in postmenopausal women)
      Combination of estrogen and androgen?
      Conjugated estrogen (most frequently 0.625 mg)
      Medroxyprogesterone (5 mg/daily)
   b. Local (topical) estrogen (Premarin cream, Estring)
      Testosterone (transdermal preparation)[*,**]

2. Sildenafil
   25–100 mg (However, double-blind study did not confirm sildenafil's usefulness)

3. Other vasoactive agents
   a. Alprostadil (topical, intravaginal cream; 0.05%, 0.1%, 0.2%)
   b. Apomorphine (suggested, but no data available)
   c. L-arginine (ArginMax)?
   d. Phentolamine (40 mg orally or locally)
   e. Yohimbine (5.4 mg; suggested, but no data available)

4. Lubricants

   See Table 19.7

5. Other modalities (mechanical)

   EROS-Clitoral Therapy Device (vacuum pump)

6. Psychotherapy and sex therapy

---

[*] Usually supraphysiologic doses; dangers expected but unknown.
[**] Risks include hirsutism, masculinization, clitoral enlargement, hypercholesterolemia, and possibly increased risk of breast cancer.

replacement also has been used for female sexual arousal disorder, especially in women who have undergone oophorectomy.

Systemic Estrogens

Systemic hormone administration solely for female sexual arousal disorder in premenopausal women has not been properly studied. Improvement of FSAD symptoms in postmenopausal women usually occurs together with improvement in systemic symptoms such as hot flashes. The most frequently used systemic oral estrogen preparation is a conjugated estrogen (Premarin, doses 0.3 mg, 0.625 mg, 0.9 mg, 1.25 mg, and 2.5 mg, with the 0.625 mg tablet probably being the most frequently used). Medroxyprogesterone 5 mg daily for 10 days every 1 to 3 months may be used in women with intact uterus who require progesterone opposition.

One study of the effect of oral estrogen replacement (1.25 mg) compared with a combination of estrogen–androgen (1.25 mg of estrogen and 2.5 mg of methyltestosterone) on sexual function in 20 postmenopausal women reported significantly greater improvement in sexual sensation and desire with the combination treatment than estrogen alone. However, the improvement in sexual arousal was not significantly greater.

Local Estrogens

Even though the practice of using various estrogen preparations, especially creams, is widespread, the evidence from rigorous studies of their efficacy is scarce. One group of researchers compared a continuous low-dose estradiol releasing vaginal ring (Estring) with conjugated equine estrogen vaginal cream (Premarin cream) in the treatment of postmenopausal urogenital atrophy in an open, parallel, comparative multicenter trial of 194 women. Both preparations were equal in efficacy and safety; however, the vaginal ring was significantly more acceptable than the cream and was preferred to it.

Topical estrogen preparations probably should be used daily and not just prior to intercourse.

Androgens and Androgen–Estrogen Combinations

The role of androgen replacement in the management of FSAD is less clear than the role of other hormones, and it is poorly understood. Hormonal imbalances may be important contributing factors to the pathophysiological mechanisms of FSAD. Androgens modulate the growth and function of female genital sexual organs, such as the labia, vagina, and clitoris.

Androgen replacement has been used commonly in women after oophorectomy. A combination of androgens and estrogens also has been used in menopausal women for various symptoms, including the lack of vaginal lubrication.

One study compared sublingual testosterone in combination with counseling versus diazepam in combination with counseling for the complaint of female sexual unresponsiveness in 32 couples. Women receiving testosterone improved in various aspects of sexual functioning, but the significance could not be confirmed in some variables, including vaginal lubrication. In another study, which compared an estrogen–androgen combination with androgen alone, estrogen alone, and placebo, testosterone was found to enhance the intensity of sexual desire and arousal.

It is important to note that the use of testosterone and other androgens in women poses some health risks, such as masculinization (including hirsutism), clitoral enlargement, hypercholesterolemia, and possible increased risk of breast cancer.

One study found that transdermal testosterone added to oral conjugated estrogens improved various aspects of sexual functioning in 75 women who had undergone oophorectomy and hysterectomy. However, the effect on arousal did not seem to be much different from the effect of placebo.

Thus it is not clear if testosterone alone or in combination with estrogens helps with impaired sexual arousal in women. Androgens seem to be helpful with impaired sexual desire and thus occasionally may be of "secondary" help in cases of impaired arousal.

Interestingly, acute oral adrenal hormone dehydroepiandrosterone (DHEA) was reported to have no substantial effect on sexual arousal in premenopausal women inspite of experts' speculations about its usefulness in this indication.

The use of hormones in patients with female sexual arousal disorder seems to be indicated only when there is clear evidence of hormonal deficiency (see algorithm by Warnock, in Table 19.8).

Sildenafil

Sildenafil has been used successfully in the management of male sexual arousal disorder. The physiological and biochemical similarities between the penis and the clitoris and the involvement of vascular congestion encouraged the use of sildenafil in women. Sildenafil acts as a cGMP-specific phosphodiesterase type V inhibitor. It increases the levels of cGMP and nitric oxide in smooth muscles of the vagina and clitoris. Since it has been suggested that some female sexual arousal dysfunction may be associated with clitoral and vaginal vascular insufficiency, using vasoactive drugs may be helpful in some cases of FSAD.

Several researchers initiated therapeutic trials of sildenafil and other vasoactive drugs in women with sexual arousal disorder. In an open-label pilot study, sildenafil 100 mg significantly improved sexual functioning in 48 women, following 6 weeks of home use of this medication. Arousal was also significantly improved. A pilot study of 16 women suggested efficacy of sildenafil for female sexual dysfunction, including vaginal lubrication (improvement with placebo, 0%; with sildenafil, 63%).

Another study, a double-blind crossover placebo-controlled investigation of 25 and 50 mg of sildenafil, reported a significant improvement of sexual arousal in 51 premenopausal women affected by sexual arousal disorder. Both doses of sildenafil were significantly better than placebo, and there was no difference between doses of sildenafil. The treatment with sildenafil was well tolerated by 84% of women. However, another large double-blind, placebo-controlled multicentric study of estrogenized women with sexual dysfunction associated with FSAD showed no difference between sildenafil (10, 50, or 100 mg) and placebo in the treatment of sexual dysfunction. Female sexual arousal disorder was diagnosed in all women in this study, but it was the primary diagnosis only in 46% of 583 women.

Interestingly, several studies reported improvement of female sexual dysfunction, including lubrication, associated with antidepressant treatment.

The side effects of sildenafil include lightheadedness, dizziness, facial flushing, mild headaches, nasal congestion, visual changes, and nausea.

Sildenafil seems to be a potentially useful treatment for FSAD in doses from 25 mg to 100 mg about 1 hour prior to intercourse. Nevertheless, its efficacy in this indication needs to be confirmed in further double-blind studies, because the results of recent double-blind studies are contradictory.

Other Agents

Alprostadil

As noted above, some cases of female sexual arousal disorder may be associated with vascular clitoral and vaginal insufficiency and possibly could be alleviated with vasoactive drugs. One study, using color-duplex sonography, demonstrated that topical alprostadil (prostaglandin E1) can cause labial and clitoral engorgement and affect peak systolic velocity and end diastolic velocity of clitoral arteries. Another group of researchers conducted a small study evaluating the efficacy and safety of three doses of topical alprostadil cream in eight patients with FSAD. Each patient was administered placebo followed by ascending doses of 0.05%, 0.1%, and 0.2% alprostadil cream intravaginally, after a photoplethysmograph gauge was inserted into the vagina. A 30-minute period was allowed to permit drug absorption, followed by 30 minutes of visual sexual stimulation (erotic videotapes). Alprostadil enhanced the subjective and physiological arousal during visual sexual stimulation. The changes were suggestive of increased arousal with alprostadil.

Further studies assessing the use of topical alprostadil during sexual activity in women with FSAD are warranted. Topical alprostadil might be a useful treatment option for this disorder. However, it remains an experimental treatment modality for FSAD at present.

Apomorphine

Apomorphine is a short-acting dopaminergic agonist that has been used for the induction of emesis. However, it also has been used in men with erectile dysfunction, and it is plausible that apomorphine may alleviate the symptoms of desire and arousal disorders. Even though several review articles touted the possible use of apomorphine in FSAD, there are no published data, to date, on its usefulness in this indication. Reportedly, apomorphine is being tested in women with various sexual dysfunctions.

Again, as with other drugs, apomorphine may be useful in FSAD in some cases. However, some of its side effects, such as nausea and vomiting, may be a hindrance. There are no commercially available preparations of apomorphine at the present time.

L-Arginine

L-arginine is a precursor of nitric oxide, one of the key mediators of relaxation in the peripheral and vascular smooth muscles. Increased L-arginine tissue levels result in increased levels of nitric oxide and thus increased smooth muscle relaxation. Increased smooth muscle relaxation may result in increased vaginal lubrication, vaginal wall engorgement and clitoral engorgement. Thus sexual arousal may increase/improve.

Some review articles suggest that, similar to apomorphine, the amino acid L-arginine (especially in combination with yohimbine) might be helpful in the management of female sexual arousal disorder. However, the only published study on the use of L-arginine in this indication describes the use of ArginMax, a proprietary nutritional supplement consisting of extracts of Korean ginseng, ginkgo biloba, damiana leaf, L-arginine, and multivitamins and minerals (calcium, iron, and zinc). ArginMax was compared to placebo in a double-blind fashion (34 women received ArginMax and 43 received placebo). After 4 weeks, 73.5% of women on ArginMax reported improvement in satisfaction with their overall sex life, while only 37.2% women on placebo reported improvement. This difference was significant. Improvement included reduction in vaginal dryness and improvement in clitoral sensation. It is difficult to assert whether this improvement was due to the administration of L-arginine. As mentioned above, ArginMax also contains ginseng, ginkgo, and damiana. All these extracts have been reported to improve sexual functioning.

Further studies examining the role of L-arginine (and other components of ArginMax) in the management of female sexual arousal disorder are warranted. This nutritional supplement could become an easy to use, well-tolerated first-line adjunct therapy for FSAD.

Phentolamine

Phentolamine is an alpha-adrenergic blocking agent (combined alpha-1 and alpha-2 adrenergic antagonist, which relaxes vascular smooth muscles). In the past, it has been used for the treatment of pheochromocytoma-induced hypertension and norepinephrine-related dermal necrosis. In addition, psychiatrists used it in the emergency management of hypertensive crisis during the use of monoamine oxidase inhibitors, and physicians used it, in combination with other drugs, for intracavernosal therapy of erectile dysfunction. Several studies demonstrated efficacy of its oral preparation in erectile dysfunction. One study, evaluating the potential use of oral phentolamine in female sexual arousal disorder, administered a single dose of 40 mg of phentolamine and placebo in a single-blind, dose-escalation design to six postmenopausal women who had a lack of lubrication and sexual arousal difficulties. The results suggested a mild positive effect of phentolamine across all measures of arousal, with significant changes in self-reported lubrication and pleasurable sensations in the vagina. The drug was fairly well tolerated. Another study of 41 postmenopausal women with FSAD found 40 mg of phentolamine, in either a vaginal solution or an oral tablet, significantly better than placebo in subjective measures of arousal in postmenopausal women who also received hormone replacement therapy. As suggested by some researchers, although these results appear promising, the role of phentolamine in clinical treatment of FSAD remains unclear, and large studies are needed.

Phentolamine is currently not available in the United States for other than research purposes. However, if larger clinical trials prove its usefulness in female sexual arousal disorder, it may become part of the expanding armamentarium for the treatment of this disorder.

Yohimbine

Yohimbine, an indolealkylamine similar to reserpine, is an alpha-adrenergic blocking agent that also blocks peripheral serotonin receptors and has a little direct effect on smooth muscle. It has been used in the treatment of erectile dysfunction, including antidepressant-induced sexual dysfunction. The results have been mixed. There have not been any reports of its efficacy in female sexual arousal disorder, though its use in this indication has been suggested. Oral yohimbine is available in the United States (5.4 mg tablets).

Lubricants

Various commercially available lubricants (see Table 19.7) and even mineral oils have been widely used when lack of lubrication and/or urogenital atrophy is present, especially in postmenopausal women. However, the use of lubricants does not address other aspects of female sexual arousal disorder, such as decreased clitoral and labial

Table 19.7   Commercially available lubricants for female sexual arousal disorder*

General Category (examples)	Positive Aspects	Negative Aspects
Petroleum-based (Vaseline, Baby Oil)	Easily available	Breaks down latex in condoms; irritation
Water-based (K-Y, Astroglide, Sex Grease, Liquid Silk, O'My)	Found in most drugstores	Often needs reapplication due to drying out over time
Silicone-based (Eros Gel, Venus & Eros)	Lasts longer	Not much information
Made from fruits (Sylk)	Natural	Irritation in some women
Suppositories (Lubrin, apply 45–60 min. prior to sexual activity)	Discreetly inserted, more natural	Less readily available; sometimes run out soon
Vaginal moisturizers (Replens)	Used daily, not necessarily associated with sexual activity	Some experience vaginal discharge; need to find out the right number of days to apply

Some women use vitamin E (takes time to dissolve) or vegetable oil, which is perceived as more natural. Some lubricants contain numerous herbal supplements (e.g., Sex Grease: marigold, myrrh, carrot, chamomile, elder). Most lubricants are applied prior to penetration; some need to be reapplied.

* Courtesy of Kathleen Segraves, Ph.D.

FEMALE SEXUAL AROUSAL DISORDER

engorgement and vaginal smooth muscle relaxation. Thus it seems plausible that lubricants will be used as an adjunct remedy in the management of FSAD, with pharmacological agents addressing the underlying pathophysiology of this disorder.

Other Modalities

Clitoral engorgement plays an important role in female sexual arousal. Difficulty or inability to achieve clitoral engorgement has been cited as one of the factors in female sexual arousal disorder. Any medication/device increasing clitoral engorgement might be useful in the management of this disorder. UroMetrics, a company in St. Paul, Minnesota, developed a small battery-powered device called EROS-Clitoral Therapy Device (EROS-CTD), designed to increase blood flow into the clitoris and thus enhance arousal and orgasm. When this device is placed over the clitoris, a gentle vacuum is created over the clitoris, using a pump. Thus blood flow into the clitoris increases and engorgement follows. In a study of 32 women (20 with female sexual dysfunction and 12 healthy volunteers), 90% of women with sexual dysfunction reported greater sensation when using the EROS-CTD, and 58% women with no dysfunction also noted increased sensation. In addition, 80% of women with sexual dysfunction and 33% of women with no dysfunction reported increased lubrication when using this device. The ability to achieve orgasm and overall sexual satisfaction also increased in some women in both groups.

EROS-CTD seems to be a promising new device for the management of FSAD and female orgasmic disorder. Its use needs to be tested in long-term studies and in studies combining this device with oral and topical pharmaceutical agents.

Combining Psychopharmacological and Psychotherapy Treatment

Female sexual arousal disorder is usually of multifactorial origin. Various psychological factors (including an undiagnosed or comorbid major psychiatric disorder) frequently play a major role in the etiology of this disorder. Relationship problems also can be a major factor in female sexual arousal disorder. Thus the use of various psychotherapies has played a major role in the management of this disorder prior to the arrival of various pharmacological preparations. The abandonment of psychotherapy in the management of FSAD is not warranted. Individual or couple psychotherapy, sensate focus strategy, and imagery techniques should probably be combined with the new pharmacological management strategies. However, no studies combining pharmacotherapy and psychotherapy in the management of FSAD have been published, to date.

Management of Medication-Related Female Sexual Arousal Disorder

Numerous medications have been found to be associated with female sexual arousal disorder. As pointed out throughout this book, baseline (i.e., pretreatment) evaluation of sexual functioning is absolutely necessary for making the diagnosis of any sexual dysfunction associated with medication. The strategies that could be implemented in the management of sexual dysfunction associated with medication (including FSAD) include (1) waiting for spontaneous remission, (2) decreasing the dose (if possible), (3) scheduling sexual activity just prior to the single daily dose of medication, (4) taking drug holidays (not always possible), (5) switching to another agent with a lower incidence of sexual dysfunction, and (6) using various antidotes. Among the antidotes, sildenafil seems to be a possibly useful antidote for female sexual dysfunction associated with antidepressants and other psychotropic medications. Typically, the starting dose is 50 mg about an hour prior to intercourse, with possible increase to 100 mg if the lower dose was not effective. A lower starting dose (25 mg) is also possible. It is important to evaluate the cardiovascular status of the patient prior to using sildenafil and to make sure that the patient is not using nitrates. For more specific information regarding the management of female sexual arousal disorder associated with particular medication(s), see the pertinent chapter of this book.

CONCLUSIONS

The pharmacology of female sexual arousal disorder is in its beginnings. Commercial lubricants, mineral oils, and even vitamin E have been a mainstay of "pharmacological" management of this disorder until fairly recently. Topical and oral hormonal replacement has been demonstrated effective in this indication, especially in postmenopausal or otherwise hormone-deficient females. Among the vasoactive agents, sildenafil seems to be the most promising, while agents such as alprostadil, apomorphine, phentolamine, and yohimbine need further studies to prove their efficacy in FSAD. These agents may address more than one aspect of female sexual arousal disorder (i.e., clitoral/vaginal engorgement and lubrication). New treatment approaches, such as the EROS-CTD, are also emerging.

Various psychotherapeutic approaches remain an important part of FSAD management. Combination of pharmacotherapy and

Table 19.8 Warnock's algorithm for treatment of FSAD (acquired, generalized)*

Step 1.
  a. Signs and symptoms of estrogen deficiency: replacement with estrogen.
  b. Signs and symptoms of androgen deficiency: replacement with androgen.
  c. Signs and symptoms due to a particular medication: consider switching to another
     medication with fewer sexual side effects, or adding an antidote (e.g., bupropion, sildenafil).

Step 2.
  Etiology unable to ascertain: Consider adding sildenafil, beginning at a low dose (25 mg)

Step 3.
  Consider the UroMetrics EROS-CTD (clitoral therapy device), which works by means of
  vacuum

* Adapted from Warnock, 2001.

psychotherapy seems to be a prudent clinical approach to the management of this disorder. Detailed evaluation of the patient, and possibly the partner, prior to treatment is essential. Table 19.8 summarizes Warnock's algorithm for treatment of female sexual arousal disorder (acquired, generalized).

Given that there are no studies suggesting the superiority of any pharmacological or other approach to FSAD, a comprehensive approach to this disorder, perhaps even using several treatment modalities (e.g., lubricant + sildenafil or EROS-CTD + individual/couple therapy), seems to be indicated. Participation and education of both partners may be warranted.

REFERENCES

American Psychiatric Association. (1994). *Diagnostic and Statistical Manual of Mental Disorders.* 4th ed. Washington, DC: American Psychiatric Association.

Ayton RA, Darling GM, Murkies AL, et al. A comparative study of safety and efficacy of continuous low-dose estradiol released from a vaginal ring compared with conjugated equine oestrogen vaginal cream in the treatment of postmenopausal urogenital atrophy. *Brit J Obstetrics Gynaecology.* 1995;103:351–358.

Basson R. A model of women's sexual arousal. *J Sex & Marital Ther.* 2002;28: 1–10.

Basson R, Berman J, Burnett A, et al. Report of the international consensus development conference on female sexual dysfunction: definitions and classifications. *J Sex & Marital Ther.* 2001;27:83–94.

Basson R, McInness R, Smith MD, Hodgson G, Spain T, Koppiker N. Efficacy and safety of Viagra in estrogenized women with sexual dysfunction associated with female sexual arousal disorder. *Obstet Gynecol.* 2000; 95(Suppl 1):S54 (abstract).

Becher EF, Bechara A, Casabe A. Clitoral hemodynamic changes after topical application of alprostadil. *J Sex & Marital Ther.* 2001;27:405–410.

Berman LA, Berman JR, Chhabra S, Goldstein I. Novel approaches to female arousal dysfunction. *Exp Opin Invest Drugs.* 2001;10:85–95.

Berman JR, Berman LA, Lin H, et al. Effect of sildenafil on subjective and physiologic parameters of the female sexual response in women with sexual arousal disorder. *J Sex & Marital Ther.* 2001;27:411–420.

Billups KL, Berman L, Berman J, Metz ME, Glennon ME, Goldstein I. A new non-pharmacological vacuum therapy for female sexual dysfunction. *J Sex & Marital Ther.* 2001;27:435–441.

Both S, Everaerd W. Comment on "The female sexual response: a different model." *J Sex & Marital Ther.* 2001;28:11–15.

Carney A, Bancroft J, Matthews A. Combination of hormonal and psychological treatment for female sexual unresponsiveness: a comparative study. *Brit J Psychiatry.* 1978;132:339–346.

Caruso S, Intelisano G, Lupo L, Agnello C. Premenopausal women affected by sexual arousal disorder treated with sildenafil: a double-blind, cross-over, placebo-controlled study. *Brit J Obstetrics and Gynaecology.* 2001;108:623–628.

Chai TC, Wong J, Berman JR. Pilot study on effectiveness of Viagra™ for treatment of female sexual dysfunction: physiologic predictors of success. *J Urol.* 2000;163:77 (abstract).

Davis A. Recent advances in female sexual dysfunction. *Curr Psychiatry Rep.* 2000;2:211–214.

Fava M, Rankin MA, Alpert JE, Nierenberg AA, Worthington JJ. An open trial of oral sildenafil in antidepressant-induced sexual dysfunction. *Psychother Psychosom.* 1998;67:328–331.

Frank E, Anderson C, Kupfer DJ. Profiles of couples seeking sex therapy and marital therapy. *Am J Psychiatry.* 1976;133:559–562.

Goldstein I. Female sexual arousal disorder: new insights. *Int J Impot Res.* 2000;12(Suppl 4):S152–S157.

Graziottin A. Clinical approach to dyspareunia. *J Sex & Marital Ther.* 2001;27:489–501.

Gwinup G. Oral phentolamine in nonspecific erectile insufficiency. *Annals of Internal Medicine.* 1988;109:162–163.

Heaton JP, Morales A, Adams MA, Johnston B, el-Rashidy R. Recovery of erectile function by the oral administration of apomorphine. *Urology.* 1995;45:200–206.

Hollander E, McCarley A. (1992). Yohimbine treatment of sexual side effects induced by serotonin reuptake inhibitors. *J Clin Psychiatry.* 1992;53:207–209.

Islam A, Mitchel J, Rosen R, et al. Topical alprostadil in the treatment of female arousal disorder: a pilot study. *J Sex & Marital Ther.* 2001;27:531–540.

Ito TY, Trant AS, Polan ML. A double-blind placebo-controlled study of ArginMax, a nutritional supplement for enhancement of female sexual dysfunction. *J Sex & Marital Ther.* 2001;27:541–549.

Khan MA, Thompson CS, Mumtaz FH, Mikhailidis DP, Morgan RJ. Urological aspects of female sexual dysfunction. *Urol Int.* 2000;65:1–8.

Laumann EO, Paik A, Rosen RC. Sexual dysfunction in the United States: prevalence and predictors. *JAMA.* 1999;281:537–544.

Meston CM, Heiman JR. Acute dehydroepiandrosterone effects on sexual arousal in premenopausal women. *J Sex & Marital Ther.* 2002;28:53–60.

Nurnberg HG, Lauriello J, Hensley PL, Parker LM, Keith SJ. Sildenafil for sexual dysfunction in women taking antidepressants. *Am J Psychiatry.* 1999;156:1664.

Park K, Goldstein I, Andry C, Siroky MB, Krane RJ, Azadzoi KM. Vasculogenic female sexual dysfunction: the hemodynamic basis for vaginal engorgement insufficiency and clitoral erectile insufficiency. *International Journal of Impotence Research.* 1997;9:26–27 (abstract).

Phillips NA. Female sexual dysfunction: evaluation and treatment. *Am Fam Physician.* 2000;62:127–136, 141–142.

Redmond GP. Hormones and sexual function. *Int J Fertil.* 1999;44:193–197.

Rosen RC, Phillips NA, Gendrano NC, Ferguson DM. Oral phentolamine and female sexual arousal disorder: a pilot study. *J Sex & Marital Ther.* 1999;25:137–144.

Rosen RC, Taylor JF, Leiblum SR, Bachmann GA. Prevalence of sexual dysfunction in women: results of a survey study of 329 women in an outpatient gynecological clinic. *J Sex & Marital Ther.* 1993;19:171–188.

Rubio-Aurioles E, Lopez M, Lipezker M, et al. Phentolamine mesylate in postmenopausal women with female sexual arousal disorder: a psychophysiological study. *J Sex & Marital Ther.* 2002;28(Suppl 1):205–215.

Salerian AJ, Deibler WE, Vittone BJ, et al. Sildenafil for psychotropic-induced sexual dysfunction in 31 women and 61 men. *J Sex & Marital Ther.* 2000;26:133–140.

Sarrel P, Dobay B, Wiita B. Estrogen and estrogen–androgen replacement in postmenopausal women dissatisfied with estrogen-only therapy. Sexual behavior and neuroendocrine responses. *J Reprod Med.* 1998;43:847–856.

Segraves RT, Bari M, Segraves K, Spirnak P. Effect of apomorphine on penile tumescence in men with psychogenic impotence. *J Urol.* 1991;145:1174–1175.

Shabsigh R. Prevalence of and recent developments in female sexual dysfunction. *Curr Psychiatry Rep.* 2001;3:188–194.

Sherwin BB, Gelfand MM, Brender W. Androgen enhances sexual motivation in females: a prospective, crossover study of sex steroids administration in the surgical menopause. *Psychosom Med.* 1985;47:339–351.

Shifren JL, Braunstein GD, Simon JA, et al. Transdermal testosterone treatment in women with impaired sexual function after oophorectomy. *N Engl J Med.* 2000;343:682–688.

Spector IP, Carey MP. Incidence and prevalence of the sexual dysfunctions: a critical review of the empirical literature. *Arch Sex Behav.* 1990;19:389–408.

Traish AM, Kim N, Min K, Munarriz R, Goldstein I. Androgens in female genital sexual arousal function: a biochemical perspective. *J Sex & Marital Ther.* 2002;28(Suppl 1):233–244.

Warnock JK. Hormonal aspects of sexual function in women: treatment advantages with hormone replacement therapy. *Primary Psychiatry.* 2001;8:60–64.

Zorgniotti AW. Experience with buccal phentolamine mesylate for impotence. *Int J Impot Res.* 1994;6:37–41.

20. Treatment of Premature Ejaculation

INTRODUCTION

Medications do not always have deleterious or unpleasant effects on sexuality. Even their sexual side effects could be utilized occasionally in the treatment of sexual problems. The most prominent example is the relatively new area of "sexual pharmacology": the treatment of premature ejaculation with some of the older and newer antidepressants.

This chapter focuses on:

- Description, epidemiology, diagnosis, and physiology of premature or rapid ejaculation
- Treatment with clomipramine
- Treatment with selective serotonin reuptake inhibitors
- Treatment with topical agents
- Potential treatment with other pharmacological agents
- Treatment with a combination of pharmacological agents
- Treatment with various pharmacological agents in combination with sildenafil
- The importance of combining psychopharmacological and psychotherapeutic treatment modalities
- Maintenance treatment
- Side effects of pharmacological treatment and their management.

Table 20.1 lists the drugs discussed in this chapter.

It is important to emphasize that none of the mentioned agents has been approved by the FDA for the treatment of premature ejaculation (probably because of the cost associated with the FDA approval process).

Table 20.1 Pharmacological agents discussed in this chapter

Generic Name	Brand Name	Dose (mg) and Form (mg/day)
	Antidepressants—Heterocyclic	
amitriptyline	Elavil	t: 10/25/75/100/150
		p: 10 mg/mL
	Endep	t: 10/25/75/100/150
clomipramine	Anafranil	c: 25/50/75
desipramine	Norpramin	t: 10/25/75/100/150
	Antidepressants—Selective Serotonin Reuptake Inhibitors	
citalopram	Celexa	t: 20/40
		o: 10 mg/5 mL
fluoxetine	Prozac	t: 10/20
		pulvules: 40
		o: 20 mg/5 mL
	Sarafem	pulvules: 10/20
fluvoxamine	Luvox	t: 25/50/100
paroxetine	Paxil	t: 10/20/30/40
		o: 10 mg/5 mL
sertraline	Zoloft	t: 25/50/100
		o: 20 mg/mL
	Antidepressants—Atypical	
nefazodone	Serzone	t: 100/150/200/250
	Antipsychotics	
thioridazine	Mellaril	t: 10/15/25/50/100/150/250
		o: 30/100 mg/mL
	Antianxiety Agents	
lorazepam	Ativan	t: 0.5/1/2
	Oral Agents for Erectile Dysfunction	
sildenafil	Viagra	t: 25/50/100
	Topical Agents	
prilocaine/lidocaine	EMLA cream	25 mg of each/g of cream

c = capsules; o = oral concentrate; p = parental concentrate; t = tablets

DESCRIPTION, EPIDEMIOLOGY, DIAGNOSIS, AND PHYSIOLOGY

Premature or rapid ejaculation is defined as a persistent or recurrent ejaculation with minimal sexual stimulation before, on, or shortly after penetration, and before the person wishes it. The disturbance must cause distress or interpersonal difficulty. The disturbance should be independent of other mental or physical conditions. The descriptors *premature* and *rapid* are used interchangeably. Premature ejaculation is divided into various types or subtypes, such as primary versus

Table 20.2   The diagnostic dimensions of premature ejaculation

1. Time
   Ejaculatory latency (*DSM:* before the person wishes; *ICD-10:* within 15 seconds after beginning of the intercourse).

2. Control
   Voluntary control is not possible

3. Distress
   Presence of marked distress or interpersonal difficulty due to premature ejaculation

4. Exclusivity
   Lack of direct effect of a substance (e.g., withdrawal from opioids)

secondary, lifelong versus acquired, generalized versus situational, and attributed to psychological factors or to combined factors.

Premature ejaculation is the most prevalent male sexual dysfunction. According to the National Health and Social Life Survey (1999), 21% of men suffer from this dysfunction. However, the estimates of its prevalence vary up to 40% or even 75%, depending on the sample and criteria used.

The diagnosis of premature ejaculation is made along four dimensions, summarized in Table 20.2.

The diagnosis of premature ejaculation is based on a clinical interview of both the individual and the couple (if possible), sexual history (erectile dysfunction also present?), review of systems (special focus on genitourinary and neurological diseases), and, in most cases, general physical examination. Laboratory examinations should include, at least, urinalysis. Standardized psychological and marital/relationship testing also could be included, but is usually not required. Table 20.3 summarizes the actions involved in diagnosing premature ejaculation.

Table 20.3   Factors to consider in establishing the diagnosis of premature ejaculation

Category	Focus
Interview	Individual + couple (if possible)
Sexual history	Erectile dysfunction also present?
	Painful ejaculation?
Review of systems	Genitourinary and neurological diseases
Physical examination	Urethral discharge? Prostatitis?
	Neurological examination—bulbocavernous reflex present? Sensation intact?
Laboratory tests	Urinalysis. Glucose level?
Psychological testing	Possible but not required
Marital/relationship testing	Possible but not required

Our understanding of the physiology and etiology of ejaculation and premature ejaculation is incomplete. Ejaculation is a complicated process that includes three components: seminal emission, ejaculation, and bladder neck closure. Though most of the theories about physiology of ejaculation and premature ejaculation have been derived from animal studies, some of the evidence also has been extrapolated from human treatment studies. Drugs that are predominantly serotonergic clearly delay or inhibit ejaculation; increased serotonergic activation seems to be associated with orgasmic inhibition in men and women. In addition, the cholinergic system seems to play a modulatory role: Ejaculation seems to be mediated by alpha-receptor activation, presumably at a peripheral level, with cholinergic fibers playing a modulatory role. Nevertheless, the main neurotransmitter of the ejaculatory response is unclear. Serotonin system involvement in ejaculation presumably occurs at the brain level.

We know very little about the physiology of ejaculation, and we know even less about the etiology and physiology of premature ejaculation. The medical literature emphasizes physiological, neurological, or urological causes. The psychiatric literature emphasizes the role of psychological factors such as anxiety, lack of control, learned behavior during adolescence, masturbation, and relationship distress. Physiological studies have not found any definite abnormalities in subjects with premature ejaculation, with the exception of a possibly shortened bulbocavernosus reflex.

Various psychotherapies and procedures—such as cognitive, dynamic, educational, and muscle relaxation—have been used in the treatment of premature ejaculation to address the presumed psychological and physiological problems. However, for a long time the standard therapy for premature ejaculation has utilized three variations of a behavioral technique: the Semans pause maneuver, the Masters and Johnson pause–squeeze technique, and the Kaplan's stop–start method. These very popular techniques are simple and usually highly effective (43–100% success rate). However, they require collaboration from the partner, lack long-term gains, and fail at times. Thus the discovery of delayed ejaculation as a side effect of some psychotropic drugs led to attempts to use these drugs in the treatment of premature ejaculation. The original drugs observed to delay ejaculation included antipsychotics, monoamine oxidase inhibitors, tricyclic antidepressants, and, later, the selective serotonin reuptake inhibitors (SSRIs). As a result of their efficacy and tolerability, SSRIs and the tricyclic antidepressant clomipramine became the most widely used pharmacological options for the treatment of premature ejaculation. However, other substances, such as benzodiazepines and topical creams, were also found effective in the management of this sexual dysfunction.

TREATMENT

Clomipramine

The possibility of treating premature ejaculation with clomipramine was inferred from case reports of delayed ejaculation with this strongly serotonergic tricyclic antidepressant. Studies of sexual side effects of antidepressants also reported a high incidence of great difficulty in achieving orgasm with clomipramine (e.g., up to 96% of those on 25 mg/day, or more). Some authors reported cases of patients with premature ejaculation who responded well to clomipramine. (Table 20.4 summarizes the success rates of clomipramine.) One researcher described five cases of men who improved significantly on low doses of clomipramine (10–25 mg) usually taken daily (two men took it as needed). Interestingly, two of these patients had failed to respond to sex therapy previously (in one case, this included stop–start and relaxation techniques).

One open study of clomipramine used to treat premature ejaculation (30–40 mg/day; in some cases, up to 75 mg/day) demonstrated a high success rate (12/13 cases = 92%). Over the last two decades, six double-blind studies addressed the efficacy of clomipramine in premature ejaculation. The first study failed to find a difference between clomipramine and placebo in 20 men during the initial double-blind crossover part of the study. The initial dose was 10 mg/day at 6 P.M., with an option to increase the dose up to 40 mg/day. Only 16 patients completed the study; 4 dropped out (3 on clomipramine, one on placebo). However, during the open follow-up part of the study, 9 of 16 patients (56%) reported some or complete beneficial effects of clomipramine. Some patients increased clomipramine to a fairly high dose (four of them to 150 mg/day, one to 200 mg/day).

The remaining five studies demonstrated a high efficacy of clomipramine in premature ejaculation. One study administered 20 mg of

Table 20.4 Success rates of clomipramine

Study	Double-Blind Design Success Rate	Open Study Design Success Rate	N
Eaton		92%	13
Goodman	0%	56%	16
Girgis et al.	40–50%		39
Segraves et al.	70% (25 mg)		20
	83% (50 mg)		
Althof et al.	100%?		15
Haensel et al.	100%?		8
Strassberg et al.	77%?		22
Kim & Seo	69.4%		36

clomipramine or placebo daily to 50 males in a double-blind crossover study. Only 39 patients completed the study. The reasons for the 11 drop-outs after the first visit were not given. The success rate ranged between 40% to 50%, depending on the order of administration of clomipramine (subjects who started on clomipramine reported higher success rates). Other researchers studied 29 men in a double-blind placebo-controlled study. Nine men dropped out and were not included in the analysis. Subjects were given 25–50 mg of clomipramine daily. The average estimated time to ejaculation after vaginal penetration increased to 6.1 minutes on 25 mg of clomipramine, compared to 51 seconds on placebo, and to 8.4 minutes on 50 mg of clomipramine/day. Ratings of libido, erections, ejaculatory timing, ejaculatory quality, and overall sexual satisfaction all significantly improved with clomipramine, but not with placebo. Success rate, defined as 2 or more minutes between penetration and ejaculation, was 70% on 25 mg, 83% on 50 mg, and 20% on placebo.

One group of researchers studied 15 couples in a variable-length, repeated measures, randomized, placebo-controlled crossover study with a 2-month follow-up period. Males were given 25 and later 50 mg of clomipramine daily. The mean time to ejaculation prior to the treatment was 81 seconds; it increased to 202 seconds (249%) with 25 mg and to 419 seconds (517%) with 50 mg of clomipramine/day. Ejaculatory latency returned to baseline levels during the follow-up period when the medication was discontinued. Men and women reported significant improvement in sexual satisfaction. Interestingly, 3 of the 5 women who reported that they had never experienced an orgasm during intercourse became coitally orgasmic. In addition, 6 of the 10 women who previously had attained orgasm during intercourse reported that orgasm occurred more frequently during the clomipramine administration. It is impossible to determine the exact success rate, but some success occurred in all couples—thus it approached 100%.

In another study, in a prospective, randomized, double-blind, placebo controlled, crossover study of 14 men (8 with primary premature ejaculation, 6 with premature ejaculation and erectile dysfunction) and 8 controls, clomipramine (25 mg as needed) significantly increased the latency to ejaculation during sexual activity (coitus or masturbation) from approximately 2 to 8 minutes in men with primary premature ejaculation. There were no significant effects in controls and men with premature ejaculation and erectile dysfunction. Interestingly, clomipramine inhibited nocturnal penile tumescence in all subjects. It is impossible to estimate the success rate; nevertheless, as in the preceding study, all men with primary premature ejaculation improved.

In an extension and elaboration of this study, another group of researchers studied 23 premature ejaculators and 11 controls in a double-blind, placebo-controlled crossover study. Subjects were given 25 mg of clomipramine 4–6 hours prior to intercourse on an as-needed basis. In premature ejaculators, the orgasmic latency during intercourse increased from 52 to 229 seconds on clomipramine. The success rate was difficult to estimate, but judging from the numbers presenting orgasmic latency in premature ejaculators on clomipramine and placebo, of the 22 subjects who had intercourse at least once during both the placebo and clomipramine period, at least 17 seemed to have longer orgasmic latency on clomipramine. Thus the success rate would be about 77%.

The success rate of clomipramine in a study comparing fluoxetine, sertraline, and clomipramine was 69.4%. Interestingly, in this double-blind, placebo-controlled study, clomipramine was found to be the most efficacious, but sertraline was nearly as effective and better tolerated.

The side effects in these studies were usually mild and dose-dependent, and included dry mouth, perspiration/sweating, drowsiness, nausea, constipation, diarrhea, headache, dizziness, feeling different, sleep disturbance, and others that were less frequent.

Clomipramine in a low dose of 25–50 mg seems to be an effective and fairly well-tolerated pharmacological modality for premature ejaculation.

Selective Serotonin Reuptake Inhibitors

The efficacy of clomipramine in treating premature ejaculation encouraged studies with other, better tolerated selective serotonin reuptake antidepressants (SSRIs) for this indication.

The SSRIs studied more frequently in regard to premature ejaculation are fluoxetine, paroxetine, and sertraline.

Fluoxetine

Two independent groups of researchers described cases of males with premature ejaculation satisfactorily responding to 20–40 mg/day of fluoxetine. In an 8-week open study by another group, the intravaginal ejaculation latency time changed significantly at a dosage of 20–40 mg/day of fluoxetine in 9 (82%) of 11 subjects (the dose was increased up to 60 mg/day in 2 subjects).

Two studies compared fluoxetine to placebo in a double-blind fashion. In one small study, fluoxetine 20 mg/day for 1 week and 40 mg/day afterward significantly prolonged the latent period of intravaginal ejaculation (from 25 to 180 seconds) in 7 subjects, when compared to 7 subjects on placebo. The other study investigated the efficacy of fluoxetine in 9 patients with premature ejaculation, 9 patients with premature ejaculation and erectile dysfunction, 7 patients with erectile dysfunction, and 15 controls; treatment consisted of 5 mg/day of fluoxetine for 2 weeks, followed by 10 mg for 2 weeks. The latency time increased significantly for the premature ejaculation and premature ejaculation/erectile dysfunction groups combined, and for the premature ejaculation/erectile dysfunction group alone, but not significantly for the premature ejaculation group alone. Of the premature ejaculation group, 6 of 7 patients reported an increase in the time to ejaculation; of the premature ejaculation/erectile dysfunction group, 6 of 8 reported an increase (overall rate of 80%).

Fluoxetine was also compared to other antidepressants in three double-blind studies. In one, researchers compared fluoxetine (40 mg/day), sertraline (100 mg/day), and clomipramine (50 mg/day) to placebo in 53 patients; however, only 36 patients completed the whole study. All patients took each drug and placebo for 4 weeks, with a washout period of at least 1 week between agents (clearly not enough time to eliminate fluoxetine with its long half-life). The mean intravaginal ejaculation latency time was significantly increased from 46 seconds to 2.27 minutes for placebo, 2.30 minutes for fluoxetine, 4.27 minutes for sertraline, and 5.75 minutes for clomipramine. Treatment with clomipramine or sertraline caused a greater increase in mean latency time than fluoxetine or placebo. The most effective drug in the prolongation of ejaculation latency time was clomipramine (69.4% of patients), followed by sertraline (33.3%) and fluoxetine (13.9%). Clomipramine was rated higher than other medications or placebo in regard to sexual satisfaction; however, it also had a higher incidence of side effects.

In a presumably double-blind but not placebo-controlled study, patients received 20 mg/day of fluoxetine for a week and 40 mg/day thereafter, or 50 mg/day of sertraline. In the fluoxetine group, 73.1% of the 26 patients were either "cured or improved"; in the sertraline group, 71% of the 31 patients were either cured or improved.

In a complicated study of 51 men with an intravaginal ejaculation latency time of less than 1 minute, researchers compared fluoxetine (20 mg/day, N = 10), fluvoxamine (100 mg/day, N = 10), paroxetine (20 mg/day, N = 11), sertraline (50 mg/day, N = 11), and placebo with regard to their ejaculation-delaying effect. During the 6-week study period, paroxetine, fluoxetine, and sertraline all delayed ejaculation to a clinically relevant extent that was significantly different from placebo. Paroxetine exerted the strongest delay (almost 600%), followed by

Table 20.5 Success rates of fluoxetine

Study	Double-Blind Design Success Rate	Open Study Design Success Rate	N
Lee et al.		82%	11
Haensel et al.	80%		15
Kim & Seo	13.9%		36
Basar et al.	73.1%		26

fluoxetine and sertraline. The slight delay in ejaculation with fluvoxamine was not clinically relevant and was not significantly different from placebo. The authors suggested that both paroxetine and sertraline 20 mg/day may be regarded as effective treatments of lifelong premature ejaculation.

Finally, researchers compared the efficacy of fluoxetine alone and fluoxetine plus lidocaine ointment in the treatment of premature ejaculation. Of the 26 patients receiving fluoxetine 20 mg/day, 73.1% were rated as "cured or improved" (30.8% as cured). Of the 17 patients receiving fluoxetine 20 mg/day plus local application of lidocaine ointment, 82.3% were rated as "cured or improved" (52.9% as cured). The combination of fluoxetine and lidocaine was more effective than fluoxetine alone.

Table 20.5 summarizes the success rates of fluoxetine reported in the literature.

The side effects with fluoxetine were mild and infrequent: gastrointestinal discomfort, dizziness, tingling, nausea, headache, insomnia, dry mouth, loose stools, and increased libido.

In several studies fluoxetine was found to be an efficacious and well-tolerated, though not the most effective SSRI, treatment for premature ejaculation.

Paroxetine

In an open study, researchers found a longer interval to ejaculation in all 32 men included in their study who were treated with 20 mg/day of paroxetine. In another open study, 61 men were treated with 20 mg/day of paroxetine, and those who responded were switched to paroxetine on demand. The remaining 33 men were treated with paroxetine on "demand only." Paroxetine prolonged the ejaculation time up to 3.9 minutes in the first group and 1.5 minutes in the on-demand group. Five patients reported anejaculation.

In a complicated single-blind "two study" design of 66 men, researchers found paroxetine up to 20 mg/day to be superior to placebo when administered on a chronic or as-needed basis.

Two studies evaluated the efficacy of paroxetine in a double-blind fashion. In a small, placebo-controlled study, 2 of 8 patients on 20 mg/day of paroxetine dropped out because of side effects. The remaining 6 patients reported remarkable prolongation of the ejaculation time (paroxetine was increased to 40 mg/day in the second week), up to 10 minutes after 6 weeks. These researchers also compared two doses of paroxetine daily (20 and 40 mg) in another study. Interestingly, both groups showed improvement in ejaculation time, and there was no statistically significant difference between groups.

Researchers compared paroxetine to other antidepressants in the treatment of premature ejaculation in two double-blind studies. The first study compared paroxetine (20 mg/day, N = 12), sertraline (50 mg/day, N = 12), nefazodone (400 mg/day, N = 12), and placebo (N = 12). Paroxetine and sertraline gradually increased the ejaculation time (to 146 and 58 seconds, respectively, from 17 and 14 seconds, respectively), whereas nefazodone did not. Furthermore, nefazodone did not differ from placebo. Paroxetine exerted the strongest delay. In a comparison of 20 mg of paroxetine and 20 mg of citalopram (15 patients in each group), paroxetine strongly increased the ejaculation latency time (8.9 times) from 18 to 170 seconds, whereas citalopram increased it only modestly (1.8 times) from 21 to 44 seconds. In a previously mentioned study by the same group, paroxetine exerted the strongest delay in ejaculation when compared to fluoxetine, fluvoxamine, and sertraline.

Table 20.6 summarizes the success rates of paroxetine reported in the literature.

The success rates in most paroxetine studies were difficult to estimate due to complicated designs or different outcome measures. Paroxetine was usually relatively well tolerated (decrease in sexual desire, anejaculation, nausea, dry mouth, fatigue, perspiration, intense yawning mentioned as side effects).

Paroxetine seems to be the most effective among the SSRIs in the treatment of premature ejaculation.

Table 20.6   Success rates of paroxetine

Study	Double-Blind Design Success Rate	Open Study Design Success Rate	N
Ludovico et al.		100%	32
McMahon & Touma		71%	94

Sertraline

Similar to other antidepressants, several case reports suggested the usefulness of 50–100 mg/day of sertraline in the treatment of premature ejaculation.

Several open studies demonstrated the efficacy of various doses of sertraline in the management of premature ejaculation. One study reported that 87.5% of their patients responded clinically to 50 mg/day of sertraline. Various doses of sertraline, 50–100 mg, daily or prn, prolonged ejaculation up to 5.9 minutes in 24 patients in another study. In a dose-ranging study of 46 men, sertraline 25 mg/day prolonged ejaculation time to 7.6 minutes, sertraline 50 mg/day to 13.1 minutes, and 100 mg/day to 16.4 minutes.

A single-blind placebo-controlled crossover study showed prolongation of ejaculation time up to 3.2 minutes in 37 men with 50 mg of sertraline. Finally, two double-blind placebo-controlled studies demonstrated the efficacy of sertraline in premature ejaculation and its superiority over placebo. In one study, sertraline 50–200 mg/day (mean dose 141 mg/day) prolonged ejaculation time to 4–5 minutes in 26 men. Sertraline 50 mg/day also significantly prolonged ejaculation time (from 41 to 325 seconds) when compared to placebo (from 44 to 115 seconds) in a study of 37 patients. Again, the success rates in some studies were difficult to estimate again.

In previously discussed studies, sertraline also demonstrated efficacy in the treatment of premature ejaculation. However, clomipramine and paroxetine seemed to be somewhat more efficacious, and fluoxetine a bit less efficacious.

Table 20.7 summarizes the success rates of sertraline reported in the literature.

Sertraline also has been relatively well tolerated, with dry mouth, nausea, diarrhea, fatigue, and failure to ejaculate being the most frequently noted among its side effects.

Sertraline appears to be another psychopharmacological treatment modality for the treatment of premature ejaculation.

Table 20.7   Success rates of sertraline

Study	Double-Blind Design Success Rate	Open Study Design Success Rate	N
Balbay et al.		87.5%	16
Kim & Seo	33.3%		36
Basar et al.	71%		31

Fluvoxamine and Citalopram

Researchers did not find a clinically relevant prolongation of ejaculation latency time in premature ejaculation subjects treated with fluvoxamine. Similarly, citalopram increased the ejaculation latency time only very modestly in another study.

Fluvoxamine and citalopram thus do not seem to be suitable for the treatment of premature ejaculation.

Topical Agents

Several topical agents—local anesthetics and herbal agents—have been used in the treatment of premature ejaculation. The rationale behind their use is the decrease or correction of the presumed heightened genital sensitivity. They have been used mostly outside the United States (Germany, Korea). One group of researchers reported a marked improvement in ejaculatory latency time in 9 of 11 men treated for premature ejaculation with prilocaine–lidocaine cream (EMLA) (2.5 g in each tube). Another group also reported a successful use of prilocaine–lidocaine cream in 15 men with premature ejaculation (ejaculation latency increased from 2 to 8 minutes). After the application of 2.5 g of the cream, patients were instructed to put on a condom, wait 10 minutes, remove the condom, wipe off the cream, and start sexual activity.

One group of researchers reported that SS-cream (a proprietary preparation consisting of extracts of nine natural products, such as ginseng, cinnamon and others; not available in the United States) is effective in the treatment of premature ejaculation, with a few local effects, and that the clinically optimal dose is 0.20 g.

Though the use of topical preparations in premature ejaculation may sound interesting, their use is probably limited: they may cause penile, vaginal, and clitoral anesthesia or numbness (lidocaine and prilocaine–lidocaine); the use of a condom is advised; and the application may be a bit cumbersome and distracting. However, they may be useful for those patients who cannot tolerate SSRIs.

It suggested that an inexpensive over-the-counter mouthwash spray, Chloraseptic, which has a local anesthetic effect, may also be useful in the management of premature ejaculation.

Table 20.8 summarizes the usefulness of topical agents reported in the literature.

Other Potential Pharmacological Agents

Several other oral psychotropic medications, such as thioridazine (25–100 mg), iproniazid and lorazepam (0.5 mg), have been effective in

Table 20.8 Summary of the usefulness of topical agents in the treatment of premature ejaculation

Preparation	Study	Design	Number of Subjects	Success Rate
Prilocaine-lidocaine	Berkovitch et al.	Open	11	81%
	Slob et al.	Open	15	from 2 min to 8 min
SS-cream	Choi et al.	Double-blind, placebo-controlled	50	from 1.35 min to 11 min, or from 30% to 84%, depending on the dose of SS-cream

premature ejaculation. In addition, the antibiotic ciprofloxacin alleviated premature ejaculation in one case report. However, these agents either have disappeared from the market (iproniazid), or could cause various side effects (thioridazine), and thus should be tried only if other agents fail to succeed.

Recently one group of researchers suggested that intracavernous injection of either prostaglandin or papaverine + fentolamine following an ejaculation/orgasm could lead to an erection presumably sufficient for intromission, which suggests that intracavernous injection may be a therapeutic option for rapid ejaculators.

Combination of Pharmacological Agents

On group of researchers found the combination of oral fluoxetine and local lidocaine ointment more efficacious than oral fluoxetine alone. Thus a combination of various premature ejaculation pharmacological modalities may be advisable in treatment-resistant cases. At the present time, combination of oral agents is not advisable, with the possible exception noted below.

Interestingly, propranolol has not been found effective in premature ejaculation.

Pharmacological Agents in Combination with Sildenafil

Surprisingly, not much has been published on the use of sildenafil as an adjunct therapy in premature ejaculation, especially in cases when premature ejaculation coexists with erectile dysfunction. Nevertheless, sildenafil may be a useful augmentation to behavioral therapy for premature ejaculation (patient gains confidence). Similarly, it is possible that the combination of SSRIs and sildenafil may be effective in the treatment of premature ejaculation alone or comorbid with erectile dysfunction. One group of researchers recently compared clomipramine, sertraline, paroxetine, sildenafil, and the

Table 20.9 Various potentially useful solo and combination agents in the treatment of premature ejaculation

Oral
  Solo
    Ciprofloxacin
    Lorazepam
    Sildenafil?
    Thioridazine
  Combination
    SSRIs + sildenafil?

Intracavernous injections
  Prostaglandine?
  Papaverine + fentolamine?

Other combinations
  Oral fluoxetine + topical lidocaine

pause–squeeze technique in the treatment of 31 men with premature ejaculation. Sildenafil was superior to other modalities in terms of ejaculation latency and satisfaction. The three antidepressants were comparable to each other in terms of efficacy. Paroxetine was superior to pause–squeeze technique in terms of efficacy. Sildenafil may either reduce performance anxiety or increase erection time and thus help prolong the ejaculation time. Sildenafil certainly deserves more trials, either alone or in combinations, in the management of premature ejaculation.

Table 20.9 summarizes the usefulness of various potential solo and combination treatments reported in the literature.

Combining Psychopharmacological and Psychotherapy Treatment Modalities

Paroxetine has been found superior to the pause–squeeze in one study so far. No other solid data comparing psychopharmacological and psychotherapeutic techniques exist. However, some drugs may facilitate the efficacy of behavioral techniques (e.g., sildenafil). However, the combination of pharmacological and behavioral modalities is advisable probably only in treatment-resistant cases. Nevertheless, psychotherapy (individual, group, and/or couple) should always be part of the management of premature ejaculation.

Maintenance Treatment

The maintenance therapy of premature ejaculation is an unresolved issue. Though some reports suggested sustained effect of the antidepressants after discontinuation, most of the studies did not address this issue. Some studies showed return of ejaculatory latency time to baseline after the treating agent was discontinued. Thus, similar to the discontinuation of behavioral techniques, the ejaculation

Table 20.10   Management strategies for side effects of drugs used in premature ejaculation

1. Decrease dose
2. Switch to a better tolerated drug (e.g., from clomipramine to SSRIs)
3. Decrease dose and add an adjunct agent (e.g., SSRIs and topical cream, or SSRIs and sildenafil?)

latency time frequently returns to the baseline level after discontinuation of the psychopharmacological agents. The therapy for premature ejaculation should continue probably indefinitely, with occasional attempts to discontinue the medication and see if the disturbance recurs.

Side Effects of Pharmacological Treatment and Their Management

Side effects of most of the agents used in the management of premature ejaculation are infrequent and usually mild. Using the agents, as needed, probably decreases the occurrence of lasting side effects. The strategies employed in the management of side effects during daily dosing of the medications include decreasing the dose, switching to an agent that is better tolerated, and using adjunctive or antidotal agents (e.g., sildenafil in cases of erectile dysfunction).

Table 20.10 summarizes the management of drug side effects.

CONCLUSIONS

1. Treatment of premature ejaculation with pharmacological agents is feasible, practical, and well tolerated.
2. Careful evaluation is indicated before medication is started.
3. No pharmacological modality for premature ejaculation has been approved by the FDA.
4. Clomipramine and three SSRIs—paroxetine, sertraline, and fluoxetine—are preferred, with paroxetine being first-rated among the SSRIs. (However, the insurance companies may not reimburse the use of these antidepressants in the treatment of premature ejaculation.)
5. As needed or regular administration of oral agents is effective.
6. The recommended daily or as-needed doses of antidepressants in the treatment of premature ejaculation are:
   - Clomipramine 25–50 mg
   - Paroxetine 20–40 mg
   - Sertraline 50–200 mg
   - Fluoxetine 20 mg

7. Topical ointments (lidocaine, prilocaine–lidocaine) could be used alone or in combination with oral agents.

8. Sildenafil might be a useful adjunct or sole treatment for premature ejaculation; however, more studies are warranted.

9. The side effects of agents used in the management of premature ejaculation are usually infrequent and mild.

10. Various treatment modalities can be combined; the combination of pharmacotherapy and psychotherapy is advisable.

11. Partners should be involved in the treatment.

12. Long-term maintenance treatment of premature ejaculation is probably indicated, with occasional trials of medication discontinuation, testing for relapse.

REFERENCES

Abdel-Hamid IA, El Naggar EA, Gilany A-HEL. Assessment of as needed use of pharmacotherapy and the pause–squeeze technique in premature ejaculation. *Int J Impot Res.* 2001;13:41–45.

Althof SE, Levine SB, Corty EW, Risen CB, Stern EB, Kurit DM. A double-blind crossover trial of clomipramine for rapid ejaculation in 15 couples. *J Clin Psychiatry.* 1995;56:402–407.

American Psychiatric Association. *Diagnostic and Statistical Manual of Mental Disorders.* 4th ed., Washington DC:American Psychiatric Association; 1994.

Assalian P. Clomipramine in the treatment of premature ejaculation. *J Sex Res.* 1988;24:213–215.

Atan A, Basar MM, Aydoganli L. Comparison of the efficacy of fluoxetine alone vs. fluoxetine plus lidocaine ointment in the treatment of premature ejaculation. *Arch Esp de Urol.* 2000;53:856–858.

Balbay MD, Yildiz M, Salvarci A, Ozsan O, Ozbek E. Treatment of premature ejaculation with sertralin. *International Urology and Nephrology.* 1998;30:81–83.

Balon R. Antidepressants in the treatment of premature ejaculation. *J Sex & Marital Ther.* 1996;22:85–96.

Balon R, (Ed.) *Practical Management of the Side Effects of Psychotropic Drugs.* New York: Marcel Dekker; 1999.

Basar MM, Atan A, Yildiz M, Baykam M, Aydoganli L. Comparison of sertraline to fluoxetine with regard to their efficacy and side effects in the treatment of premature ejaculation. *Arch Esp de Urol.* 1999;52:1008–1011.

Baum N, Spieler B. Medical management of premature ejaculation. *Medical Aspects of Human Sexuality.* 2001;4(1):15–18, 23–25.

Beaumont G. Sexual side effects of clomipramine (Anafranil). *J Int Med Res.* 1973;1:469–472.

Bennett D. Treatment of ejaculation praecox with monoamine-oxidase inhibitors. *Lancet.* 1961;2:1309.

Berkovitch M, Keresteci AG, Koren G. Efficacy of prilocaine–lidocaine cream in the treatment of premature ejaculation. *J Urol.* 1995;154:1360–1361.

Biri H, Isen K, Sinik Z, Onaran M, Kupeli B, Bozkirli I. Sertraline in the treatment of premature ejaculation: a double-blind placebo controlled study. *Int Urol Nephrol.* 1998;30:611–615.

Brown AJ. Ciprofloxacin as cure of premature ejaculation. *J Sex & Marit Ther.* 2000;26:351–352.

Choi HK, Jung GW, Moon KH, et al. Clinical study of SS-cream in patients with lifelong premature ejaculation. *Urol.* 2000;55:257–261.

Choi HK, Xin ZC, Lee WH, Mah SY, Kim DK. Safety and efficacy study with various doses of SS-cream in patients with premature ejaculation in a double-blind, randomized, placebo-controlled clinical study. *Int J Impot Res.* 1999;11:261–264.

Cooper AJ, Cernovsky ZZ, Colussi K. Some clinical and psychometric characteristics of primary and secondary premature ejaculators. *J Sex & Marit Ther.* 1993;19:276–288.

Cooper AJ, Magnus RV. A clinical trial of the beta blocker propranolol in premature ejaculation. *J Psychosom Res.* 1984;28:331–336.

Eaton H. Clomipramine (Anafranil) in the treatment of premature ejaculation. *J Int Med Res.* 1973;1:213–215.

Forster P, King J. Fluoxetine for premature ejaculation. *Am J Psychiatry.* 1994;151:1523.

Girgis SM, El-Haggar S, El-Hermouzy S. A double-blind trial of clomipramine in premature ejaculation. *Andrologia.* 1982;14:364–368.

Godpodinoff ML. Premature ejaculation: clinical subgroups and etiology. *J Sex & Marit Ther.* 1999;15:130–134.

Goodman RE. An assessment of clomipramine (Anafranil) in the treatment of premature ejaculation. *J Int Med Res.* 1980;1:432–434.

Haensel SM, Rowland DL, Kallan KTHK, Slob AK. Clomipramine and sexual function in men with premature ejaculation. *J Urol.* 1996;156:1310–1315.

Haensel SM, Klem TMAL, Hop WCJ, Slob AK. Fluoxetine and premature ejaculation: a double-blind, crossover, placebo-controlled study. *J Clin Psychopharmacol.* 1998;18:72–77.

Kaplan PM. The use of serotonergic uptake inhibitors in the treatment of premature ejaculation. *J Sex & Marit Ther.* 1994;20:321–324.

Kara H, Aydin S, Agargun MY, Odabas O, Yilmaz Y. The efficacy of fluoxetine in the treatment of premature ejaculation: a double-blind placebo-controlled study. *J Urol.* 1996;156:1631–1632.

Kim SC, Seo KK. Efficacy and safety of fluoxetine, sertraline and clomipramine in patients with premature ejaculation: a double-blind, placebo-controlled study. *J Urol.* 1998;159:425–427.

Kim SW, Paick J-S. Short-term analysis of the effects of as-needed use of sertraline at 5 P.M. for the treatment of premature ejaculation. *Urology.* 1999;54:544–547.

Klug B. Clomipramine in premature ejaculation. *Med J Aust.* 1984;141:71.

Kotler M, Cohen H, Aizenberg D, et al. Sexual dysfunction in male post-traumatic stress disorder patients *Psychother Psychosom.* 2000;69:309–315.

Laumann EO, Paik A, Rosen RC. Sexual dysfunction in the United States: prevalence and predictors. *JAMA.* 1999;281:537–544.

Lee HS, Song DH, Kim C-H, Choi HK. An open clinical trial of fluoxetine in the treatment of premature ejaculation. *J Clin Psychopharmacol.* 1996;16:379–382.

Ludovico GM, Corvasce A, Pagliarulo G, Cirillo-Maruco E, Marano A, Pagliarulo A. Paroxetine in the treatment of premature ejaculation. *Br J Urol.* 1996;77:881–882.

McMahon CG. Treatment of premature ejaculation with sertraline hydrochloride: a single-blind, placebo-controlled crossover study. *J Urol.* 1998a;159:1935–1938.

McMahon CG. Treatment of premature ejaculation with sertraline hydrochloride. *Int J Impot Res.* 1998b;10:181–184.

McMahon CG, Touma K. Treatment of premature ejaculation with paroxetine hydrochloride as needed: two single-blind placebo-controlled crossover studies. *J Urol.* 1999a;161:1826–1830.

McMahon CG, Touma K. Treatment of premature ejaculation with paroxetine hydrochloride.*Int J Impot Res.* 1999b;11:241–246.

Mellgren A. Treatment of ejaculation praecox with thioridazine. *Psychother Psychosom.* 1967;15:454–460.

Mendels J, Camera A, Sikes C. Sertraline treatment for premature ejaculation. *J Clin Psychopharmacol.* 1995;15:341–346.

Metz ME, Pryor JL. Premature ejaculation: a psychophysiological approach for assessment and management. *J Sex & Marit Ther.* 2000;26:293–320.

Monteiro WO, Noshirvani HF, Marks IM, Lelliott PT. Anorgasmia from clomipramine in obsessive–compulsive disorder: a controlled trial. *Brit J Psychiatry.* 1987;151:107–112.

Morales A. Developmental status of topical therapies for erectile and ejaculatory dysfunction. *Int J Impot Res.* 2000;12 (Suppl 4):S80–S85.

Quirk KC, Einarson RT. Sexual dysfunction and clomipramine. *Can J Psychiatry.* 1982;27:228–231.

Rowland DL, Strassberg DS, de Gouveia Brazao CA, Slob AK. Ejaculatory latency and control in men with premature ejaculation: an analysis across sexual activities using multiple sources of information. *J Psychosom Res.* 2000;48:69–77.

Seftel AD, Althof SE. Rapid ejaculation. *Sexual Dysfunction in Medicine.* 2000;2:10–13.

Segraves RT. Treatment of premature ejaculation with lorazepam. *Am J Psychiatry.* 1987;144:1240.

Segraves RT. Effects of psychotropic drugs on human erection and ejaculation. *Arch Gen Psychiatry.* 1989;46:275–284.

Segraves RT. Two additional uses for sildenafil in psychiatric patients. *J Sex & Marital Ther.* 1999;25:265–266.

Segraves RT, Saran A, Segraves K, Maguire E. Clomipramine versus placebo in the treatment of premature ejaculation: a pilot study. *J Sex & Marital Ther.* 1993;19:198–200.

Singh R. Therapeutic use of thioridazine in premature ejaculation. *Am J Psychiatry.* 1963;119:891.

Slob AK, van Berkel A, van der Werff ten Bosch JJ. Premature ejaculation treated by local penile anaesthesia in an uncontrolled clinical replication study. *J Sex Res.* 2000;37:244–247.

Slob AK, Verhulst ACM, Gijs L, Maksimovic PA, van der Werff ten Bosch JJ. Intracavernous injection during diagnostic screening for erectile dysfunction: five-year experience with over 600 patients. *J Sex & Marital Ther.* 2001;28:61–70.

St. Lawrence JS, Madakasira S. Evaluation and treatment of premature ejaculation: a critical review. *Int J Psychiatry Med.* 1992;22:77–97.

Strassberg DS, de Gouveia CA, Rowland DL, Tan P, Slob AK. Clomipramine in the treatment of rapid (premature) ejaculation. *J Sex & Marital Ther.* 1999;25:89–101.

Stratta P, Mancini F, Cupillari M, Rossi A, Casacchia M. Fluoxetine in premature ejaculation. *Human Psychopharmacology.* 1993;8:61–62.

Waldinger MD, Berendsen HHG, Blok BFM, Olivier B, Holstege G. Premature ejaculation and serotonergic antidepressants-induced delayed ejaculation. *Behav Brain Res.* 1998;92:111–118.

Waldinger MD, Hengeveld MW, Zwinderman AH. Paroxetine treatment of premature ejaculation: a double-blind, randomized, placebo-controlled study. *Am J Psychiatry.* 1994;151:1377–1379.

Waldinger MD, Hengeveld MW, Zwinderman AH. Ejaculation-retarding properties of paroxetine in patients with primary premature ejaculation: a double-blind, randomized, dose-response study. *Br J Urol.* 1997;79:592–595.

Waldinger MD, Hengeveld MW, Zwinderman AH, Olivier B. Effect of SSRI antidepressants on ejaculation: a double-blind, randomized, placebo-controlled study with fluoxetine, fluvoxamine, paroxetine, and sertraline. *J Clin Psychopharmacol.* 1998;18:274–281.

Waldinger MD, Zwinderman AH, Olivier B. Antidepressants and ejaculation: a double-blind, randomized, placebo-controlled, fixed-dose study with paroxetine, sertraline, and nefazodone. *J Clin Psychopharmacol.* 2001a;21:283–297.

Waldinger MD, Zwinderman AH, Olivier B. SSRIs and ejaculation: a double-blind, randomized, fixed-dose study with paroxetine and citalopram. *J Clin Psychopharmacol.* 2001b;21:556–560.

Wise TN. Sertraline as a treatment for premature ejaculation. *J Clin Psychiatry.* 1994;55:417.

21. Treatment of Paraphilias and Sexual Offenders

INTRODUCTION

Treatment of sexual offenders is a very difficult task. Sexual offenders and persons with sexual or nonsexual paraphilias are known to be fairly resistant to "psychological" treatments, and as various psychotherapies and behavioral treatments. Treatment of paraphilias and sexual offenders has been controversial, with other than strictly medical issues involved, such as legal and ethical ones. In addition, the attention of the mass media and the society as a whole could complicate the treatment issues further.

Pharmacological treatment of sex offenders is based on several assumptions. One assumption is that suppression of sexual drive will decrease paraphilic behavior, sexual fantasies, and urges. Another assumption is that these behaviors are part of either the obsessive–compulsive spectrum disorders or impulse control disorders and that if control of compulsion or impulses is exerted, paraphilic behavior will become extinct. Based on these assumptions and clinical observations, various hormones, hormone-releasing hormones, hormone antagonists and agonists, antidepressants, antipsychotics, mood stabilizers, and other drugs have been used with varying degrees of success in the management of sex offenders. This chapter reviews the available treatments for paraphilias and their practical applications. Severe sexual offenders are usually treated in special facilities and under court order. However, many paraphilias are treated in routine clinical practice.

Though numerous articles have addressed the issues involved in the treatment of paraphilia and sex offenders, solid, hard evidence is scarce. The majority of earlier reports on the treatment of paraphilias and sex offenders were single case reports, and treatment studies of paraphilias and sex offenders have been marred by poor methodology. Kilmann and colleagues (1982) published the most comprehensive review of methodological issues in the outcome research of the paraphilias. Treatment studies of paraphilias and sex offenders are difficult to conduct for the following reasons:

1. Paraphilias are rare, and thus it is difficult to get a large enough and homogeneous study sample.

2. Paraphilias are not socially acceptable, and paraphilias and/or sex offenders usually do not seek treatment voluntarily.

3. Comorbidity rates, especially for personality disorders and substance abuse, among serious sex offenders are high.

4. Ethical considerations frequently do not allow for double-blind placebo-controlled study, especially with violent sex offenders.

This chapter discusses the available pharmacological treatment of sex offenders and paraphilias. Other biological treatments, such as surgical castration and stereotactic neurosurgery, used usually only in the most serious offenders, are beyond the scope of this chapter. This chapter focuses on:

- Description, epidemiology, physiology, and diagnosis of paraphilias
- Treatment of paraphilias and sex offenders with antidepressants (clomipramine) and selective serotonin reuptake inhibitors (SSRIs)
- Treatment with antipsychotics
- Treatment with mood stabilizers
- Treatment with hormonal preparations
- Treatment with other psychotropic agents
- Treatment with a combination of agents
- The importance of combining psychopharmacological and psychotherapeutic treatment modalities
- Legal issues
- Clinical guidelines.

Table 21.1 lists the pharmacological agents discussed in this chapter.

It is important to emphasize that none of the mentioned agents has been approved by the Food and Drug Administration (FDA) for the treatment of sex offenders or paraphilias (probably because of the cost associated with the FDA approval process).

Table 21.1   Pharmacological agents discussed in this chapter

Generic	Brand	Route	Dose (mg/day)
Antiandrogens and Other Hormonal Preparations			
cyproterone acetate		PO	50–150
(CPA)***		IM*	300–600
leuprolide acetate	Lupron Depot	IM	3.75–7.5 monthly
	Lupron Injections	IM	?
	Trenantone***	SC	11.25/3 months
medroxyprogesterone acetate	Provera	Oral	20–150
(MPA)	Depo-Provera	IM*	100–800
	Premphase	Oral	
	Prempro	Oral	
triptorelin***	Decapeptyl	IM	3.75/month
Antidepressants—Heterocyclic			
clomipramine	Anafranil	Oral	50–250
desipramine	Norpramin	Oral	25–250
Antidepressants—Selective Serotonin Reuptake Inhibitors			
citalopram	Celexa	Oral	10–50
fluoxetine	Prozac	Oral	10–80
fluvoxamine	Luvox	Oral	50–300
paroxetine	Paxil	Oral	10–60
sertraline	Zoloft	Oral	50–200
Antidepressants—Atypical			
nefazodone	Serzone	Oral	50–400
Anxiolytics—Azaspirones			
buspirone hydrochloride	BuSpar	Oral	20–30
Antipsychotics			
benperidol***		Oral	0.5–1.0
chlorpromazine	Thorazine	Oral	50–125
clozapine	Clozaril	Oral	50
fluphenazine enanthate***	Prolixin enanthate	IM	25 mg**
fluphenazine decanoate	Prolixin decanoate	IM	?
oxyprothepine decanoate***		IM	12.5–25/2–4 weeks
risperidone	Risperdal	Oral	6
Mood Stabilizers			
carbamazepine	Tegretol	Oral	1200++
lithium carbonate	Eskalith	Oral	600–1800++
valproic acid	Depakote	Oral	?2000 mg++
Others			
cimetidine	Tagamet	Oral	600–1600

* Administered once every 1–3 weeks.
** Administered every 2 weeks.
*** Not available in the United States.
++ Level monitoring recommended.

DEFINITION, DESCRIPTION, EPIDEMIOLOGY, PHYSIOLOGY, AND DIAGNOSIS

Paraphilia means love (*philia*) beyond the usual (*para*). The essential features of paraphilias are recurrent, intense, sexually arousing fantasies, sexual urges or behaviors generally involving (1) nonhuman objects, (2) the suffering or humiliation of oneself or one's partner, or (3) children or other nonconsenting persons, that occur over a period of at least 6 months. The major categories of paraphilias include exhibitionism, fetishism, frotteurism, pedophilia, sexual masochism, sexual sadism, transvestic fetishism, and voyeurism. Further paraphilias, classified in the DSM-IV as "not otherwise specified," include telephone scatologia, necrophilia, partialism, coprophilia, klismaphilia, zoophilia, urophilia, hypoxiphilia. There are about 30 (many quite rare) paraphilias; those discussed in this chapter are listed in Table 21.2.

Table 21.2   Paraphilias discussed in this chapter

Paraphilia	Description or Focus of Paraphilia
Autoerotic asphyxiation (hypoxyphilia)	Altered state of mind and enhanced orgasm secondary to hypoxia (via strangulation, volatile nitrite, or nitrous oxide) during masturbation.
Coprophilia	Sexual pleasure associated with the desire to defecate on a partner, to be defecated on, or to eat feces.
Exhibitionism	Exposure of one's genitals to a stranger (with or without masturbation).
Fetishism	Sexual pleasure associated with the use of nonliving objects (e.g., underpants, bras, shoes) while masturbating or during regular sexual activity.
Frotteurism	Touching and rubbing against a nonconsenting person.
Klismaphilia	Use of enemas as a part of sexual stimulation.
Necrophilia	Sexual gratification from cadavers.
Partialism	Exclusive focus on part of body; could involve oral–genital contact, if this is the sole source of sexual gratification.
Pedophilia	Sexual activity with a prepubescent child (13 years or younger); the individual with pedophilia must be at least 16 years old and at least 5 years older than the child.
Sexual masochism	Involves the act (real, not simulated) of being humiliated, beaten, bound, or otherwise made to suffer during sexual activity.
Sexual sadism	Involves acts (real, not simulated) in which the individual derives sexual excitement from the psychological or physical suffering (including humiliation) of the victim.
Telephone/computer scatologia	Sexual pleasure associated with making obscene phone calls to unsuspecting persons.
Transvestic fetishism	Involves cross-dressing; while cross-dressed, the person usually masturbates, imagining himself to be both the male subject and female object of his sexual fantasy.
Voyeurism	Involves observing unsuspecting individuals, usually strangers, who are naked, in the process of disrobing, or engaging in sexual activity.
Urophilia	Desire to urinate on a partner or to be urinated on.
Zoophilia	Intercourse, masturbation, or oral–genital contact with animals.

The actual incidence and prevalence of paraphilias are unknown. Para-philias are rarely diagnosed in a general clinical setting. However, the prevalence of paraphilias in the general population is probably higher than in the clinical setting, as suggested by the large commercial market for pornography and paraphiliac paraphernalia. Nevertheless, it is important to note that true paraphilias are practiced by a rela-tively small percentage of the population and that buying or watching pornographic movies does not a constitute paraphilia. Paraphilias are much more frequent among men (except for sexual masochism), and some of them occur exclusively among men. The most common para-philias seen in clinics specializing in the treatment of these disorders are pedophilia, voyeurism, and exhibitionism. Sexual masochism and sadism are less common. Interestingly, about half of those with para-philias seen clinically are married. Paraphiliac behavior declines with age.

The etiology of paraphilias is unknown. Various psychological (e.g., Freud's theories), developmental, environmental, genetic, and organic factors have been entertained as contributing to or explaining the etiology of paraphilia. Nevertheless, none of them has fully explained any of the paraphilias. Some theorists consider paraphilias a part of the obsessive–compulsive spectrum. For example, Bradford poin-ted out clinical similarities between obsessive–compulsive disorder (OCD) and sexual disorders, both paraphilic and nonparaphilic (e.g., hypersexuality):

1. Obsessions are similar to sexual fantasies, both paraphilic and non-paraphilic.

2. Compulsions are similar to compulsive sexual behavior, which can be paraphilic or nonparaphilic.

3. There is a crossover of comorbidity between OCD and sexual disor-ders, with depression and anxiety disorders being common in both groups.

4. At the neurobiological and neuropharmacological levels, there is a significant overlap between these disorders.

The fact that serotonergic drugs such as clomipramine and the SSRIs alleviate symptomatology in both groups of disorders (OCD spectrum and paraphilias) could be considered as another piece of supporting evidence. However, there is no consensus as to whether paraphil-ias and compulsive sexual behavior (nonparaphilic hypersexuality) should be included in the OCD spectrum disorders. Other authors point out the high comorbidity rates of paraphilias with other Axis-I disorders, such as mood, anxiety, and substance abuse disorders, and the frequent comorbid personality disorder traits or definite personality disorder diagnoses among this population.

The physiology and neurobiology of paraphilias are also unclear. It is known that various neurotransmitters and hormones have different effects on sexuality (e.g., dopamine could stimulate, serotonin could decrease, sexual urges); however, their manipulation and abnormalities do not explain particular paraphilias. Various serotonergic antidepressants and antiandrogens have been successfully used in the treatment of people with paraphilias, but their effect is nonspecific. Similarly, lesions of certain areas of the brain (e.g., frontal lobe) could lead to sexual disinhibition. Nevertheless, these lesions do not lead to disinhibition specific for paraphilias and do not fully explain their content. The origins of paraphilias are probably multifactorial.

The basis for making the diagnosis of paraphilia is a detailed clinical interview, including all the parts of a good psychiatric evaluation (present illness, past history, family history, social history, mental status examination, review of systems). The diagnosis of paraphilia(s) is made along four or more dimensions, listed in Table 21.3.

Some paraphilias have other specific features; for example, people with pedophilia must be at least 16 and at least 5 years older than the child abused.

A person can suffer from more than one paraphilia. Some paraphilias could be more or less acceptable in different cultures.

The technique of penile phaloplethysmography during various visual stimuli has been used to asses some paraphilias or confirm the diagnosis. However, its validity and reliability are not clear, and thus it should be considered an adjunctive or research tool.

Table 21.3 The diagnostic dimensions of paraphilias

1. Pathological fantasies, behaviors, urges
   Presence of recurrent, intense, sexually arousing fantasies, sexual urges, or behaviors generally involving either:
   a) nonhuman objects,
   b) suffering or humiliation of oneself or one's partner,
   c) children or nonconsenting adults.

2. Distress
   The fantasies, sexual urges, or behaviors cause clinically significant distress or impairment in social, occupational, or other important areas of functioning.

3. Time
   The disturbance last for at least 6 months.

4. Exclusivity
   Nonpathological fantasies, mental retardation, dementia, personality change due to a general medical condition, substance intoxication, manic episode, and schizophrenia must be ruled out.

Because frequent unprotected sex may lead to sexually transmitted diseases, good evaluation of paraphilia(s) should usually include an evaluation for these diseases.

TREATMENT

Clomipramine and Selective Serotonin Reuptake Inhibitors

Several authors hypothesized the usefulness of serotonergic antidepressants in the treatment of paraphilias and sex offenders, based on the phenomenological similarity of paraphilias and obsessive–compulsive and impulse control disorders and the efficacy of serotonergic drugs in these conditions.

Most of the evidence on the efficacy of antidepressants comes from case reports, case series, and retrospective studies. Shortly after the introduction of fluoxetine, the first case reports on its usefulness in paraphilias appeared. In 1990, one researcher reported on the successful treatment of compulsive cross-dressing with fluoxetine 20 mg/day, and another described a man suffering from exhibitionism who improved on fluoxetine 40 mg/day (after unsuccessful treatment with medroxyprogesterone and, later, fluphenazine). These cases were followed by case reports of fluoxetine's effectiveness, at 20–60 mg/day, in voyeurism, fetishism, and still another investigator described a 16-year-old male whose paraphilia (not otherwise specified) improved on fluoxetine, up to 60 mg/day. Interestingly, his testosterone level decreased by 24% from 613 ng/dL to 466 ng/dL during fluoxetine treatment. Other researchers successfully treated three males suffering from various paraphilias (pedophilia, exhibitionism, and voyeurism–frotteurism) with fluoxetine 20–80 mg/day.

Cases of other SSRIs' and clomipramine's effectiveness in treating paraphilias and other sexual disorders also have been reported: fluvoxamine in compulsive exhibitionism, sertraline and lithium in transvestic fetishism, sertraline in sexual addiction, paroxetine in voyeurism, exhibitionism and sexual addiction, and clomipramine in sexual preoccupation, sexual addiction (voyeurism with nonparaphilic sexual addiction and paraphilic [not otherwise specified] compulsive masturbation), and paraphilic behavior (exhibitionism, public masturbation) in dementia.

In addition, four larger case series confirmed the efficacy of serotonergic drugs in treating paraphilias and other sexual disorders. One researcher treated 10 men suffering from paraphilias and nonparaphilic sexual addictions with fluoxetine, lithium, or imipramine. Another researcher reported that patients with various paraphilias (mostly pedophilia) responded well to fluoxetine, either alone or in combination with lithium, carbamazepine, or imipramine. A chart review study reported various success levels with fluoxetine, fluvoxamine, and clomipramine. Paraphilia patients in this review study did not report improvement in sexual symptoms, but their OCD symptoms improved. The researchers felt that paraphilias may be less responsive than sexual obsessions to serotonergic drugs. A large retrospective chart review study of 94 patients treated with either fluoxetine, fluvoxamine, or sertraline for various paraphilias (mostly pedophilia, 74%). The severity of sexual fantasies decreased with all three drugs, and there were no significant differences in efficacy between the drugs.

Finally, several studies demonstrated the efficacy of serotonergic antidepressants in treating paraphilias, paraphilia-related disorders, and nonparaphilic sexual addictions. Fluoxetine was successful in 9 men with paraphilia and 7 men with nonparaphilic sexual addictions in one study. Sertraline (mean dose 100 mg/day) was efficacious in about half the men treated for various paraphilias and paraphilia-related disorders. Nine of those who failed to respond to sertraline were subsequently treated with fluoxetine up to 50 mg/day, and six of them improved. The overall success rate with SSRIs was 71%. Some patients required augmentation with methylphenidate or other drugs. Augmentation with psychostimulants in men with paraphilias and a history of attention-deficit disorder was advocated in one report. Interestingly, two researchers described an improvement of paraphilias with both clomipramine and desipramine in their double-blind crossover comparison in 15 men.

The results of a small retrospective study suggest that nefazodone might be helpful in nonparaphilic compulsive sexual behavior, while not producing the undesired sexual side effects of SSRIs.

It is important to note that most of the patients discussed in these cases, case series, and studies suffered from comorbid conditions, such as mood, anxiety, and substance abuse disorders. When reported, the majority of patients also described improvement in "normal" sexual behavior. Antidepressants, especially serotonergic ones, seem to be a useful treatment modality for paraphilias, especially in cases of comorbid mood and anxiety disorders.

Based on the discussed studies, some authors argued that paraphilias are part of the OCD spectrum because of the treatment effect of serotonergic drugs. Even though this is possible, the argument is flawed—one cannot assume that anxiety disorders are psychotic disorders because antipsychotics reduce anxiety.

Table 21.4   Antidepressants successfully used in treating paraphilias

Case reports

Antidepressant	Dosage	Type of Paraphilia
Clomipramine	up to 200 mg/day	compulsive masturbation exhibitionism, voyeurism
Fluvoxamine	up to 300 mg/day	exhibitionism
Fluoxetine	up to 80 mg/day	cross-dressing, exhibitionism, fetishism, frotteurism, masochism, voyeurism, mixed paraphilias
Paroxetine	up to 40 mg/day	exhibitionism, voyeurism
Sertraline	up to 200 mg/day	fetishism

Case-series, studies
  (antidepressants usually used in various paraphilias and their combinations)

Antidepressant	Dosage
Clomipramine	up to 400 mg/day
Desipramine	up to 250 mg/day
Fluvoxamine	up to 300 mg/day
Fluoxetine	up to 80 mg/day
Imipramine	up to 225 mg/day
Nefazodone	up to 400 mg/day
Setraline	up to 250 mg/day

Due to their better tolerability, serotonergic antidepressants, especially SSRIs, provide two major advantages over other preparations in the treatment of paraphilias. First, their use is much less threatening and less complicated (no pretreatment tests, no monitoring) to an average psychiatrist, and therefore paraphilias can be treated more frequently by average psychiatrists. Second, they can be used safely in adolescents, the age group most affected by the onset of many paraphilias. However, these drugs may disrupt "normal" sexual functioning through various deleterious effects, such as delayed ejaculation or anorgasmia. Interestingly, there is a possibility that SSRIs not only decrease the obsessive–compulsive symptomatology but also decrease testosterone levels. Table 21.4 summarizes the use of clomipramine and the SSRIs in treating paraphilias.

Antipsychotics

Antipsychotics have been used occasionally in the treatment of paraphilias since the 1960s. One study treated 26 sexually deviant individuals with 1 ml intramuscular fluphenazine enanthate (25 mg) every 2 weeks and reported a reduction of sexual drive and performance, with no "undue side effects" when antiparkinsonian drugs were also given. Fluphenazine enanthate is not available in the United States, but fluphenazine decanoate (1 ml = 25 mg) is, and it could be useful, theoretically.

Another researcher described the successful treatment of 28 sexual offenders (some imprisoned, some outpatients on probation) with oral benperidol 0.5–1.0 mg, a butyrophenone not available in the United States. Others compared benperidol and chlorpromazine in a double-blind placebo-controlled study of 12 pedophiliac sexual offenders. There were no significant differences between benperidol, chlorpromazine, and placebo, except in the self-rating of sexual thoughts, which was lower on benperidol. The researchers felt that the libido-reducing effect of benperidol was weak and unlikely to control serious anti-social sexual behavior.

Two studies from Czechoslovakia reported successful treatment of deviant sexual behavior with another long-acting antipsychotic, oxyprothepine decanoate (not available in the United States). In an open study comparison of this preparation with cyproterone acetate and lithium, cyproterone acetate fared the best. However, the authors felt that oxyprothepine decanoate was probably more suitable for uncooperative patients.

Two case reports published during the 1990s confirmed the usefulness of antipsychotics in special cases of paraphilia. The first described a case of a pedophile with comorbid dysthymia, who reported being free of the problematic sexual thoughts for the first time in his life, only when risperidone 6 mg/day was added to fluoxetine 80 mg/day. The second study used a low dose of clozapine (50 mg/day) in a case of zoophilia that developed subsequent to treatment of Parkinson's disease with dopaminergic agents in a 79-year-old male.

Since the use of antipsychotic agents has become more restricted during the last few decades, due to the risk of tardive dyskinesia, their use in paraphilias probably should be restricted to treatment-resistant cases or in cases of comorbidity with major mental disorders (e.g., schizophrenia). Table 21.5 summarizes the use of antipsychotic agents in treating paraphilias.

Table 21.5   Antipsychotics successfully used in treating paraphilias

Antipsychotic	Dosage	Type of Paraphilia
Benperidol	up to 1.25 mg/day	pedophilia
Chlorpromazine*	up to 125 mg/day	pedophilia
Clozapine*	50 mg/day	zoophilia
Fluphenazine enanthate	25 mg i.m./2 weeks	mixed (pedophilia, exhibitionism, etc.)
Oxyprothepine decanoate	25 mg i.m./2–4 weeks	mixed (pedophilia, exhibitionism, voyeurism)
Risperidone* (added to fluoxetine)	6 mg/day	pedophilia

* Available in the United States.

Table 21.6   Mood stabilizers used in treating paraphilias

Report	Drug(s)	Format	Dose	Paraphilia
Ward, 1975	lithium	single case	1800 mg/day	transvestism
Bártová et al., 1979	lithium DES*	open 24 on lithium 25 on DES	up to 1200 mg/day	exhibitionism pedophilia fetishism
Cesnik & Coleman, 1979	lithium	single case	up to 1200 mg/day	autoerotic asphyxia
Kolomazník et al., 1983	lithium	single case	1500 mg/day	pedophilia
Goldberg & Buongiorno, 1983	carbamazepine	single case	1200 mg/day	pedophilia, voyeurism
Coleman & Cesnik, 1990	lithium	two cases	300–900 mg/day	gender dysphoria
Coleman et al., 1992	lithium	four cases (one with added fluoxetine)	not available	pedophilia
Nelson et al., 2001	divalproex sodium	case-series retrospective 17 patients with bipolar disorder	2103 mg/day (mean daily dose)	pedophilia, frotteurism, paraphilia, NOS

* Diethylstilbestrol.

Mood Stabilizers

Several reports suggested the usefulness of mood stabilizers in the management of paraphilias. Most of them focused on lithium. The efficacy of mood stabilizers in pure paraphilia is unclear. Most of the patients whose paraphilia symptomatology was reported to have improved with mood stabilizers suffered from comorbid mood disorders. Mood stabilizers should not be used as first-line treatment of paraphilias and should probably be reserved for paraphilias comorbid with mood disorders. Table 21.6 summarizes the research on the use of mood stabilizers in treating paraphilias.

Hormonal Preparations

As we pointed out, one of the assumptions underlying treatment of paraphilias is that reduction of sex drive also will reduce paraphilic behavior. Because androgens seem to be essential for normal sexual behavior and sex drive, blocking them or administering antiandrogens seems to be a logical approach to the management of paraphilias and sex offenders. Originally, estrogens were used to reduce sex drive. However successful, estrogens have many unpleasant side effects, such as nausea, vomiting, feminization, and breast carcinoma. Thus their use has been limited.

The two main hormonal preparations used in the treatment of paraphilias are medroxyprogesterone acetate (MPA) and cyproterone acetate (CPA). These are progestogens or antiandrogens (actually, CPA is a true antiandrogen, MPA is not; see below). Their use has been summarized in several comprehensive reviews. Cumulative totals of over 200 and 500 sex offenders treated with either MPA or CPA, respectively, have been reported in the literature.

MPA

MPA probably has been the most common hormonal pharmacological treatment of paraphilias in the United States, partially because of lack of alternatives such as CPA (not available in the United States). MPA has been used in the treatment of sex offenders since the late 1950s. It induces testosterone reductase in the liver and thus decreases the levels of circulating testosterone. MPA also blocks follicle stimulating hormone and luteinizing hormone, but does not compete with androgens on the androgen receptor level, and thus it is not a true antiandrogen. It also affects the binding of testosterone to the plasma testosterone-binding globulin. MPA reduces sexual drive, erotic fantasies, sexual activity, possibly aggressiveness, as well as nocturnal penile tumescence.

MPA has been found effective in various paraphilias and sex offenders. Table 21.7 summarizes this research. MPA also has been compared to other treatment modalities, such as assertiveness training (not possible to draw a definite conclusion from this study because the drop-out rate was very high) and imaginal desensitization. Interestingly, MPA was not significantly different from imaginal desensitization alone or imaginal desensitization plus MPA in 24 males with anomalous sexual urges or behaviors. In a small, double-blind study, MPA was superior to placebo in reduction of sexual fantasies. MPA appeared to be a useful

Table 21.7 Medroxyprogesterone acetate (MPA) in paraphilias

Report	Format	Dosage	Paraphilia
Pinta, 1978	single case	400 mg/10 days	homosexual pedophilia
Kiersch, 1990	case series, 8 cases case-controlled vs. saline	100–400 mg/week	mostly pedophilia, rape
Meyer et al., 1992	open (23 cases) control group (21 cases)*	400 mg/week	pedophilia, rape, exhibitionism
Kravitz et al., 1995	open naturalistic (29 cases)	300–900 mg/week	pedophilia, exhibitionism, frotteurism

* 18% reoffended while on MPA; 35% reoffended after stopping MPA; 58% controls reoffended.

sex-drive reducing medication, but attaining compliance in taking the drug was a major obstacle.

MPA was compared to CPA and placebo in a double-blind study with seven pedophiles. Both drugs performed equally, reducing sexual thoughts and fantasies, the frequency of erections on awakening, the frequency and pleasure of masturbation, and level of sexual frustration. Serum testosterone, follicle stimulating hormone and luteinizing hormone all declined during drug administration but returned to pretreatment values by the end of the final placebo phase. It is important to note that many patients relapse after MPA discontinuation.

The side effects of MPA include weight gain, deep venous thrombosis, nausea, vomiting, salivation, depression, headaches, decreased sperm production, and decrease in "normal" sexual functioning.

The doses of MPA used in the treatment of paraphilias vary from 100 mg to 400 mg either weekly or less frequently (every 2–4 weeks) during the acute phase, and 100–400 mg/week during the maintenance phase (depending on the study, the length of acute phase varied). Usually, it has been applied intramuscularly, though it could be given orally. For instance, in one open study, researchers administered MPA 60 mg/day orally, for 15 months, to 7 subjects with paraphilias.

Laboratory tests and other measures that should be obtained prior to starting treatment with MPA (see also Tables 21.8 and 21.14) include serum testosterone level, follicle stimulating hormone, luteinizing hormone, prolactin, complete blood count, liver function tests, blood glucose, blood pressure and determination of weight. The pretreatment testosterone level may be one of the determinants of treatment length—patients with low pretreatment testosterone levels received MPA for longer periods of time in one study. Table 21.8 summarizes side effects, doses, and laboratory tests.

Table 21.8 Medroxyprogesterone acetate (MPA) treatment issues in paraphilias

Side Effects	Doses/Phases	Tests Prior Treatment
Decreased sperm production	Acute phase:	Blood glucose
Decreased sexual functioning	100–400 mg/week or less	Blood pressure
Deep venous thrombosis	frequently (q 2–4 weeks)	Complete blood count
Depression	Maintenance phase:	FSH, LH
Diabetes mellitus	100–400 mg/week	Liver function tests
Headaches		Serum prolactin
Hypertension		Serum testosterone
Nausea		Weight
Salivation		
Vomiting		
Weight gain		

CPA

CPA is considered a true antiandrogen. It has been used widely in the treatment of paraphilias since the 1960s, mainly in Europe and Canada (it is not available in the U.S.). CPA blocks the intracellular uptake of testosterone and the intracellular metabolism of the androgen. It reduces the levels of testosterone, follicle stimulating hormone, and luteinizing hormone. It also decreases erection, ejaculation, and spermatogenesis. Interestingly, CPA seems to reduce anxiety and irritability as well.

CPA has been found effective in treating various paraphilias and deviant sexual behavior. Table 21.9 summarizes this research.

Table 21.9   Cyproterone acetate (CPA)* in paraphilias

Doses	Paraphilias Treated
Oral: 5–100 mg/day	Exhibitionism, pedophilia, sexual sadism, fetishism, frotteurism, rape, multiple paraphilias
Intramuscularly: 300 mg/ every 2 weeks Pretreatment recidivism rates: 50–100% Posttreatment recidivism rates: 0–16.7%	

* CPA acts to decrease levels of circulating sex hormones.

The side effects of CPA include liver damage, feminization (manifested mainly by gynecomastia), loss of body hair, reduction of sebum production, and adrenal suppression.

The doses of CPA range from 50–200 mg/day orally or 200–600 mg/ weekly or biweekly intramuscularly.

Laboratory tests and other measures that should be obtained prior to starting treatment with CPA (see also Tables 21.10 and 21.14) include serum testosterone level, follicle stimulating hormone, luteinizing hormone, prolactin, complete blood count, liver function tests, blood glucose, blood pressure, body weight, and ECG. Table 21.10 lists side effects of, and laboratory tests for, CPA.

LHRH Agonists and Flutamide

Because MPA and CPA have considerable side effects, various other hormonal preparations with similar properties have been tried in the treatment of paraphilias. These include mainly gonadotropin hormone-releasing hormone agonists and pure antiandrogen flutamide. The luteinizing hormone-releasing hormone agonists (LHRH agonists) overstimulate the hypothalamus, then reduce gonadotropin-releasing hormone secretion, and consequently the secretion of testosterone

Table 21.10 Cyproterone acetate (CPA) treatment issues in paraphilias

Side Effects	Tests Prior Treatment
Adrenal suppression	Blood glucose
Decreased activity	Blood pressure
Decreased body hair	Body weight
Decreased ejaculate, sperm count	Complete blood count
Decreased sexual functioning	ECG
Decreased testosterone	FSH, LH
Depression	Liver function tests
Fatigue	Serum prolactin
Feminization (gynecomastia)	Serum testosterone
Liver damage	
Reduction of sebrum production	

and dihydrotestosterone decreases to almost zero. These preparations are usually given intramuscularly.

Rousseau and colleagues (1990) reported a reduction of severe exhibitionism with LHRH agonist and flutamide. Dickey (1992) described an improvement of severe paraphilias in a male treated with long-acting LHRH agonist. Long-lasting GnRH hormone agonist was effective in 5 of 6 patients with severe pedophilias and exhibitionism (Thibault et al., 1993; 1995). Triptorelin, a long-acting analogue of gonadotropin releasing hormone, 3.75 mg/monthly, together with supportive psychotherapy, decreased deviant sexual fantasies and desires in 30 men (25 with pedophilia) in a study by Rosler and Witztum (1998).

Leuprolide Acetate

Three reports, summarized in Table 21.11, suggest that leuprolide acetate (Lupron) could be helpful in the management of paraphilias.

The side effects mainly include erectile failure, hot flashes, and decreased bone mineral density.

The doses of leuprolide acetate probably should be 3.75–7.5 mg/month applied intramuscularly. Pretreatment laboratory and other tests include serum testosterone, follicle stimulating hormone, luteinizing

Table 21.11 Leuprolide acetate in paraphilias

Report	Format	Dose	Paraphilia in Which Successful
Rich & Ovsiew, 1994	single case	7.5 mg i.m./month	exhibitionism (in Huntington)
Briken et al., 2001	case-series retrospective 11 cases	11.25 mg subcutaneous	pedophilia, rape, sadism, combined paraphilias
Krueger & Kaplan, 2001	case-series 12 cases	3.75–7.5 mg i.m./monthly	pedophilia, exhibitionism, masochism, voyeurism, frotteurism

Table 21.12   Leuprolide acetate treatment issues in paraphilias

Main Side Effects	Tests Prior Treatment
Decreased body hair	Bone density measurement
Decreased bone mineral density	BUN, creatinine
Erectile failure	Complete blood count
Hot flashes	ECG
	FSH, LH
	Serum testosterone
	1 mg test dose of leuprolide (anaphylaxis?)

hormone, BUN and creatinine, complete blood count, bone density measurement, ECG and 1 mg test dose of leuprolide to observe for anaphylactic reaction or allergy. Table 21.12 summarizes side effects and laboratory tests.

Hormonal preparations are definitely a useful part of the management of paraphilias and sexual offenders. However, they should probably not be used as a first-line treatment of mild paraphilias (see below), but clearly should be used in severe cases. The advantage, in addition to their efficacy, is their intramuscular route of administration, which may be helpful when treating noncompliant patients. At the present time, MPA and leuprolide acetate are the only two preparations available in the United States.

Buspirone, Cimetidine

One researcher reported two cases of successfully treated paraphilia (transvestic fetishism with generalized anxiety disorder and alcohol dependence; and atypical paraphilia and transvestic fetishism) with 20 mg/day of buspirone. Another report described the case of a man with obscene telephoning and exhibitionistic behavior, who responded to 25 mg/day of buspirone.

Buspirone may be an alternative treatment for some cases of paraphilia, especially in cases of comorbid substance abuse. It has a low side effect profile and is especially void of sexual side effects.

Theoretically interesting is the case of decreased libido and hypersexual behavior in patients with dementia who were administered cimetidine (600–1600 mg), a histamine H_2-receptor antagonist. Cimetidine is a nonhormonal antiandrogen that is not indicated in paraphilia but could be used as an adjunct agent in some cases.

Combination of Agents

Various combinations of different psychotropic and hormonal preparations have been used in the treatment of paraphilias and sexual offenders. Examples include combining sertraline and lithium, fluoxetine and risperidone, LHRH agonist and flutamide, and others combining hormonal preparations and antidepressants may allow for a lower dose of hormones, thus decreasing the probability of potentially serious side effects. Based on published data creativity is probably the rule.

Combining Psychopharmacological and Psychotherapeutic Treatment Modalities

Though it is known that sex offenders are particularly resistant to psychological treatment, the combination of pharmacological treatment and various psychotherapies appears to be superior to drugs alone, although solid research evaluating this approach is still lacking. Various reports suggested the usefulness of combining lithium with psychotherapy, triptorelin with supportive psychotherapy, and a combination of other pharmacological agents with various therapies. Psychotherapy also may enhance compliance with the pharmacological treatment. Thus it is recommended that people with paraphilias and sex offenders be treated with various pharmacological agents (see guidelines below) in combination with various psychotherapies.

Legal Issues

The treatment of paraphilias frequently implicates psychiatric, legal, and societal versus individual interests. One researcher pointed out the differences between states in reporting sexual involvement with children. Another discussed the aftermath of laws mandating compulsory hormonal treatments of people with paraphilias, and the constitutionality of the civil commitment of sexual predators to treatment until they are safe to be released into the society. According to one group of researchers, there is considerable variation as to who is subject to MPA (and other substances) treatment laws, and how such laws—including specific provisions, such as clinical criteria, if any, required for treatment, type and period of treatment plans, informed consent—are implemented, because sentencing laws vary widely from state to state. They also emphasized that sentencing laws may have remarkably little relation to what is widely considered effective treatment for pedophilia.

All these articles and debates underscore the importance of an appropriate informed consent and solid knowledge of local legal regulations regarding reporting such crimes and enforcing commitment.

CLINICAL GUIDELINES

Depending on the treatment agent and its legal status (voluntary vs. court-ordered), the provision of informed consent for the treatment of paraphilias could raise special concerns. Some of the potential medical complications of treatment with hormonal preparations (and antipsychotics) are serious and their long-term effects are not well known. Patients should have a clear understanding that, in addition to other side effects, they may permanently lose fertility and sex drive. The optimal doses of hormonal preparations (and, in fact, of all pharmacological treatments) have not been established, and these doses may vary greatly from patient to patient. Similarly, the appropriate length of treatment for paraphilias has not been established and may be indefinite.

Patients should be carefully diagnosed and screened for comorbid conditions, which may affect the pharmacotherapy selected. Doses of medications do not always have to be high, as suggested by some, but they should be individualized. Medication effects and side effects should be considered in the selection of pharmacotherapy and regularly monitored. Medications should be increased gradually, usually not sooner than 1 month from initiation or previous increase. Various combinations could be considered in treatment-resistant cases.

Bradford suggested a practical six-level algorithm for the treatment of paraphilias. This treatment algorithm uses an enhanced version of the *DSM-III–R*'s three categories of paraphilias: *mild* (i.e., the person is markedly distressed by the recurrent paraphilic urges but has never acted on them); *moderate* (i.e., the person has occasionally acted on the paraphilic urge; and *severe* (i.e., the person has repeatedly acted on the paraphilic urge). Bradford adds a fourth category: *catastrophic*. According to him, this category would be indicated by clear evidence of sexual sadism in terms of fantasies, urges, history, and behavior. The presence of victimization would render this the highest level of risk in all categories. In the absence of victimization, this designation would result from evidence of predatory stalking behavior with sadistic or homicidal urges, or urges to torture. Bradford's six proposed levels of treatment are presented in Table 21.13.

Whereas antidepressants are usually contraindicated only in cases of known sensitivity to the particular drug or in combination with an inhibitor of monoamine oxidase, hormonal preparations are contraindicated in cases of active pituitary pathology (all), thromboembolic disorders (MPA and CPA), liver failure (MPA and CPA), and osteoporosis (leuprolide). Antipsychotics can have special contraindications, depending on the drug used (e.g., clozapine: myeloproliferative disorders or uncontrolled epilepsy).

Antidepressants do not usually require any special monitoring during treatment. Hormonal preparations require various pretreatment tests and monitoring during the treatment, which are detailed in Table 21.14.

Table 21.13 Bradford's algorithm for the treatment of paraphilias*

Level 1
  Regardless of the severity level of paraphilia, cognitive-behavioral treatment and relapse prevention should be always administered.
Level 2
  Pharmacological treatment would start with SSRIs (our recommendation: or with clomipramine). This prescription would be indicated in all cases of mild paraphilia.
Level 3
  If the SSRIs (or clomipramine) were not effective in 4–6 weeks at adequate doses, a small dose of antiandrogen should be added (e.g., sertraline 200 mg/day with 50 mg of MPA or 50 mg of CPA daily.
Level 4
  The full antiandrogen or hormonal treatment should be given orally. This treatment would involve 50–300 mg of MPA/day or 50–300 mg of CPA/day. This regime would be used in most moderate cases and in some severe cases.
Level 5
  The full antiandrogen or hormonal treatment should be given intramuscularly. This treatment would involve 300 mg of MPA given each week ort 200 mg of CPA every 2 weeks. This regime would be used in severe cases and some catastrophic cases.
Level 6
  A complete suppression of androgens and sex drive should be sought. Administer CPA 200–400 mg i.m. weekly or provide LHRH agonist. This regime should be used for some severe paraphilias and would be the treatment of choice for catastrophic paraphilias.

* Adapted from Bradford, 2000; Bradford, 2001.
†Antipsychotics could probably be used in higher levels, too, especially when hormonal preparations are contraindicated.

Table 21.14 Recommended pretreatment tests and monitoring during hormonal treatment of paraphilias

Preparation	Pretreatment Tests	Monitoring during Treatment
medroxyprogesterone (MPA)	1. Serum testosterone, FSH, LH, and prolactin 2. Liver function tests 3. Complete blood count 4. Serum glucose 5. Blood pressure 6. Weight	1. Serum testosterone monthly for 4 months, then every 6 months 2. Serum LH and prolactin every 6 months 3. Changes in blood pressure and weight 4. If testosterone suppressed significantly, bone mineral density at baseline and yearly 5. If hepatotoxicity suspected, liver function tests
cyproterone (CPA)	1. Steps 1–6 same as for medroxyprogesterone 2. ECG	1. Steps 1–5 same as for medroxyprogesterone
leuprolide	1. Serum testosterone, FSH, and LH 2. BUN and creatinine 3. Complete blood count 4. Bone mineral density 5. ECG 6. Test dose: leuprolide 1 mg subcutaneously, with observation for allergy and anaphylaxis	1. Serum testosterone and complete blood count monthly for 4 months, then every 6 months 2. Serum LH every 6 months 3. BUN and creatinine every 6 months 4. Bone mineral density yearly

* Modified from Reilly et al., 2000.

Antipsychotics require monitoring for abnormal movements and/or for the development of tardive dyskinesia.

Patients must be able to acknowledge that they are ultimately responsible for controlling their sexual behavior, knowing that help is available. Success is certainly more probable in motivated patients. Combining treatment approaches—namely, psychopharmacology, psychotherapy, and behavioral approaches—appears to be superior to medications alone.

Knowledge is lacking regarding the length of treatment for paraphilic behavior (indefinite?) and the long-term side effects of some medications used in this indication (hormonal preparations). Periodic monitoring, evaluation of compliance and efficacy, and in stable, voluntary patients, occasional decrease or discontinuation of medication and observation for symptoms of relapse are recommended.

CONCLUSIONS

Pharmacotherapy of people with paraphilias and sex offenders has undergone significant developments. Still, no ideal medication for paraphilia is available, and thus a careful selection from the available armamentarium, based on symptoms, level of paraphilia, legal requirements, medical status, and possible side effects, is recommended. The serotonergic antidepressants and hormonal preparations seem to be the medications of choice, which should be used in combination with various psychotherapies. Other psychotropic and nonpsychotropic medications (e.g., antipsychotics, mood stabilizers, anxiolytics, H_2 blockers,) could be used in special cases of treatment resistance or when comorbidity of psychiatric disorders is an issue.

REFERENCES

Abouesch A, Clayton A. Compulsive voyeurism and exhibitionism: a clinical response to paroxetine. *Arch Sex Behav.* 1999;28:23–30.

Aguirre B. Fluoxetine and compulsive sexual behavior. *J Am Acad Child Adolesc Psychiatry.* 1999;38:943.

American Psychiatric Association. *Diagnostic and Statistical Manual of Mental Disorders* 3rd ed.- rev. Washington DC: American Psychiatric Association; 1987.

American Psychiatric Association. *Diagnostic and Statistical Manual of Mental Disorders* 4th ed. Washington DC: American Psychiatric Association; 1994.

Azhar MZ, Varma SL. Response to clomipramine in sexual addiction. *Eur Psychiatry.* 1995;10:263–265.

Balon R. Pharmacological treatment of paraphilias with focus on antidepressants. *J Sex & Marital Ther.* 1998;24:241–254.

Bancroft J, Tennent G, Loucas, K, Cass J. The control of deviant sexual behaviour by drugs: I. Behavioural changes following oestrogens and anti-androgens. *Brit J Psychiatry.* 1974;125:310–315.

Bancroft J, Wu FCW. Changes in erectile responsiveness during androgen replacement therapy. *Arch Sex Behav.* 1983;12:59–66.

Bartholomew AA. Some side effects of thioridazine. *Med J Australia.* 1964;1:57.

Bartholomew AA. A long-term phenothiazine as a possible agent to control deviant sexual behavior. *Am J Psychiatry.* 1968;124:917–923.

Bártová D, Náhunek K, Švestka J, Hajnová R. Comparative study of prophylactic lithium and diethylstilbestrol in sexual deviants. *Activ Nerv Sup (Praha).* 1979;21:163–164.

Bártová D, Hajnová R, Náhunek K, Švestka J. Oxyprothepin decanoate in the treatment of deviant sexual behaviour. *Activ Nerv Sup (Praha).* 1981;23:248–249.

Bártová D, Burešová A, Hajnová R, Švestka J, Tichý P. [Effect of oxyprothepine decanoate, lithium and cyproterone acetate on deviant sexual behavior.] *Čs Psychiatrie.* 1986;82:355–360.

Berlin FS. The paraphilias and Depo-Provera: some medical, ethical and legal considerations. *Bull Am Acad Psychiatry Law.* 1989;17:233–239.

Berlin FS, Meinecke CF. Treatment of sex offenders with antiandrogenic medication: conceptualization, review of treatment modalities and preliminary findings. *Am J Psychiatry.* 1981;138:601–607.

Bianchi MD. Fluoxetine treatment of exhibitionism. *Am J Psychiatry.* 1990;147:1089–1990.

Bourgeois JA, Klein M. Risperidone and fluoxetine in the treatment of pedophilia with comorbid dysthymia. *J Clin Psychopharmacol.* 1996;16:257–258.

Bradford JMW. The paraphilias, obsessive–compulsive spectrum disorders, and the treatment of sexually deviant behaviour. *Psychiatric Quarterly.* 1999;70:209–219.

Bradford JMW. The treatment of sexual deviation using a pharmacological approach. *J Sex Res.* 2000;37:248–257.

Bradford JMW. The neurobiology, neuropharmacology, and pharmacological treatment of the paraphilias and compulsive sexual behaviour. *Can J Psychiatry.* 2001;46:26–34.

Bradford JMW, Pawlak A. Double-blind placebo crossover study of cyproterone acetate in the treatment of paraphilias. *Arch Sex Behav.* 1993a;22:383–402.

Bradford JMW, Pawlak A. Effects of cyproterone acetate on sexual arousal patterns of pedophiles. *Arch Sex Behav.* 1993b;22:629–641.

Bradford JMW, Pawlak A. Sadistic homosexual pedophilia: treatment with cyproterone acetate: a single case study. *Can J Psychiatry.* 1987;32:22–31.

Brantley JT, Wise TN. Antiandrogenic treatment of a gender-dysphoric transvestite. *J Sex & Marital Ther.* 1985;11:109–112.

Briken P, Nika E, Berner W. Treatment of paraphilia with luteinizing hormone-releasing hormone agonist. *J Sex & Marital Ther.* 2001;27:45–55.

Cesnik JA, Coleman E. Use of lithium carbonate in the treatment of autoerotic asphyxia. *Am J Psychotherapy.* 1989;43:277–286.

Clayton AH. Fetishism and clomipramine. *Am J Psychiatry.* 1993;150:673–674.

Coleman E, Cesnik J. Skoptic syndrome: the treatment of an obsessional gender dysphoria with lithium carbonate and psychotherapy. *Am J Psychotherapy.* 1990;44:204–217.

Coleman E, Cesnik J, Moore A-M, Dwyer SM. An exploratory study of the role of psychotropic medication in the treatment of sex offenders. *J Offender Rehab.* 1992;18:75–88.

Coleman E, Gratzer T, Nesvacil L, Raymond NC. Nefazodone and the treatment of nonparaphilic compulsive sexual behavior: a retrospective study. *J Clin Psychiatry.* 2000;61:282–284.

Cooper AJ. A placebo-controlled trial of the antiandrogen cyproterone acetate in deviant hypersexuality. *Compr Psychiatry.* 1981;22:458–465.

Cooper AJ. Progestogens in the treatment of male sex offenders: a review. *Can J Psychiatry.* 1986;31:73–79.

Cooper AJ. Sadistic homosexual pedophilia treatment with cyproterone acetate. *Can J Psychiatry.* 1987;32:738–740.

Cooper AJ, Losztyn S, Cernovsky Z. Medroxyprogesterone acetate, nocturnal penile tumescence, laboratory arousal, and sexual acting out in a male with schizophrenia. *Arch Sex Behav.* 1990;19:361–371.

Cooper AJ, Sadhu S, Losztyn S, Cernovsky Z. A double-blind placebo-controlled trial of medroxyprogesterone acetate and cyproterone acetate with seven pedophiles. *Can J Psychiatry.* 1992;37:687–693.

Cordoba OA, Chapel JL. Medroxyprogesterone acetate antiandrogen treatment of hypersexuality in a pedophiliac sex offender. *Am J Psychiatry.* 1983;140:1036–1039.

Davies TS. Cyproterone acetate for male hypersexuality. *J Int Med Res.* 1974;2:159–163.

Dickey R. The management of a case of treatment-resistant paraphilia with a long acting LHRH agonist. *Can J Psychiatry.* 1992;37:567–569.

Elmore JL. SSRI reduction of nonparaphilic sexual addiction. *CNS Spectrums.* 2000;11:53–56.

Emmanuel NP, Lydiard RB, Ballenger JC. Fluoxetine treatment of voyeurism. *Am J Psychiatry.* 1991;148:950.

Fedoroff JP. Buspirone hydrochloride in the treatment of transvestic fetishism. *J Clin Psychiatry.* 1988;49:408–409.

Fedoroff JP. Buspirone hydrochloride in the treatment of an atypical paraphilia. *Arch Sex Behav.* 1992;21:401–406.

Fedoroff JP. Serotonergic drug treatment of deviant sexual interests. *Ann Sex Res.* 1993;6:105–121.

Fernandez HH, Durso R. Clozapine for dopaminergic-induced paraphilias in Parkinson's disease. *Mov Disord.* 1998;13:597–598.

Field LH. Benperidol in the treatment of sexual offenders. *Med Sci Law.* 1973;13:195–196.

Fischbain DA. Buspirone and transvestic fetishism. *J Clin Psychiatry.* 1989;50:436–437.

Goldberg RL, Buongiorno PA. The use of carbamazepine for the treatment of paraphilias in a brain-damaged patient. *Intl J Psychiatry in Medicine.* 1983;12:275–279.

Greenberg DM, Bradford JMW, Curry S, O'Rourke A. A comparison of treatment of paraphilias with three serotonin reuptake inhibitors: a retrospective study. *Bull Am Acad Psychiatry Law.* 1996;24:525–532.

Heller CG, Laidlaw WM, Harvey HT, Nelson DL. Effects of Progestational compounds on the reproductive processes of the human male. *Ann NY Acad Sci.* 1958;71:649–665.

Hucker S, Langevin R, Bain J. A double blind trial of sex drive reducing medication in pedophiles. *Ann Sex Res.* 1988;1:227–242.

Jorgensen VT. Cross-dressing successfully treated with fluoxetine. *NY State J Med.* 1990;90:566–567.

Kafka MP. Successful treatment of paraphilic coercive disorder (a rapist) with fluoxetine hydrochloride. *Br J Psychiatry.* 1991a;158:844–847.

Kafka MP. Successful antidepressant treatment of nonparaphilic sexual addictions and paraphilias in men. *J Clin Psychiatry.* 1991b;52:60–65.

Kafka MP. Sertraline pharmacotherapy for paraphilias and paraphilia-related disorders: an open trial. *Ann Clin Psychiatry.* 1994;6:189–195.

Kafka MP. Psychopharmacologic treatments for nonparaphilic compulsive sexual behaviors. *CNS Spectrums.* 2000;5:49–59.

Kafka MR, Hennen J. Psychostimulant augmentation during treatment with selective serotonin reuptake inhibitors in men with paraphilias and paraphilia-related disorders: a case series. *J Clin Psychiatry.* 2000;61:664–670.

Kafka MP, Prentky R. Fluoxetine treatment of nonparaphilic sexual addictions and paraphilias in men. *J Clin Psychiatry.* 1992;53:351–358.

Kiersch TA. Treatment of sex offenders with Depo-Provera. *Bull Am Acad Psychiatry Law.* 1990;18:179–187.

Kilmann PR, Sabalis RF, Gearing II, ML, Bukstel LH, Scovern AW. The treatment of sexual paraphilias: a review of outcome research. *J Sex Res.* 1982;18:193–252.

Kolomazník M, Sůva J, Švejnohová D, Janoušek I, Hronek J. [Case history of pedophil incestuous action treated with lithium: sexuological aspects.] *Čs Psychiatrie.* 1983;79:217–222.

Kravitz HM, Haywood TW, Kelly J, Liles S, Cavanaugh Jr. JL. Medroxyprogesterone and paraphiles: do testosterone levels matter? *Bull Am Acad Psychiatry Law.* 1996;24:73–83.

Kravitz HM, Haywood TW, Kelly J, Wahlstrom C, Liles S, Cavanaugh Jr. JL. Medroxyprogesterone treatment for paraphiliacs. *Bull Am Acad Psychiatry Law.* 1995;23:19–33.

Krueger RB, Kaplan MS. Depot-leuprolide acetate for treatment of paraphilias: a report of twelve cases. *Arch Sex Behav.* 2001a;30:409–422.

Krueger RB, Kaplan MS. The paraphilic and hypersexual disorders: an overview. *Journal of Psychiatric Practice.* 2001b;7:391–403.

Krucsi MJP, Fine S, Valladares L, Phillips Jr. RA, Rapoport JL. Paraphilias: a double-blind crossover comparison of clomipramine versus desipramine. *Arch Sex Behav.* 1992;21:587–593.

Langevin R, Paitich D, Hucker S, et al. The effects of assertiveness training, provera, and sex of therapist in the treatment of genital exhibitionism. *J Behav Ther Exp Psychiatry.* 1979;10:275–282.

Laschet U, Laschet L. Psychopharmacotherapy of sex offenders with cyproterone acetate. *Pharmakopsychiatrie Neuropsychopharmakologie.* 1971;4:99–104.

Leo RJ, Kim KY. Clomipramine treatment of paraphilias in elderly demented patients. *J Geriatr Psychiatry Neurol.* 1995;8:123–124.

Litkey LJ, Feniczy P. An approach to the control of homosexual practices. *Int J Neuropsychiatry.* 1967;3:20–23.

Lorefice LS. Fluoxetine treatment of a fetish. *J Clin Psychiatry.* 1991;52:41.

McConaghy N, Blaszczynski A, Kidson W. Treatment of sex offenders with imaginal desensitization and/or medroxyprogesterone. *Acta Psychiatr Scand.* 1988;77:199–206.

Meyer III, WJ, Cole C, Emory E. Depo Provera treatment for sex offending behavior: an evaluation of outcome. *Behav Sci Law.* 1992;18:83–110.

Money J. Paraphilias: phenomenology and classification. *Am J Psychotherapy.* 1984;38:164–179.

Money J, Wiedekind C, Walker P, Migeon C, Meyer W, Borgaonkar D. 47, XYY and 46, XY males with antisocial and/or sex-offending behavior: antiandrogen therapy plus counseling. *Psychoneuroendocrinology.* 1975;1:165–178.

Murray MAF, Bancroft JHJ, Anderson DC, Tennent TG, Carr PJ. Endocrine changes in male sexual deviants after treatment with anti-androgens, oestrogens or tranquillizers. *J Endocr.* 1975;67:179–188.

Nelson E, Brusman L, Holcomb J, et al. Divalproex sodium in sex offenders with bipolar disorders and comorbid paraphilias: an open retrospective study. *J Affect Disord.* 2001;64:249–255.

Pearson HJ, Marshall WL, Barbaree HE, Southmayd S. Treatment of a compulsive paraphiliac with buspirone. *Ann Sex Res.* 1992;5:239–246.

Perilstein RD, Lipper S, Friedman LJ. Three cases of paraphilias responsive to fluoxetine treatment. *J Clin Psychiatry.* 1991;52:169–170.

Pinta ER. Treatment of obsessive homosexual pedophilic fantasies with medroxyprogesterone acetate. *Biol Psychiatry.* 1978;13:369–373.

Reilly DR, Delva NJ, Hudson RW. Protocols for the use of cyproterone, medroxyprogesterone, and leuprolide in the treatment of paraphilias. *Can J Psychiatry.* 2000;45:559–563.

Rich SS, Ovsiew F. Leuprolide acetate for exhibitionism in Huntington's disease. *Mov Disord.* 1994;9:353–357.

Rosler A, Witztum E. Pharmacotherapy of paraphilias in the next millennium. *Behav Sci Law.* 2000;18:43–56.

Ross LA, Bland WP, Ruskin P, Bacher N. Antiandrogen treatment of aberrant sexual activity. *Am J Psychiatry.* 1987;144:1511.

Rousseau L, Couture M, Dupont A, Labrie F, Couture N. Effects of combined androgen blockade with LHRH agonist and flutamide in one severe case of male exhibitionism. *Can J Psychiatry.* 1990;35:338–341.

Rubenstein EB, Engel NL. Successful treatment of transvestic fetishism with sertraline and lithium. *J Clin Psychiatry.* 1996;57:92.

Rubey R, Brady KT, Norris GT. Clomipramine treatment of sexual preoccupation. *J Clin Psychopharmacol.* 1993;13:158–159.

Snaith RP, Collins SA. Five exhibitionists and a method of treatment. *Brit J Psychiatry.* 1981;138:126–130.

Stein DJ, Hollander E, Anthony DT, et al. Serotonergic medications for sexual obsessions, sexual addictions, and paraphilias. *J Clin Psychiatry.* 1992;53:267–271.

Stone TH, Winslade WJ, Klugman CM. Sex offenders, sentencing laws and pharmaceutical treatment: a prescription for failure. *Behav Sci Law.* 2000;18:83–110.

Tennent G, Bancroft J, Cass J. The control of deviant sexual behavior by drugs: A double-blind controlled study of benperidol, chlorpromazine, and placebo. *Arch Sex Behav.* 1974;3:261–271.

Thibault F, Cordier B, Kuhn J-M. Effects of long-lasting gonadotropin hormone-releasing hormone agonist in six cases of severe male paraphilia. *Acta Psychiatr Scand.* 1993;87:445–450.

Thibault F, Cordier B, Kuhn J-M. Gonadotropin hormone releasing hormone agonist in cases of severe paraphilia: a lifetime treatment. *Psychoneuroendocrinology.* 1996;21:411–419.

Ward N. Successful lithium treatment of transvestitism associated with manic depression. *J Nerv Mental Dis.* 1975;161:204–206.

Wincze JP, Bansal S, Malamud M. Effects of medroxyprogesterone acetate on subjective arousal, arousal to erotic stimulation, and nocturnal penile tumescence in male sex offenders. *Arch Sex Behav.* 1986;15:293–305.

Wiseman SV, McAuley JW, Freidenberg GR, Freidenberg DL. Hypersexuality in patients with dementia: possible response to cimetidine. *Neurology.* 2000;54:20–24.

Zohar J, Kaplan Z, Benjamin J. Compulsive exhibitionism successfully treated with fluvoxamine: a controlled case study. *J Clin Psychiatry.* 1994;55:86–88.

Index

adrenergic (agents/processes):
 alpha/beta blockers, 103
 atypical antipsychotics, effects on, 33
 blockers, 102, 116
 sexual function and, 17, 18, 110–11
 stimulants, 102–3, 112
 typical antipsychotics, effects on, 31
age, erectile function affected by, 4
alcohol, sexual side effects of, 184–86
alfuzosin, 96–97
alkylating agents, 123, 124, 125, 127
alpha-adrenoceptor blockers, 96–97
alprostadil, for female sexual arousal
 disorder, 258–59, 263
Althof, S. E., 271
American Psychiatric Association, 250
American Urological Association,
 234, 235
amphetamines, sexual side effects of,
 184, 186–87
androgens (androgenic
 agents/processes):
 basic facts of, 222
 deficiency syndrome, 207
 effects in oral contraceptives, 139
 exogenous, treating postmenopausal
 women, 204–6
 masculinizing effects of, 143, 205, 206,
 207, 209, 255, 257
 menopausal levels of, 143–44, 148,
 206–7
 replacement, 129, 187
 -supressing drugs, 130
 treating female low libido, 202, 207,
 208–10
 treating male low libido/erectile
 dysfunction, 224, 237–39
 see also testosterone
angiotensin converting enzyme (ACE)
 inhibitors, 103, 111, 115, 116

angiotensin-2 receptor antagonists, 103
anorgasmia, see orgasm
antacid agents, 88–90
antiandrogen(ic):
 disorders, 149
 drugs/therapy, 124, 137, 149–50, 220,
 292, 302
antianxiety drugs, sexual side effects
 associated with, 30–40
antiarrythmics, 103–4, 112, 192
antibiotics, 194
anticonvulsants:
 available in the United States, 74,
 158
 sexual dysfunction associated with,
 78–79, 161–65
 see also mood stabilizers
antidepressants:
 for bipolar disorder, 83–84
 diagnostic criteria for sexual
 dysfunction associated with, 56
 forms and doses of, 47–48
 interplay of, 54–55
 overview of, 45–46
 sexual dysfunction and, 50–56, 258
 see also selective serotonin reuptake
 inhibitors
antidiarrhetic agents, 87
antidotes:
 to anticonvulsant-induced sexual
 dysfunction (epilepsy), 166, 167
 to antidepressant-induced sexual
 dysfunction, 48, 58–59, 60–61
 to antipsychotic-induced sexual
 dysfunction, 34
 in general, 263
 to mood stabilizer-induced sexual
 dysfunction (bipolar), 81, 82, 83
antiemetic agents, 87–88
antiepileptics, see anticonvulsants

INDEX

313

I
N
D
E
X